John Tung.

John Tung.

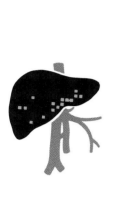

ATLAS
OF
LIVER
PATHOLOGY

ATLASES IN
DIAGNOSTIC SURGICAL PATHOLOGY

Consulting Editor
Gerald M. Bordin, M.D.
Department of Pathology
Scripps Clinic and Research Foundation

Published:

WOLD, McLEOD, SIM, AND UNNI:
ATLAS OF ORTHOPEDIC PATHOLOGY

COLBY, LOMBARD, YOUSEM, AND KITAICHI:
ATLAS OF PULMONARY SURGICAL PATHOLOGY

Forthcoming Titles:

WENIG: **Atlas of Head and Neck Pathology**

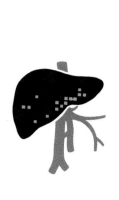

ATLAS OF LIVER PATHOLOGY

Gary C. Kanel, M.D.
Associate Professor of Pathology
University of Southern California School of Medicine
Associate Pathologist
Rancho and USC Liver Unit Laboratories
Downey, California

Jacob Korula, M.D.
Associate Professor of Clinical Medicine
University of Southern California School of Medicine
Attending Physician, USC Liver Unit
Rancho Los Amigos Medical Center
Downey, California

W. B. SAUNDERS COMPANY
Harcourt Brace Jovanovich, Inc.

Philadelphia ■ London ■ Toronto ■ Montreal ■ Sydney ■ Tokyo

W. B. SAUNDERS COMPANY
Harcourt Brace Jovanovich, Inc.

The Curtis Center
Independence Square West
Philadelphia, Pennsylvania 19106

Kanel, Gary C.
   Atlas of liver pathology / Gary C. Kanel, Jacob Korula.
     p. cm.
   ISBN 0-7216-2657-2
   1. Liver—Diseases—Atlases. I. Korula, Jacob. II. Title.
   [DNLM: 1. Liver Diseases—atlases. WI 17 K16a]
  RC846.9.K35 1992
  616.3'6207—dc20
  DNLM/DLC   91-43137

Editor: Jennifer Mitchell
Designer: W. B. Saunders Staff
Production Manager: Carolyn Naylor
Manuscript Editor: Jeanne Carper
Illustration Specialist: Peg Shaw
Indexer: Nancy Matthews

Atlas of Liver Pathology   ISBN 0-7216-2657-2

Printed in the United States of America.

Last digit is the print number: 9   8   7   6   5   4   3   2   1

TO OUR MENTORS

Telfer B. Reynolds, M.D.
Allan G. Redeker, M.D.

and
in memoriam

Robert L. Peters, M.D.

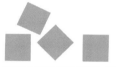

FOREWORD

This volume, *Atlas of Liver Pathology,* is designed to provide the practicing pathologist easy access to the vast information in hepatic pathology. The text covers a wide range of liver diseases and in some sections reflects views based on observations of disease entities seen at the USC Liver Unit. The presentation of the histologic material includes major and minor morphologic features seen on needle or wedge liver biopsy, differential diagnoses, special stains, and, where appropriate, immunohistochemistry and aspiration cytology. We try to present the clinical and biologic behavior in as concise a manner as possible, fully recognizing that we may not have done full justice to topics such as viral hepatitis, alcoholic liver disease, and hepatocellular carcinoma, about which volumes have been written. The photomicrographs are derived from the enormous collection of biopsy specimens acquired at this Unit during the past three decades.

We have been greatly enriched from our experience in compiling this volume and hope that our efforts will prove worthwhile. Our reward can be only the satisfaction of the reader, whether it be the student of pathology grappling with the basics of the subject, the clinician interested in liver disease, or the academic pathologist who values this *Atlas* as a useful reference and teaching resource.

GARY C. KANEL, M.D.
JACOB KORULA, M.D.
Downey, California

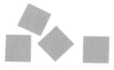

CONTENTS

■ CHAPTER 7

Nonviral Infectious Disorders 107

■ CHAPTER 8

Developmental, Familial, and Metabolic Disorders 135

■ **CHAPTER 10**

Miscellaneous Conditions

CHAPTER 1

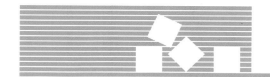

General Aspects of the Liver and Liver Diseases

■ **Basic Architecture and Histologic Features**

For proper assessment of the morphology of liver biopsy specimens the following features must be individually examined:

Simple Acinus (Functional Unit)
Portal Tract
1. Portal vein
2. Hepatic arteriole
3. Interlobular bile duct and cholangiole
4. Inflammatory cells
5. Connective tissue
6. Limiting plate

Parenchyma
1. Hepatocyte
2. Canaliculus
3. Kupffer cells and endothelial cells
4. Sinusoid
5. Terminal hepatic (central) venule

■ **Nonspecific Changes**

The following morphologic features may be characteristic, but are not diagnostic, of a whole variety of physiologic and pathophysiologic changes in the liver:
1. Portal tract with lymphocytic infiltration and hyperplasia

2. Focal hepatocytolysis
3. Kupffer cell hyperplasia and hypertrophy
4. Glycogen nuclei
5. Fatty change: macrovesicular and microvesicular
6. Nuclear anisocytosis and dysplasia

■ **General Clinical Features of Acute and Chronic Liver Disease**

Diseases affecting the liver present as either an acute process or a chronic process in which progressive damage leads to steady deterioration in hepatic function, eventually resulting in hepatic failure and death.

Acute Hepatic Injury

1. Acute hepatic injury manifests as hepatocellular injury, impairment in bile flow (cholestasis), or fatty infiltration.
2. Hepatocellular injury is characterized by elevations of serum transaminase, the degree of elevation depending on the severity or type of injury.
3. Cholestasis presents with elevation of serum bilirubin, approximately half of which is conjugated, with or without an elevation in alkaline phosphatase.
4. Fatty infiltration occurs acutely with toxin or drug exposure or is idiopathic (e.g., Reye's syndrome, acute fatty liver of pregnancy). Necrosis and inflam-

Presence of Pigments and Their Characteristics

	Bile	Hemosiderin	Lipochrome	Dubin-Johnson
Distribution	Perivenular	Periportal	Perivenular	Perivenular
Color	Yellow-green	Golden-brown, refractile	Light to dark brown	Dark brown
Iron Stain	Negative	Positive	Negative	Negative
Ziehl-Neelson Acid-fast Stain	Negative	Negative	Usually positive	Occasionally positive

1

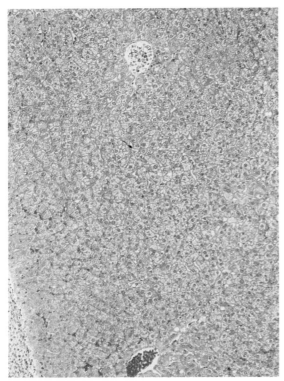

Figure 1–1. Normal liver. Blood enters the lobule by way of the portal vein and hepatic arterioles located in the portal tract (*top*), circulates through the sinusoids, and exits the lobule through the terminal hepatic venule (*bottom*).

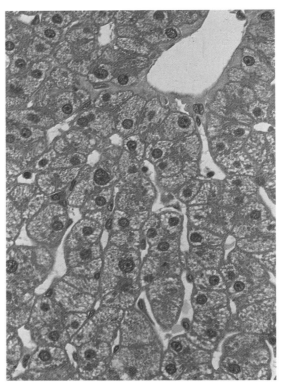

Figure 1–3. Normal liver. The parenchyma is composed of hepatocytes forming trabeculae one to two cells thick and lined by thin Kupffer and endothelial cells.

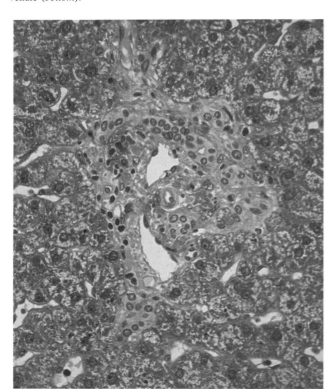

Figure 1–2. Normal liver. A normal portal tract consists of the portal vein, hepatic arteriole, one to two interlobular bile ducts, and occasional peripherally located ductules. These components are present within a collagen network often containing scanty numbers of lymphocytes.

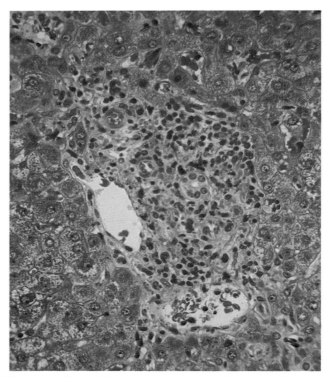

Figure 1–4. Nonspecific changes. *Lymphocytic infiltration and hyperplasia* of portal tracts can at times be fairly prominent. These cells may be limited to the portal tracts (e.g., reactive change) or may infiltrate into the parenchyma (e.g., acute viral hepatitis, chronic active hepatitis).

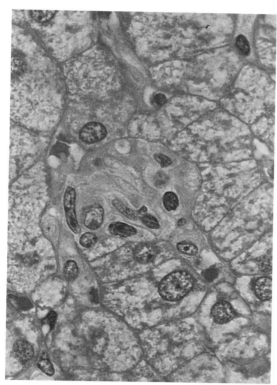

Figure 1–5. Nonspecific changes. *Hepatocytolysis* is a type of liver cell necrosis with complete dropout of hepatocytes and replacement by Kupffer cells and macrophages.

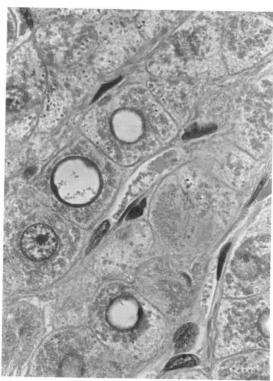

Figure 1–7. Nonspecific changes. *Glycogen nuclei* have a distinct vacuolated appearance. The glycogen may be identified to variable degrees by a periodic acid–Schiff stain on frozen sections.

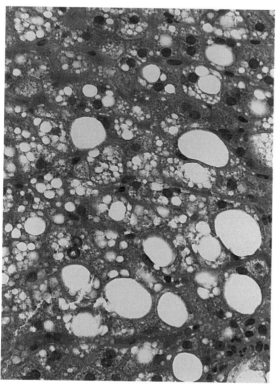

Figure 1–6. Nonspecific changes. *Fatty change* of hepatocytes may be present as *macrovesicles* (fat globules larger than nuclei) and/or *microvesicles* (globules equal to or smaller than nuclei).

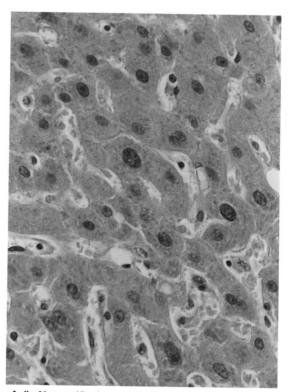

Figure 1–8. Nonspecific changes. *Nuclear anisocytosis* exhibits variation in the size of nuclei. This feature is common in the perivenular zone of elderly patients.

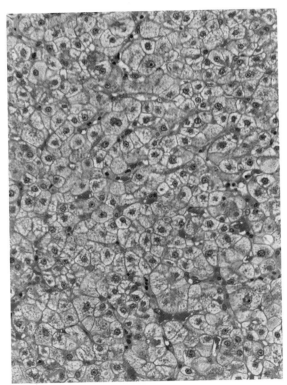

Figure 1–9. Nonspecific changes. *Regenerative activity* is characterized by proliferation of uniformly sized hepatocytes having a clear cytoplasm. Sinusoids are difficult to appreciate. Of importance is the virtual absence of inflammatory infiltration, with minimal to absent Kupffer cell reaction.

mation are minimal, and consequently serum transaminases are only mildly elevated.

5. Varying combinations of types of injury may be present. Fatty infiltration and cholestasis may accompany hepatocellular necrosis, which occurs in certain types of drug or toxin exposure.

Clinical Features of Acute Hepatic Injury

1. Depending on the severity of the acute injury, patients can be asymptomatic or develop malaise, nausea, vomiting, and anorexia.
2. Recovery is usually heralded by the rapid return of appetite, absence of gastrointestinal symptoms, and improved energy levels.
3. *Hepatic failure* is characterized by the presence of encephalopathy or renal failure (provided renal injury is not directly induced by the agent producing the hepatic injury).
4. *Fulminant hepatic failure* or massive hepatic necrosis (regardless of cause) is defined when the duration from onset of injury or infection to hepatic failure is 6 weeks or less. *Submassive hepatic necrosis* is defined when the duration exceeds 6 weeks.
5. *Serum transaminase (aspartate aminotransferase and alanine aminotransferase) levels* are moderately to markedly elevated (1000 to >10,000 IU/L), depending on the severity of the injury; the degree of

transaminase elevation does not predict the outcome of hepatitis.
6. Mild to moderate elevation of the serum total *bilirubin* level is usually noted, but may be markedly elevated (20–25 mg/dL) in the cholestatic phase of viral hepatitis.
7. The serum *alkaline phosphatase* level is usually mildly to moderately elevated.
8. *Prothrombin activity* is decreased (prothrombin time prolonged) in acute hepatic injury, with the severity of the abnormality depending on the severity of the injury. Persistent and marked decrease in prothrombin activity (less than 10%) in acute hepatic injury carries a poor prognosis, with mortality exceeding 80%.

Chronic Hepatic Injury

1. The injurious process continues unabated, resulting in repetitive phases of injury and repair.
2. Elevation of serum transaminase levels usually signifies hepatocellular injury.
3. Fibrosis laid down as part of the reparative process leads to hepatic fibrosis and eventually cirrhosis over a period of years.

Clinical Features of Chronic Hepatic Injury

1. Clinical features of chronic liver disease depend on the extent of progression of the liver disease.
2. Symptoms may be related to the activity of the underlying etiology (e.g., in autoimmune chronic active hepatitis, fatigue, malaise, arthritis, and rash may reflect the immune disturbance). If cirrhosis is present, decompensation with ascites, hepatic encephalopathy, or variceal hemorrhage may accompany such episodes.
3. Patients with significant chronic liver disease present with stigmata such as *vascular "spiders"* or *"spider" angiomas, palmar erythema, clubbing, leukonychia* (white nails), *Dupuytren's contracture,* or *parotid enlargement,* which may not all be present in a given patient. Rarely, patients with advanced cirrhosis may not demonstrate any of these features.
4. *Gynecomastia* and *testicular atrophy* occur in some male patients with chronic liver disease.
5. *Abdominal collateral vessels* develop as a result of portal hypertension.
6. *Muscle wasting* is caused by significant impairment in protein synthesis by the liver, characteristically involves the face and extremities, and is usually seen in patients with advanced liver disease.
7. *Hypoalbuminemia* may be present because of decreased synthetic hepatic function.
8. In established cirrhosis, complications such as ascites, variceal hemorrhage, and hepatic encephalopathy may develop.
9. *Ascites* results from impaired renal excretion of sodium and from portal hypertension.

10. Ascites resistant to diuretic therapy is termed *refractory ascites*.
11. *Spontaneous bacterial peritonitis* or infected ascites occurs frequently in patients with decompensated liver disease and prominent ascites.
12. *Hepatic encephalopathy* develops as a result of hepatic dysfunction with or without portosystemic shunting.
13. *Hemorrhage from esophageal and gastric varices* is a lethal complication with increased mortality (50%) in patients with severe liver disease.
14. *Hepatic transplantation* is offered to patients with fulminant hepatic failure who are not likely to survive and to those with advanced cirrhosis.

General References

Edmondson HA, Peters RL. Liver. In: Kissane JM, Anderson WAD, eds. Pathology, 8th ed. St. Louis: C.V. Mosby, 1985:1096–1111.

MacSween RNM, Scothorne RJ. Developmental anatomy and normal structures. In: MacSween RNM, Anthony PP, Scheuer PJ, eds. Pathology of the Liver, 2nd ed. Edinburgh: Churchill Livingstone, 1987:1–45.

Peters RL. Introduction. In: Peters RL, Craig JR, eds. Liver Pathology. New York: Churchill Livingstone, 1986:1–11.

Scheuer PJ. Liver Biopsy Interpretation, 3rd ed. London: Baillière Tindall, 1980:1–35.

Schiff L, Schiff ER, eds. Diseases of the Liver, 6th ed. Philadelphia: J.B. Lippincott, 1987.

Zakim D, Boyer TD, eds. Hepatology: A Textbook of Liver Disease. Philadelphia: W.B. Saunders, 1982.

CHAPTER 2

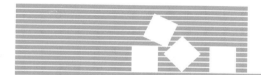

Viral Hepatitis

Major Hepatotropic Viruses: A, B, Delta (HDV), and Non-A, Non-B (HCV)

Acute Viral Hepatitis

TYPICAL FORM (SPOTTY NECROSIS)

Major Morphologic Features

1. Portal tract shows lymphocytic infiltration and hyperplasia.
2. Hydropic hepatocytes, with focal necrosis (hepatocytolysis) involving all zones of the lobule, are often accentuated in the perivenular region (Rappaport zone 3).
3. Variable degrees of lymphocytic inflammatory infiltration exist within the parenchyma.
4. Kupffer cell hyperplasia is prominent.

Other Features

1. Lobular architecture is intact; collapse in the perivenular zone may be present in early stages.
2. Spillover of lymphocytes from portal tract into parenchyma (often resembling "piecemeal" necrosis) may be present but mild.
3. Mild bile duct reduplication occurs.
4. Neutrophils are scattered in portal tracts in early stages.
5. Degree of portal inflammatory reaction may vary from different portal tracts within the same biopsy specimen.
6. *Acidophil bodies:* Liver cells with shrunken, eosinophilic cytoplasm with or without pyknotic nuclei are usually present, either within trabeculae or phagocytized by Kupffer cells.

7. Cholestasis may be present, often with perivenular accentuation.
8. *Regenerative activity:* Aggregates of clustered hydropic hepatocytes without inflammatory change are scattered throughout the parenchyma, first seen in periportal regions.
9. Scattered macrovesicular and microvesicular fat may be present in acute hepatitis B with acute delta infection.
10. All types of hepatitis secondary to hepatotropic viruses exhibit similar morphologic features, with the following exceptions:
    a. Non-A, non-B (HCV) hepatitis may exhibit atypical bile ducts (flattened epithelium, minimal to absent lumen, infiltration by lymphocytes).
    b. Acinar changes of liver cells are characteristic of epidemic waterborne non-A, non-B (hepatitis E virus).
    c. Acute hepatitis B with acute delta infection is often associated with a more severe degree of liver cell necrosis than acute hepatitis B alone.
    d. In acute hepatitis A, plasma cells are often increased in portal tracts.

Differential Diagnosis

1. *Drug-induced injury* (e.g., isoniazid, alpha-methyldopa, halothane): Morphologic features similar to those of acute viral hepatitis are present, although in general portal inflammatory changes in viral hepatitis are more prominent.
2. *Early stages of chronic active hepatitis:* Both early and relatively active stages of chronic active liver disease may resemble acute viral hepatitis, especially in small biopsy specimens without portal tracts or with only segments of portal areas. Hepatitis B virus antigens (HBsAg, HBcAg), shown by immunoper-

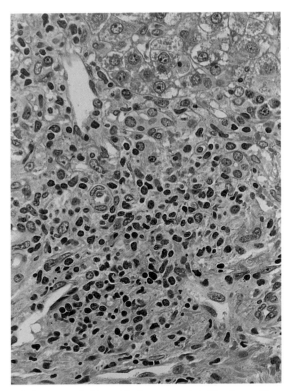

Figure 2–1. Acute viral hepatitis. Lymphocytic infiltration and hyperplasia, often with mild spillover of lymphocytes into the periportal parenchyma, is a common feature. Variation in the degree of inflammatory change between portal tracts may be present in the same biopsy specimen. Bile duct proliferation is present but not prominent.

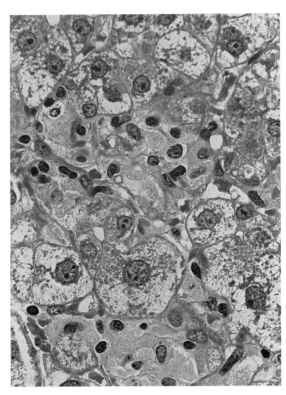

Figure 2–3. Acute viral hepatitis. In areas of necrosis, the hepatocytes are replaced by aggregates of Kupffer cells, lymphocytes, and macrophages. Adjacent liver cells exhibit variable degrees of hydropic changes.

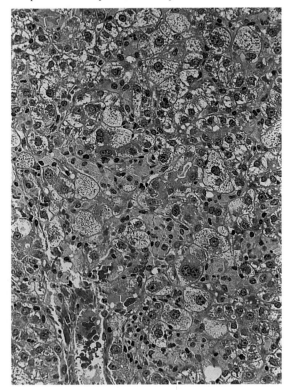

Figure 2–2. Acute viral hepatitis. The cord–sinusoid pattern is distorted as a result of focal necrosis and swelling of liver cells, most prominent in the perivenular zone. Kupffer cell hyperplasia is also present.

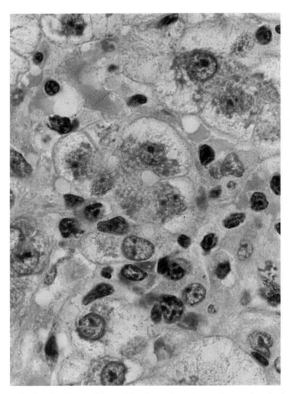

Figure 2–4. Acute viral hepatitis. Lymphocytes and occasional plasma cells are present within the sinusoids and often infiltrate into the hepatic cords. Biliary canaliculi may be dilated and filled with bile.

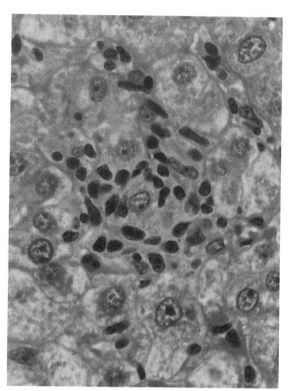

Figure 2–5. Acute viral hepatitis. In some areas lymphocytes appear to attack the hepatocytes, surrounding and infiltrating into the cytoplasm *(emperipolesis).*

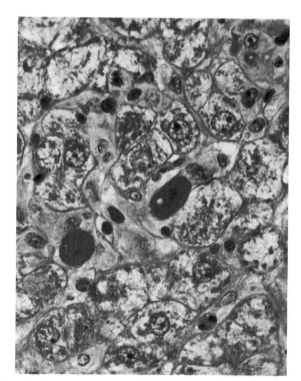

Figure 2–6. Acute viral hepatitis. *Acidophil bodies* are often common. These hepatocytes do not immediately drop out but instead undergo a shrinkage of both the nucleus and cytoplasm. The nucleus is eventually extruded into the sinusoid, with phagocytosis of the dying cell by adjacent hyperplastic Kupffer cells.

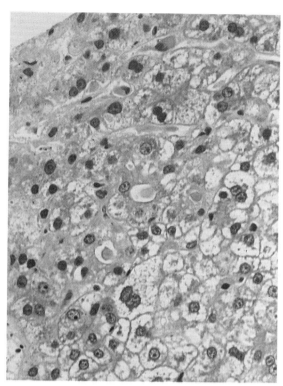

Figure 2–7. Acute viral hepatitis, non-A, non-B waterborne. The morphology of this type of acute viral hepatitis, also termed *type E,* for the most part resembles that seen with virus types A and B; however, the hepatitis is somewhat milder in its degree of inflammatory infiltration. In addition, canalicular dilatation with bile stasis, seen in this photomicrograph, may be quite prominent.

oxidase staining, are usually present in chronic, but not acute, hepatitis B.

Special Stains

1. *Periodic acid–Schiff after diastase:* Cytoplasmic lysosomal granules in macrophages and Kupffer cells are prominent in areas of hepatocytolysis and portal macrophages.
2. *Reticulin:* Condensation of black-staining fibers in perivenular zones may be present as a result of cell necrosis and dropout.

Immunohistochemistry

1. *HBsAg, HBcAg:* Surface and core antigen staining in acute hepatitis B is always negative. Positive staining for either antigen in biopsy specimens exhibiting changes of acute hepatitis is indicative of either:
   a. Replicative (active) phase of chronic active hepatitis B or
   b. Acute hepatitis (types A, non-A non-B [HCV] and drug-induced) superimposed on chronic hepatitis B (persistent or chronic active).

2. *Delta antigen:* In acute hepatitis B with acute delta infection, liver cell nuclei exhibit variable degrees of positive staining.

Clinical and Biologic Behavior (Tables 2–1 and 2–2)

1. In general, significant elevations of serum transaminase levels occur with acute viral hepatitis, sometimes to levels of more than 10,000 IU/L.
2. Children usually tend to be anicteric and asymptomatic, and adults, especially elderly patients, may develop a severe course.
3. Although serum transaminase levels are lower in anicteric or asymptomatic forms of hepatitis, the degree of transaminase elevation does not correlate with outcome or prognosis.
4. Recovery is observed with absence of gastrointestinal symptoms and improvement in prothrombin activity and sense of well-being.
5. A cholestatic phase may follow acute hepatitis, is more frequently seen with hepatitis A, and is characterized by jaundice and pruritus that may last weeks or months.
6. Persistence of serum transaminase elevations for more than 6 months should raise the possibility of chronic hepatitis.
7. In hepatitis A, relapses may occur 30 to 90 days after initial illness and mimic a biphasic hepatitic illness.
8. Chronic hepatitis and carrier state occur less frequently (0.2%) following acute symptomatic (icteric) hepatitis B.
9. In acute delta *co-infection,* resolution of acute hepatitis B is followed by a second episode of hepatitis, presenting as a biphasic illness. The synthesis of the delta virus is limited by transient HBs antigenemia, and hepatitis is mainly due to HBV infection.
10. In delta *superinfection* of chronic HBV carriers, the ensuing hepatitis may have a severe course; delta superinfection may also lead to accelerated progression of chronic hepatitis B.
11. The type of preexisting HBV infection may be important in determining the outcome of delta superinfection. Active HBV infection with viral replication (HBeAg+, HBV-DNA+) appears more likely to be associated with severe acute illness. The propensity to develop chronic Δ infection is more likely when nonreplicative HBV infection (HBeAb+, HBV-DNA−) occurs.

Prognosis

1. The development of fulminant or submassive necrosis is associated with a poor prognosis and decreased survival (10%–20%).

References

Bradley DW, Maynard JE. Etiology and natural history of post-transfusion and enterically-transmitted non-A, non-B hepatitis. Semin Liver Dis 1986;6:56–66.

DeCock KM, Jones B, Govindarajan S, et al. Prevalence of hepatitis delta virus infection: A seroepidemiologic study. West J Med 1988;148:307–309.

Lefkowitz JH, Apfelbaum TF. Non-A, non-B hepatitis: Characteristics of liver biopsy pathology. J Clin Gastroenterol 1989;11:225–232.

Okuno T, Sano A, Deguchi T, et al. Pathology of acute hepatitis A in humans: Comparison with acute hepatitis B. Am J Clin Pathol 1984;81:162–169.

Uchida T, Kronborg I, Peters RL. Acute viral hepatitis: Morphologic and functional correlations in human livers. Hum Pathol 1984;15:267–277.

Table 2–1
CLINICAL AND BIOLOGIC BEHAVIOR OF HEPATOTROPIC VIRUSES

	Hepatitis A	Hepatitis B	Hepatitis C (non-A, non-B)	Hepatitis D	Hepatitis E
Virus Type	RNA	DNA	RNA*	Defective RNA	RNA
Size	27 nm	42 nm Dane particle	32–36 nm	35–37 nm Associated with HBsAg	27–30 nm
Incubation Period (days)	15–45	40–180	15–150	28–150	15
Transmission	Fecal-oral†	Parenteral Sexual	Parenteral ? Sexual	Parenteral ? Sexual	Fecal-oral
Chronicity	None	5%–10%	50%	<1% with acute HBV 90% with chronic HBV	None
Fulminant Course	<1%	<1%	<1%	30% acute delta infection with acute hepatitis B	<1%‡

*May be two agents, short and long incubation associated with plasma and red blood cell transfusion, respectively.

†Recently, parenteral drug addicts have been reported to develop acute hepatitis A, presumably from contamination of heroin, (black tar) heroin, amphetamines, and cocaine.

‡During epidemics, mortality of infected pregnant women is 10% to 20%.

Table 2–2
SEROLOGIC DIAGNOSIS OF HEPATITIS

Type A Hepatitis
    Acute: HAV IgM positive (HAV IgG positive)
  Immunity: HAV IgG positive
Type C Hepatitis
(non-A, non-B)
    Acute: HCV antibody (positive in 15%–28% cases)
  Chronic: HCV antibody (positive in 70%–80% cases)
Type E Hepatitis
(enteric non-A, non-B)
    Acute: No antibody test available*
        Virus-like particles in stool agglutinated by acute and convalescent sera

Type B and D Hepatitis:

	Clinical State	HBsAg	HBcAb IgM	HBcAb IgG	HBV-DNA	HBsAb	HDV IgM	HDV IgG
H B V	Acute	+	+	+†	–	++‡	–	–
	Chronic (nonreplicating)	+	–	+	–	–	–	–
	Chronic (replicating)	+	–	+	++	–	–	–
	Reactivation	+	+	+	+++	–	–	–
	Immunization	–	–	–	–	++	–	–
H D V	Acute	+§	+	+	–	–	++	+
	Chronic	+	–	+	–	–	+	++

*Antibody test being developed.
†HBcAb IgG (total) reflects prior infection to HBV and not immunity; absent with immunization.
‡HBsAb positive at recovery and with clearance of HBsAg.
§HBsAg may be suppressed during acute HDV hepatitis (HBV background infection with HDV infection).

SEVERE AND FULMINANT HEPATITIS

Major Morphologic Features

1. There are three subtypes:
    a. *Confluent hepatic necrosis:* Portal and parenchymal changes are similar to acute viral hepatitis, but with prominent perivenular cell necrosis, cell dropout, and bridging of necrotic regions between adjacent lobules.
    b. *Submassive hepatic necrosis:* Striking hepatocellular necrosis occurs with dropout of majority of hepatocytes, leaving at least a rim of intact liver cells surrounding many of the portal structures.
    c. *Massive hepatic necrosis:* Total necrosis and dropout of virtually all liver cells are noted.

Other Features

1. Lobular architecture is intact in very early stages, but with extensive perivenular and midzonal collapse of the parenchymal reticulin framework.

2. Portal tracts have mild to moderate lymphocytic infiltration and hyperplasia, often not as striking as seen in typical acute viral hepatitis.
3. Mild to moderate proliferation of bile ducts occurs, often with transformation of hepatocytes into duct-like structures in periportal regions.
4. Cholestasis is almost always present.
5. Kupffer cell hyperplasia is prominent.
6. Cobblestoning pattern of hydropic hepatocytes (regeneration) occurs in patients who survive the early acute phase; these regenerative areas are unevenly distributed throughout the liver and may form nodular regions mimicking cirrhosis.
7. Acute hepatitis A, B, and non-A, non-B (HCV) show similar morphologic features; however, acute hepatitis B with acute delta infection is more often associated with these severe forms of liver cell necrosis than other viral infections alone.

Differential Diagnosis

1. *Drug-induced injury* (e.g., isoniazid, alpha-methyldopa, halothane): Morphologic features are quite

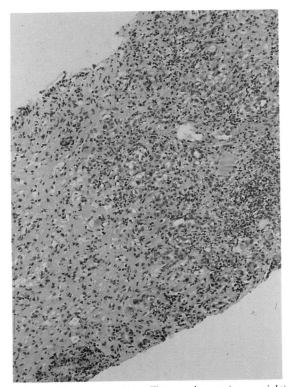

Figure 2–8. Fulminant hepatitis. The portal tract *(upper right)* and perivenular zone *(lower left)* maintain their basic architectural pattern; however, on low power, inflammatory infiltration and liver cell dropout within the parenchyma are evident.

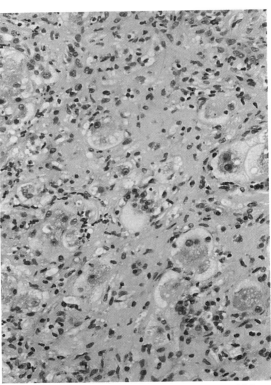

Figure 2–10. Fulminant hepatitis. The perivenular zone exhibits striking dropout of hepatocytes, with prominent Kupffer cell hyperplasia. Lymphocytes as well as plasma cells are present. The liver cells that can be identified are hydropic.

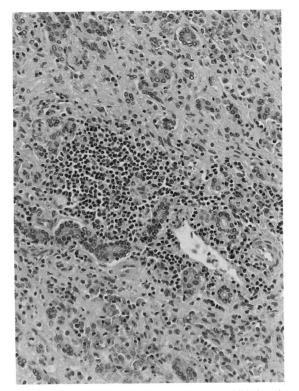

Figure 2–9. Fulminant hepatitis. The portal tracts exhibit lymphocytic infiltration and hyperplasia, with variable degrees of bile duct proliferation. The portal tracts may also appear somewhat enlarged as a result of cholangiolar proliferation.

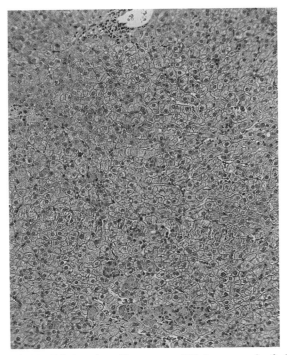

Figure 2–11. Fulminant hepatitis, recovery. This is an example of a liver biopsy specimen obtained 1 year after a clinical episode of fulminant hepatitis. Although the mortality in fulminant hepatitis is quite high, cirrhosis does *not* develop in those patients who recover. The liver in this example demonstrates a normal portal tract and an intact cord arrangement of the hepatocytes. Numerous Kupffer cells are seen containing pigment (lipochrome) that has remained from previously damaged hepatocytes.

similar to a viral-induced etiology; the degree of portal inflammatory activity is not helpful in differentiation.

Special Stains

1. *Periodic acid–Schiff after diastase:* Cytoplasmic lysosomal granules are quite prominent in mononuclear and Kupffer cells in areas of necrosis secondary to phagocytosis of necrotic liver cells.
2. *Reticulin:* The areas of extensive collapse are accentuated; in the regenerative phase, nodules are easily identified.

Immunohistochemistry

1. *HBsAg, HBcAg:* Tests for surface and core antigens in acute viral hepatitis B are always negative.
2. *Delta antigen:* In cases of acute delta infection, the delta antigen is usually present in the nuclei of many viable cells; however, these cells may be sparse or even absent in submassive and massive hepatic necrosis.

Clinical and Biologic Behavior

1. A severe course of acute hepatitis (either fulminant or submassive necrosis [see Chapter 1]) is heralded by the persistence of gastrointestinal symptoms (e.g., nausea, vomiting, dyspepsia), decreased prothrombin activity (<20%), and features of encephalopathy (drowsiness, lethargy, and asterixis).
2. The prevalence of fulminant and submassive hepatic necrosis from viral hepatitis (types A, B, C, and E) is less than 1%. There is an increased probability of fulminant hepatitis developing in hepatitis B, especially with concomitant acute hepatitis D, than with either hepatitis A or hepatitis non-A, non-B (HCV) alone.
3. A high prevalence rate (21%–50%) of HDV markers among patients with fulminant hepatitis B likely indicates that the severe hepatitis results from cumulative damage of the two viruses.
4. Established chronic hepatitis B (e.g., HBV carriers) allows full pathogenic expression of HDV, leading to fulminant hepatic failure.
5. Acute hepatitis superimposed on cirrhosis may result in a severe clinical course and increased mortality.
6. Biopsies are generally not performed in these patients because of low prothrombin activity (usually <20%) except by the transjugular route.
7. In fulminant hepatitis B, significant exponential elevations of alpha-fetoprotein are more often associated with improved survival.
8. Ascites, lower extremity or generalized edema, renal failure, gastrointestinal bleeding, disseminated intra-vascular coagulation, hypoglycemia, sepsis, and hypovolemia may complicate the course of fulminant hepatitis.
9. No patients who recover develop any form of chronic liver disease.

Prognosis

1. The prognosis and outcome depends on the type of hepatitis, presence of underlying liver disease, and age. For example, hepatitis B and delta infection have a greater probability of a severe course and a consequent poor prognosis than hepatitis B alone.
2. Older persons tend to have a more protracted and severe illness than younger patients. No patient older than 40 years of age survives fulminant hepatitis (see Impaired Regeneration Syndrome).
3. The overall mortality in fulminant hepatitis with submassive hepatic necrosis is 70% to 80%.

References

Govindarajan S, Chin KP, Redeker AG, et al. Fulminant B viral hepatitis: Role of delta agent. Gastroenterology 1984;86:1417–1420.

Karvountzis GG, Redeker AG, Peters RL. Long-term follow-up studies of patients surviving fulminant viral hepatitis. Gastroenterology 1974;67:870–877.

Yanda RJ. Fulminant hepatic failure. West J Med 1988;149:586–591.

IMPAIRED REGENERATION SYNDROME

Major Morphologic Features

1. Prominent perivenular hepatocellular dropout and collapse occurs.
2. Cord-sinusoid pattern within the midzonal and periportal regions is straight, with little to no regenerative activity.

Other Features

1. Very early features are those of typical acute viral hepatitis.
2. Portal areas are normal to slightly expanded with mild to moderate mononuclear inflammatory infiltration.
3. Interlobular bile ducts are normal to only slightly increased in number; however, cholangiolar proliferation at margins of portal tracts is present and the ductules are often dilated, contain bile plugs, and are surrounded by neutrophils.
4. Cholestasis is usually present within the parenchyma.
5. Mild focal hepatocytolysis occurs within the midzonal and periportal regions, with little inflammatory infiltration.
6. Kupffer cell hyperplasia is mild to moderate.

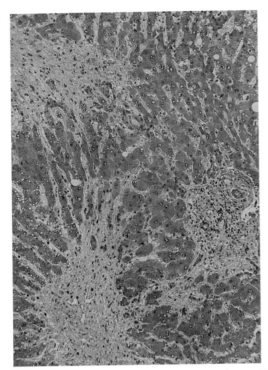

Figure 2–12. Impaired regeneration. The portal tract exhibits mild fibrosis but little inflammatory change. The two terminal hepatic venules exhibit striking dropout of liver cells, with collapse of the reticulin framework, and resemble fibrosis on routine hematoxylin and eosin staining. The adjacent hepatocytes are eosinophilic and form straight cords with no regenerative activity.

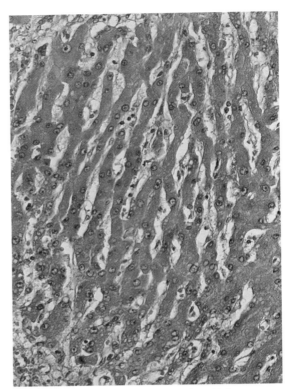

Figure 2–14. Impaired regeneration. The cords on higher power are usually straight and only one cell thick, with an *absence* of regenerative activity.

Differential Diagnosis

1. *Mechanical duct obstruction:* Cholestasis and cholangiolar proliferation with neutrophilic infiltration are also seen in large duct obstruction but without perivenular collapse and a straight cord-sinusoid pattern.

Clinical and Biologic Behavior

1. This form of viral hepatitis is typically seen in the elderly patient after a bout of a usually mild form of acute hepatitis; patients younger than 40 years of age seldom develop impaired regeneration.
2. Enzyme levels will return to normal; however, the bilirubin stays elevated or continues to rise in association with decreased prothrombin activity.
3. Although residual hepatocytes may not appear morphologically injured, the cells are poorly functional, with little to no capacity for regeneration.
4. The incidence of impaired regeneration is approximately the same for each of the hepatitis viruses and may also be seen in elderly patients after any type of severe liver cell injury.
5. The clinical course may be protracted following viral hepatitis, and resolution may occur after 6 to 12 months.

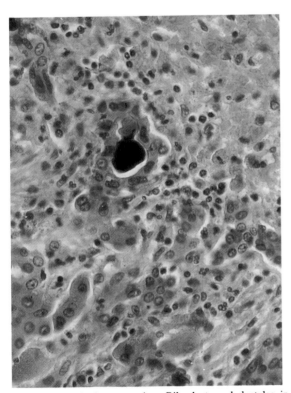

Figure 2–13. Impaired regeneration. Bile ducts and ductules in the periportal regions often are dilated, are surrounded by lymphocytes and neutrophils, and contain bile.

Prognosis

1. If patients continue to deteriorate with signs of hepatic failure, the prognosis is poor and transplantation should be considered. Associated dysfunction in other organ systems related to the age of the patient makes these patients less optimal candidates.

References

Edmondson HA, Peters RL. Liver. In: Kissane JM, Anderson WAD, eds. Pathology, 8th ed. St. Louis: C.V. Mosby, 1985:1096–1212.
Peters RL. Viral inflammatory diseases. In: Peters RL, Craig JR, eds. Liver Pathology. New York: Churchill Livingstone, 1986:86–87.

Chronic Viral Hepatitis

LOBULAR HEPATITIS

Major Morphologic Features

1. Portal tracts are expanded by lymphocytic infiltration and hyperplasia; fibrosis is *not* present.
2. Variable degrees of focal hepatocytolysis are evenly distributed throughout all lobules.

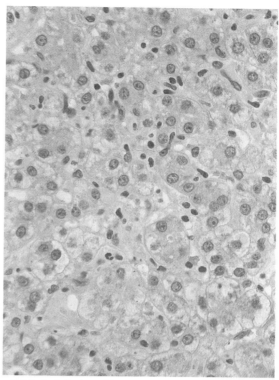

Figure 2–16. Lobular hepatitis. The parenchyma exhibits a mild distortion of the cord-sinusoid pattern. Focal necrosis, hydropic change of the hepatocytes, and Kupffer cell hyperplasia are present but mild. These changes uniformly involve all zones of the lobules, without perivenular accentuation.

Other Features

1. Kupffer cell hyperplasia is mild to moderate.
2. Acidophil bodies are occasionally evident.
3. Cholestasis is rare.
4. Spillover of inflammatory cells from portal tract into periportal region is minimal.
5. Regenerative changes are scanty to absent.
6. Ground-glass cells (HBsAg within liver cell cytoplasm) and intrasinusoidal collagen are not present.

Differential Diagnosis

1. *Acute viral hepatitis:* Perivenular accentuation in the peak phase and regenerative activity in the resolving stages are present in acute viral, but not lobular, hepatitis.
2. *Persistent viral hepatitis:* Inflammatory parenchymal activity is more prominent in lobular hepatitis; in addition, ground-glass cells are present in the majority of cases of persistent hepatitis B but absent in lobular hepatitis.
3. *Chronic active hepatitis, early stages:* Unlike chronic active hepatitis, portal fibrosis is not present in lobular hepatitis, and parenchymal necroinflam-

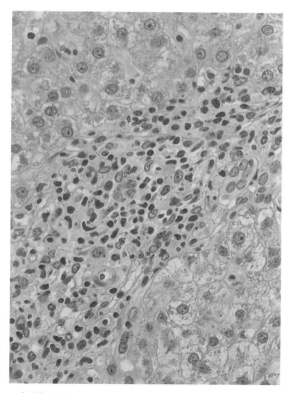

Figure 2–15. Lobular hepatitis. The portal tract is normal in size and exhibits a mild lymphocytic infiltration and hyperplasia, with minimal spillover of the inflammatory cells into the adjacent periportal region.

matory changes are *regularly* distributed throughout the biopsy specimen. However, in very early stages of chronic active liver disease, portal fibrosis may be minimal to absent. In these instances, the *irregular* degree of parenchymal inflammatory change and regeneration from one lobule to another is characteristic of chronic active hepatitis.

Immunohistochemistry

1. *HBsAg, HBcAg:* Lobular hepatitis does *not* exhibit an antigenic staining pattern in HBV infection, while the presence of cytoplasmic HBsAg and/or nuclear HBcAg staining is indicative of either persistent or chronic active hepatitis B.

Clinical and Biologic Behavior

1. *Chronic lobular hepatitis* represents a slowly resolving form of acute viral hepatitis in which the enzymes remain elevated for up to 6 months after the onset of the acute episode.
2. This rare form of chronic hepatitis may occur more often in patients with other disorders associated with immunosuppression (e.g., renal dialysis, chemotherapy).
3. Liver biopsy specimens obtained at least 6 months after initial enzyme elevations show features of a mild acute viral hepatitis; because the disorder is rare, persistent or chronic active hepatitis is usually clinically suspected.
4. Definitive diagnosis can be established only at follow up when complete resolution of the disease occurs within 1 to 2 years.
5. This form may develop after acute hepatitis B and non A, non-B (HCV) hepatitis but is exceptionally rare after acute hepatitis A.
6. The diagnosis is certain in instances in which serology confirms recovery from acute viral hepatitis (e.g., in serologically proven acute hepatitis B, the subsequent clearance of HBsAg and immunity with the development of HBsAb makes a delayed diagnosis of lobular hepatitis).

References

Peters RL. Viral inflammatory diseases. In: Peters RL, Craig JR, eds. Liver Pathology. New York: Churchill Livingstone, 1986:87–89.

Popper H. Changing concepts of the evolution of chronic hepatitis and the role of piecemeal necrosis. Hepatology 1983;3:758–762.

Popper H, Schaffner F. The vocabulary of chronic hepatitis. N Engl J Med 1971;284:1154–1156.

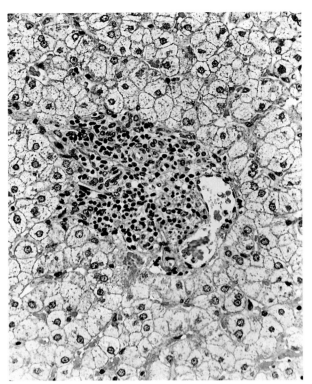

Figure 2–17. Persistent viral hepatitis. Lymphocytic infiltration and hyperplasia are present and may be prominent but are often seen to this degree in only one third of the portal structures within the same biopsy specimen. These inflammatory cells do *not* infiltrate into the periportal zone.

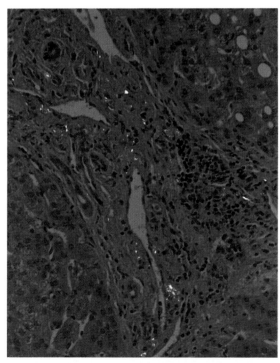

Figure 2–18. Persistent viral hepatitis, intravenous drug user (polarized light). The minority of long-term intravenous drug users may exhibit injected foreign material (e.g., talc) most prominently in macrophages in portal tracts and rarely in Kupffer cells. Granulomas and multinucleated histiocytes containing this material are typically absent.

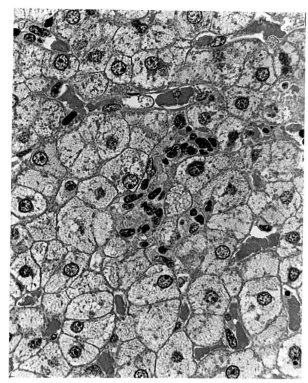

Figure 2–19. Persistent viral hepatitis. Focal necrosis with aggregates of lymphocytes, Kupffer cells, and histiocytes is often present but usually minimal. Adjacent liver cells are hydropic, and Kupffer cell hyperplasia is minimal in type B infection.

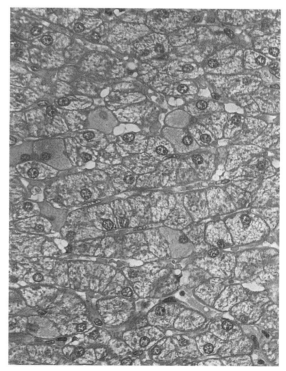

Figure 2–20. Persistent viral hepatitis—type B. Scattered ground-glass hepatocytes, representing proliferation of endoplasmic reticulum and the HBsAg, are seen in the majority of patients with chronic hepatitis B. These cells are *regularly* distributed throughout the lobule and from one lobule to the next in persistent hepatitis B.

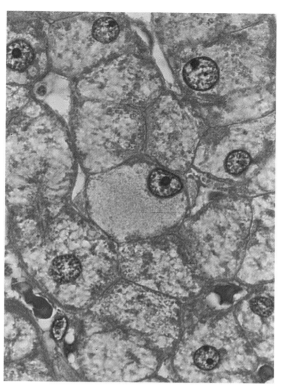

Figure 2–21. Ground-glass hepatocytes. The ground-glass cell contains finely granular eosinophilic cytoplasm, sometimes with a peripheral thin clear zone. The nucleus is often present at the cell margin. Special stains such as Shikata (orcein) and immunoperoxidase confirm the presence of HBsAg in the cytoplasm. Other disorders (e.g., drug-induced) may also produce ground-glass–like cells (negative on special stains for the surface antigen).

CHRONIC PERSISTENT (PERSISTENT VIRAL) HEPATITIS

Major Morphologic Features

1. Portal tracts are normal in size to slightly expanded, with variable degrees of lymphocytic infiltration and hyperplasia.
2. Parenchyma shows mild focal mononuclear inflammatory infiltration and focal hepatocytolysis, with no zonal distribution.
3. In hepatitis B:
   a. *Ground-glass cells:* Hepatocytes with eosinophilic granular cytoplasm, peripheral halo staining pattern, and nucleus at cell margin are present in approximately one half to three fourths of cases; these cells are *evenly* distributed both within the lobule and from one lobule to another.
   b. *Cobblestoning:* Uniform hydropic change of large clusters of hepatocytes, without a well-defined cord-sinusoid pattern, is present in two thirds of cases.
4. In *non-A, non-B (HCV)* hepatitis:
   a. The degree of focal hepatocytolysis and Kupffer cell hyperplasia is greater than in hepatitis B, without cobblestoning and ground-glass cells.

b. Fatty change and sinusoidal collagen may be present (these features are also seen in chronic active hepatitis).

c. Differentiation from relatively inactive chronic active hepatitis may not be possible; therefore, chronic non-A, non-B (HCV) hepatitis is not morphologically placed in the "persistent" category but is termed either *chronic hepatitis* alone, or *chronic active hepatitis*.

Other Features

1. Bile ducts are normal to only slightly increased in number.
2. Kupffer cell hyperplasia is minimal in hepatitis B.
3. In liver biopsy specimens of parenteral drug addicts, portal areas exhibit variable lymphocytic hyperplasia; polarizable material from particulate material used in the injectant is present in portal macrophages and rarely in Kupffer cells.

Differential Diagnosis

1. *Nonspecific reactive changes:* Intra-abdominal infections and generalized sepsis often produce portal inflammation and mild parenchymal necrosis that may resemble persistent hepatitis, predominantly of non-A, non-B (HCV) type. Features of sepsis such as neutrophilic infiltration within the portal tracts and parenchyma are not seen in persistent hepatitis, whereas ground-glass cells and cobblestoning are not features of sepsis.
2. *Drug-induced liver injury:* Many drugs may produce nonspecific reactions and resemble persistent hepatitis; occasionally cobblestoning (phenytoin) and ground-glass–like cells (phenobarbital) may be present, but these cells will be negative on both orcein and immunoperoxidase stains for HBsAg.
3. *Chronic active hepatitis:* Fairly quiescent and early stages of chronic active hepatitis may be difficult to distinguish from persistent hepatitis; necrosis, inflammation, regenerative change, and ground-glass cells (hepatitis B) *irregularly* distributed within the biopsy specimen indicate chronic active liver disease.

Special Stains

1. In chronic hepatitis B, uniform cytoplasmic staining of HBsAg in ground-glass cells is shown with the following:
   a. *Orcein (Shikata)*—brown
   b. *Victoria blue*—blue
   c. *Aldehyde fuchsin*—purple

Immunohistochemistry

1. *HBsAg:* This antigen uniformly stains the cytoplasm of ground-glass cells in chronic hepatitis B and also identifies antigen in the cytoplasm of cells that do not exhibit the characteristic ground-glass appearance on hematoxylin and eosin stain. Staining of liver cell membranes may also occur, although this pattern is more common in chronic active hepatitis.
2. *HBcAg:* This antigen is present within nuclei in chronic hepatitis B and only rarely in cytoplasm; it is often seen in abundance in patients who are immunosuppressed (e.g., owing to renal dialysis, chemotherapy, or acquired immunodeficiency syndrome).

Clinical and Biologic Behavior

1. An apparently normal biopsy specimen associated with normal liver test results in a patient who is HBsAg positive for longer than 6 months is indicative of a hepatitis B "carrier" state. Since serologic testing for chronic non-A, non-B (HCV) hepatitis is only recently available, "carrier" state status of non-A, non-B hepatitis is not known.
2. Persistent viral hepatitis has *not* been reported to develop after acute hepatitis A or hepatitis E (enteric non-A, non-B).
3. Chronic persistent hepatitis, also termed *persistent viral hepatitis,* occurs in approximately 5% to 10% of patients with asymptomatic hepatitis B.
4. The frequency of non-A, non-B chronic hepatitis is not known but is estimated to be 50% when acquired from transfusions; in sporadic forms the frequency is estimated to be 20%.
5. Elevations in serum transaminase levels generally range from 50 to 500 IU/L, although levels are usually higher in non-A, non-B hepatitis. In the latter, the serum bilirubin value is rarely increased and serum transaminase levels characteristically fluctuate, with intervening normal values that may occasionally be mistaken for a resolved hepatitis.
6. In cases of persistent hepatitis B, approximately 1% of the patients clear HBsAg per year, seroconverting with immunity and a return of liver test abnormalities to normal.
7. *Ground-glass cells* represent an admixture of proliferating rough endoplasmic reticulum and HBsAg particles throughout the cytoplasm. These cells are diagnostic of chronic hepatitis (persistent or chronic active type) and are never seen in acute hepatitis B.
8. The number of ground-glass cells does not correlate with the severity of disease; it is important to note that these cells do *not* cluster but show an even distribution throughout the lobules.
9. Persistent hepatitis type B does not develop portal fibrosis or convert to chronic active hepatitis, except in instances of delta superinfection, when con-

version to an aggressive disease occurs in 90% of the cases.

10. Most patients are asymptomatic, while a few present with malaise and nondescript symptoms. The serum albumin level and prothrombin activity are normal, confirming the absence of significant derangement in synthetic function.

11. The liver may be mildly enlarged, but no stigmata of chronic liver disease are observed, and ascites, variceal hemorrhage, and encephalopathy do not develop.

Prognosis

1. Since persistent hepatitis is a benign lesion without progression to active hepatitis or cirrhosis, the prognosis is good.

2. In the case of type B hepatitis, persistent hepatitis is seen in chronic carriers (HBsAg-positive individuals). Although there is no risk of serious liver disease, the risk of development of hepatocellular carcinoma is slightly increased. Although HCV antibody is present in approximately 70% of patients with hepatocellular carcinoma, the risk of developing this malignancy from chronic HCV infection is not known.

References

Bianchi L, Spichtin HP, Gudat F. Chronic hepatitis. In: MacSween RNM, Anthony PP, Scheuer PJ, eds. Pathology of the Liver, 2nd ed. Edinburgh: Churchill Livingstone, 1987:320–322.

Hoofnagle JH, Shafritz DA, Popper H. Chronic type B hepatitis and the "healthy" HBsAg carrier state. Hepatology 1987;7:758–763.

Peters RL. Viral inflammatory diseases. In: Peters RL, Craig JR, eds. Liver Pathology. New York: Churchill Livingstone, 1986:90–93.

CHRONIC ACTIVE HEPATITIS

Major Morphologic Features

1. Lymphocytic inflammatory infiltration and hyperplasia of portal tracts, with spillover of inflammatory cells into periportal regions, often surround individual and small groups of hepatocytes ("piecemeal" necrosis, "cuffing").

2. Variable degrees of portal fibrosis eventually lead to formation of fibrous septa and regenerative nodules ("cirrhosis").

3. Mononuclear inflammatory infiltration, hepatocellular necrosis, and regenerative changes are *irregularly* distributed within the lobules or regenerative nodules.

Other Features

1. Degree of inflammatory change is variable from one portal region to another; plasma cells may be

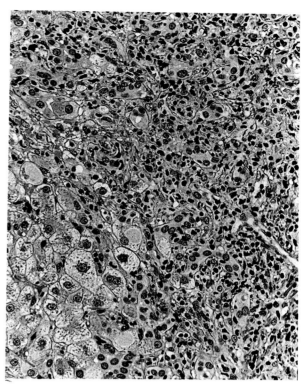

Figure 2–22. Chronic active hepatitis—type B. The portal tract is fibrotic, with moderate lymphocytic infiltration and bile duct proliferation. Scattered neutrophils are also present. Occasional ground-glass hepatocytes are present in the periportal zone.

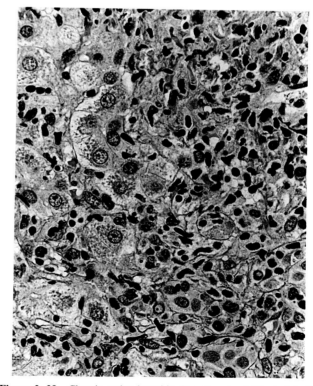

Figure 2–23. Chronic active hepatitis. Lymphocytes infiltrate into the periseptal region, surrounding individual and small groups of hepatocytes ("piecemeal" necrosis or "cuffing").

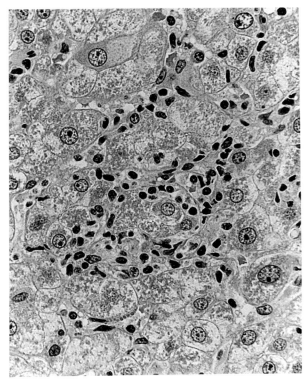

Figure 2–24. Chronic active hepatitis. Focal necrosis and aggregates of Kupffer cells, lymphocytes, and histiocytes are seen. In addition, lymphocytes surround small groups of liver cells within the parenchyma ("cuffing").

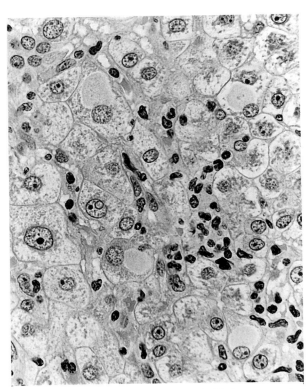

Figure 2–26. Chronic active hepatitis—type B. Numerous ground-glass cells, with typical peripheral nuclei and thin intracytoplasmic clear zones surrounding eosinophilic inclusions, are present. Ground-glass cells are *irregularly* distributed within lobules and regenerative nodules in chronic active hepatitis, in contrast to persistent hepatitis B, which typically exhibits a *uniform* distribution pattern of this cell type.

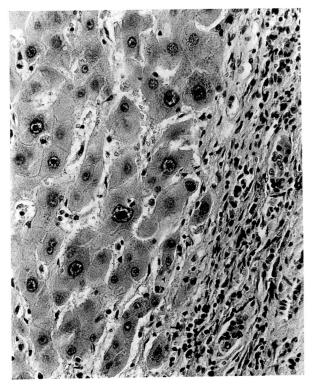

Figure 2–25. Chronic active hepatitis. In this high power view of cirrhosis, groups of periseptal hepatocytes contain large hyperchromatic nuclei with prominent nucleoli *(dysplasia)*. Aggregates of normal-sized liver cells are also present.

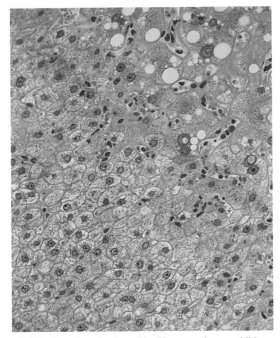

Figure 2–27. Chronic active hepatitis. The parenchyma exhibits variation in cell size and degree of inflammatory change within the same lobule. The cells *(top)* are large, contain fat, and exhibit prominent numbers of sinusoidal lymphocytes and Kupffer cell hyperplasia. The hepatocytes *(bottom)* are small with hydropic change and virtual *absence* of inflammatory cells or Kupffer cell hyperplasia.

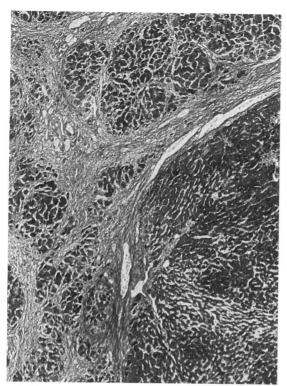

Figure 2–28. Chronic active hepatitis, cirrhotic stage (trichrome). The fibrous septa on low power surround both small as well as large regenerative nodules.

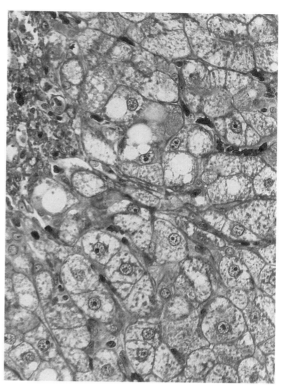

Figure 2–30. Chronic active hepatitis—HCV infection (trichrome). Sinusoidal collagen is shown as thin strands in the periportal region. Macrovesicular fat within hepatocytes is also present.

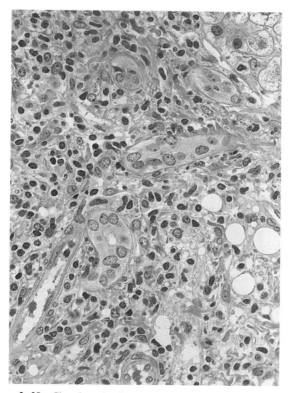

Figure 2–29. Chronic active hepatitis—HCV infection. Duct structures within this portal region are atypical, in some areas exhibiting flattened lumina and occasional infiltration by lymphocytes.

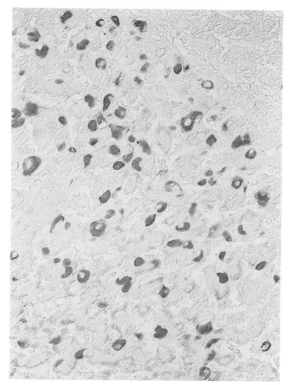

Figure 2–31. Chronic active hepatitis—HBsAg (immunoperoxidase). The surface antigen is cytoplasmic, often filling the entire cell but sparing the nucleus. In the fibrotic and cirrhotic stages, abundant numbers of hepatocytes may contain virus located within a lobule or nodule, with sparing of liver cells in the immediately adjacent regions.

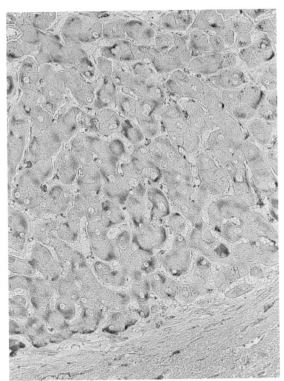

Figure 2–32. Chronic active hepatitis—HBsAg (immunoperoxidase). Membrane-associated deposition of HBsAg is much less common than diffuse cytoplasmic involvement and is believed to be a marker of hepatitis B replication. This feature may be noted in renal transplant patients.

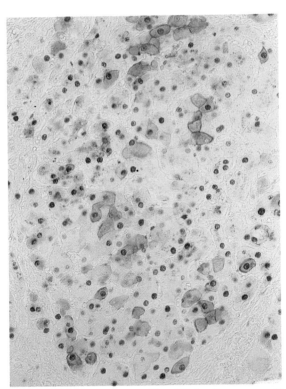

Figure 2–34. Chronic active hepatitis—HBcAg (immunoperoxidase). Staining of the core antigen is usually limited to the nucleus but is rarely seen in the cytoplasm. The delta antigen exhibits nuclear staining in both acute and chronic delta infection.

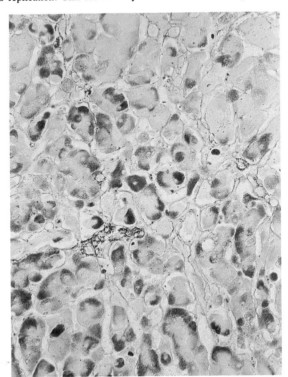

Figure 2–33. Chronic active hepatitis—HBsAg (orcein). Surface antigen in ground-glass cells is confirmed by positive cytoplasmic orcein (Shikata) staining. Orcein is typically used to stain elastic fibers but also stains both HBsAg and copper-binding protein because of their increase in disulfide bonds.

present (if abundant, an autoimmune rather than a viral etiology is often considered).

2. In very quiescent stages, and in cases of subclinical illness ("occult" chronic active hepatitis), "piecemeal" necrosis may be absent.

3. Bile duct proliferation is variable.

4. Acidophil bodies are occasionally evident.

5. Cholestasis occurs in the more active cases.

6. "Reactivation" is associated with severe necroinflammatory change and focal collapse of the lobular framework.

7. Kupffer cell hyperplasia is variable.

8. In cases secondary to HBV infection:

   a. *Ground-glass cells:* Hepatocytes with eosinophilic granular cytoplasm, peripheral halo staining pattern, and nucleus at cell margin are present in 50% to 75% of cases, with an *irregular* distribution both within the lobules or regenerative nodules and from one lobule/nodule to another.

   b. Groups of cells with variable degrees of nuclear and cytoplasmic anisocytosis and nuclear dysplasia are predominantly periportal or periseptal.

   c. In chronic delta infection, the degree of portal/septal and parenchymal inflammatory change and necrosis is usually more severe than in hepatitis B without delta infection.

9. In cases secondary to *non-A, non-B (HCV)* infection:
   a. Variability in inflammatory changes from one lobule to another may be minimal.
   b. Atypical ductular changes (flattened epithelium, minimal to absent lumina, infiltration by lymphocytes) are occasionally present.
   c. Macrovesicular fatty change is mild (1 to 2+), with no zonal distribution (20%–50% of cases).
   d. Intrasinusoidal presence of collagen is mild (30%–60% of cases).
   e. Glycogen nuclei may be present.
10. In the cirrhotic stages the regenerative nodules are of varying size, often with macronodules (>0.5 cm); in advanced cirrhosis, the specimen usually shows a mixture of both macronodules and micronodules.

Differential Diagnosis

1. *Acute viral hepatitis:* Portal fibrosis is not present in acute viral hepatitis alone, with the necroinflammatory change uniform from one lobule to another. In chronic active hepatitis, variable degrees of portal fibrosis are usually present and the inflammatory change is irregularly distributed throughout the biopsy specimen.
2. *Persistent viral hepatitis:* Cases of subclinical, occult, and early chronic active hepatitis may resemble persistent hepatitis. Irregular distribution of ground-glass cells in hepatitis B and irregular regenerative activity favor chronic active liver disease.
3. *Primary biliary cirrhosis:* The parenchymal changes in approximately 12% of cases of primary biliary cirrhosis resemble those in chronic active hepatitis. Nonsuppurative inflammatory and destructive bile duct lesions, decreased number of ducts, epithelioid granuloma formation, and proliferation of atypical ductules are strong indicators of primary biliary cirrhosis.
4. *Drug-induced injury* (e.g., oxyphenisatin, alpha-methyldopa): The morphologic changes may be virtually indistinguishable from those of chronic active hepatitis of viral etiology. Ground-glass–like cells that are positive on orcein stain in chronic hepatitis B are not present in drug-induced liver disease.

Special Stains

1. In chronic hepatitis B, uniform cytoplasmic staining of HBsAg in ground-glass cells is shown by the following:
   a. *Orcein (Shikata)*—brown
   b. *Victoria blue*—blue
   c. *Aldehyde fuchsin*—purple
2. *Masson trichrome:* This stain accentuates the portal fibrosis in cases of any etiology and intrasinusoidal collagen deposition in non-A, non-B (HCV) hepatitis.

Immunohistochemistry

1. *HBsAg:* This antigen uniformly stains the cytoplasm of ground-glass cells in hepatitis B and is also identified in cytoplasm of cells without the characteristic ground-glass appearance on hematoxylin and eosin staining. Staining of liver cell membranes may also occur.
2. *HBcAg:* This antigen is present within nuclei and only very rarely in cytoplasm in chronic hepatitis B. It is often seen in abundance in immunosuppressed patients (e.g., those on renal dialysis or chemotherapy or with the acquired immunodeficiency syndrome).
3. *Delta antigen:*
   a. In *acute* delta infection superimposed on chronic hepatitis B, variable degrees of nuclear staining are present with an even distribution from one lobule to another, often suppressing expression of both HBsAg and HBcAg.
   b. In *chronic* delta infection, variable nuclear staining with an *irregular* distribution from one lobule to another is characteristic; suppression of HBcAg, *not* HBsAg, commonly occurs.

Clinical and Biologic Behavior

1. Chronic active hepatitis and cirrhosis do *not* develop following hepatitis A and hepatitis E (enteric non-A, non-B).
2. Chronic active hepatitis occurs in approximately 1% of all cases following acute hepatitis B. The incidence of non-A, non-B (HCV) chronic active hepatitis ranges from 20% (sporadic) to 50% (post transfusion).
3. As cirrhosis develops, transaminase levels tend to be lower and may be within the normal range in advanced cirrhosis. Serum bilirubin and alkaline phosphatase levels may be mildly elevated with necroinflammatory activity. Serum albumin and prothrombin activity decrease as liver disease progresses and cirrhosis develops.
4. Symptoms associated with chronic active hepatitis are not specific. Fatigue is the most common symptom. As the disease advances, anorexia may develop with weight loss.
5. Splenomegaly is present in about 50% of the cases and is almost always present when cirrhosis and portal hypertension develop.
6. The liver may be enlarged, firm, and nontender with chronic active hepatitis and becomes impalpable when cirrhosis occurs. Cirrhosis is usually macronodular.
7. Since approximately 85% of all cases of acute viral hepatitis are subclinical, it is common for patients without a prior history of hepatitis to initially present with symptoms and signs of advanced liver disease.

8. In chronic active hepatitis B, reactivation may lead to marked increase in serum transaminase levels, hyperbilirubinemia, and hepatic failure if cirrhosis has developed. Reactivation may be spontaneous or precipitated by withdrawal of immunosuppressive therapy, as occurs in patients with hepatitis B who receive cyclical chemotherapy for lymphoproliferative disorders.

9. The duration from acquisition of hepatitis B or non-A, non-B (HCV) to the development of cirrhosis ranges from 2 to 20 years (average 8–11 years).

10. Approximately 7% of patients with chronic active hepatitis B may have HBsAg and HBcAg demonstrable in the liver by immunoperoxidase staining despite being serum HBsAg negative.

11. There is an increased frequency of hepatocellular carcinoma in B-viral cirrhosis as compared with alcoholic cirrhosis (48% vs. 6%). The integration of HBV-DNA into the genome of the host hepatocyte nucleus may play an oncogenic role in the genesis of malignant transformation.

12. Fine-needle aspiration of mass lesions detected on liver scans in patients with cirrhosis as a result of hepatitis B or non-A, non-B (HCV) is important to confirm the diagnosis of hepatocellular carcinoma.

Treatment

1. Management of complications of cirrhosis (see Chapter 1) is basically the same regardless of the specific viral-induced etiology.

References

Baptista A, Bianchi L, De Groote J, et al. The diagnostic significance of periportal hepatic necrosis and inflammation. Histopathology 1988;12:569–579.

Bianchi L, Spichtin HP, Gudat F. Chronic hepatitis. In: MacSween RNM, Anthony PP, Scheuer PJ, eds. Pathology of the Liver, 2nd ed. Edinburgh: Churchill Livingstone, 1987:322–328.

Lefkowitz JH, Apfelbaum TF. Non-A, non-B hepatitis: Characterization of liver biopsy pathology. J Clin Gastroenterol 1989;11:225–232.

Peters RL. Viral inflammatory diseases. In: Peters RL, Craig JR, eds. Liver Pathology. New York: Churchill Livingstone, 1986:93–103.

Thorne CH, Higgins GR, Ulich TR, et al. A histologic comparison of hepatitis B with non-A, non-B chronic active hepatitis. Arch Pathol Lab Med 1982;106:433–436.

Williams R, Alexander GJM. Natural history of chronic hepatitis B virus–related liver disease and its relationship to serum markers of viral replication. J Hepatol 1986;3:53–58.

■ Systemic Viral Infections With Hepatic Involvement

Epstein-Barr Virus (EBV) Infection

Major Morphologic Features

1. Portal tract expansion occurs by marked lymphocytic infiltration and hyperplasia; some of the lymphocytes are large and atypical; fibrosis is *not* present.

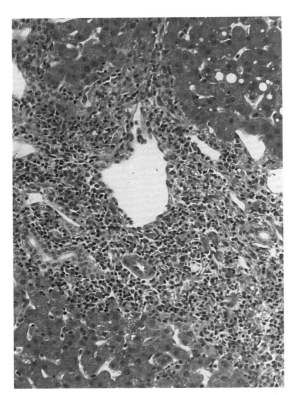

Figure 2–35. Epstein-Barr virus infection. Portal tracts are often expanded and markedly infiltrated by lymphocytes, some of which are large and atypical. Bile ducts are only slightly increased in number.

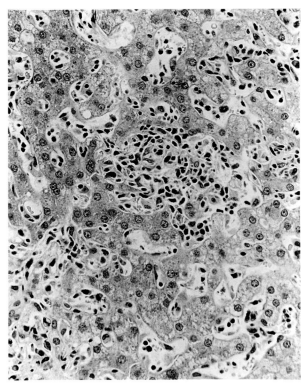

Figure 2–36. Epstein-Barr virus infection. Aggregates of lymphocytes, histiocytes, and Kupffer cells form poorly defined granulomatous lesions within the parenchyma. The surrounding hepatocytes are normal in size without hydropic change or disruption of the cord-sinusoid pattern.

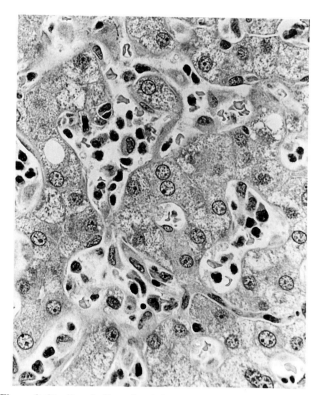

Figure 2–37. Epstein-Barr virus infection. High power exhibits prominent numbers of variously sized atypical lymphocytes within the sinusoids. Individual hepatocytes are relatively unremarkable.

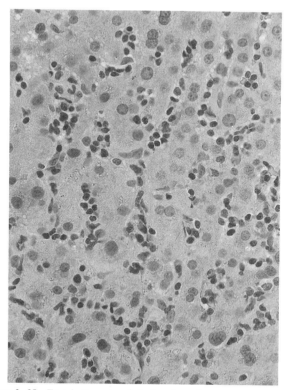

Figure 2–38. Epstein-Barr virus infection. Lymphocytes are seen crowding the sinusoids, forming a single-file "beading" appearance. The adjacent liver cell cords are intact, with hepatocytes of normal size containing eosinophilic cytoplasm.

2. Generally the cord-sinusoid pattern is intact, with focal hepatocytolysis but minimal hydropic changes of the liver cells.
3. Circulating atypical lymphocytes are increased within sinusoids, with a tendency of cells to line up in a beaded ("Indian file") pattern.

Other Features

1. Kupffer cell hyperplasia is moderate to marked.
2. Areas of parenchymal necrosis may have an ill-defined granulomatous appearance.
3. There is no zonal accentuation of changes.
4. Spillover of inflammatory cells from portal tracts into parenchyma (often resembling "piecemeal" necrosis) may be present but mild.

Differential Diagnosis

1. *Acute viral hepatitis:* Mild acute hepatitis from A, B, or non-A, non-B (HCV) viruses may exhibit a pattern similar to EBV infection.
2. *Cytomegalovirus (CMV) hepatitis:* Granulomatous necrosis tends to be somewhat more pronounced in CMV infections. Nuclear and cytoplasmic viral inclusions may be identified in hepatocytes, biliary epithelium, and Kupffer cells in immunocompromised patients.
3. *Drug-induced* (e.g., phenytoin): Morphologic features may be similar, although drugs tend to exhibit less of a portal inflammatory exudate.
4. *Lymphocytic leukemia:* Although lymphocytes within portal tracts and sinusoids may be quite prominent in EBV infection, the lymphocytes are polymorphous in type and shape, while in lymphocytic leukemia the infiltrates are monomorphic. In addition, granulomatous necrosis is not a feature of leukemia.

Clinical and Biologic Behavior

1. Epstein-Barr virus is the recognized agent causing infectious mononucleosis, with an incidence of approximately 100,000 cases per year (twice that of acute viral hepatitis).
2. The incubation period is approximately 5 weeks, after which fever, acute pharyngitis, splenomegaly, and lymphocytosis (atypical lymphocytes) develop; however, one half to two thirds of the cases are subclinical.
3. The liver is involved in over 90% of cases. Hepatomegaly is present in 10% to 15%, splenomegaly is seen in 50%, and jaundice occurs in only 5%.
4. Patients with liver involvement take longer to recover, and liver test abnormalities consist of elevated serum transaminase levels (usually ~500 IU/L and

generally less than seen in acute viral hepatitis). Alkaline phosphatase elevation may be pronounced (~1000 IU/L) and associated with moderate hyperbilirubinemia.

5. The "monospot" test is sensitive (80%) and specific (99%) but may be initially negative in 15% of patients. Elevation of EBV specific antibody, and absent or low titer antibody to EBV-associated nuclear antigen, confirm the diagnosis of acute EBV infection. A single high viral capsid antigen (VCA) antibody titer does not distinguish current from previous infection.

6. EBV infects B lymphocytes, with antigenic expression on the surface of the cell eliciting a response by T lymphocytes; their interaction produces the characteristic "atypical" lymphocyte seen in the peripheral blood and liver biopsy specimens.

7. In immunocompromised patients (e.g., those with acquired immunodeficiency syndrome), chronic enzyme elevations and morphologic changes may persist for years; however, progression of the disease into a fibrotic or cirrhotic stage has *not* been reported.

8. Other associated conditions include Guillain-Barré syndrome, pulmonary infiltrations, pericarditis and myocarditis, and splenic rupture.

References

Gowing NFC. Infectious mononucleosis: Histopathologic aspects. Pathol Annu 1975;10:1–20.

Lloyd-Still JD, Scott JP, Crussi F. The spectrum of Epstein-Barr virus hepatitis in children. Pediatr Pathol 1986;5:337–351.

Markin RS, Linder J, Zuerlein K, et al. Hepatitis in fatal infectious mononucleosis. Gastroenterology 1987;93:1210–1217.

White NJ, Juel-Jensen BE. Infectious mononucleosis hepatitis. Semin Liver Dis 1984;4:301–306.

Cytomegalovirus (CMV) Infection

Major Morphologic Features

1. Portal tracts show lymphocytic infiltration and hyperplasia; many of the lymphocytes are atypical.
2. Generally intact cord-sinusoid pattern, with focal hepatocytolysis and occasional ill-defined granuloma formation

Other Features

1. Large intranuclear, and in some instances intracytoplasmic, amphophilic inclusions with a surrounding halo ("owl's eye") in hepatocytes, bile ducts, or Kupffer cells are diagnostic but rare; inclusions are seen most often in immunocompromised patients.
2. Occasional but mild degree of macrovesicular fatty change occurs.
3. Cholestasis is evident in severe cases.
4. Portal fibrosis does not occur in the adult; however,

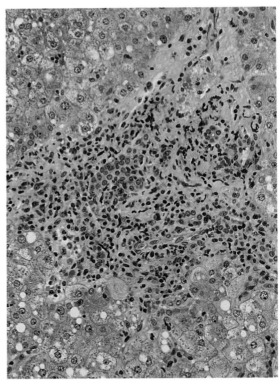

Figure 2–39. Cytomegalovirus infection. Portal areas exhibit variable degrees of lymphocytic infiltration and hyperplasia. Bile ducts are slightly increased in number. Inflammatory cells only occasionally spill over into the adjacent parenchyma.

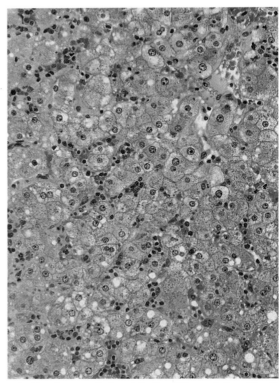

Figure 2–40. Cytomegalovirus infection. The cord-sinusoid pattern is basically maintained. Increased numbers of lymphocytes are identified within the sinusoids, with only minimal liver cell injury. Occasional hepatocytes contain mild fatty change.

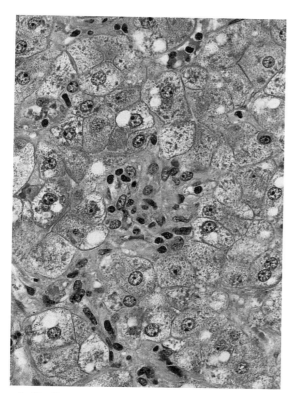

Figure 2–41. Cytomegalovirus infection. Focal necrosis with aggregates of Kupffer cells, lymphocytes, and macrophages may at times form ill-defined granulomatous lesions. Kupffer cell hyperplasia and mild fatty change are also present.

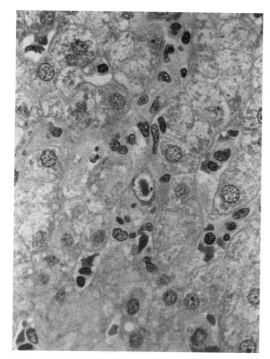

Figure 2–42. Cytomegalovirus infection and acquired immunodeficiency syndrome. In immunocompromised patients, cytomegalovirus is occasionally identified as large eosinophilic nuclear inclusions surrounded by a clear zone. Adjacent inflammatory infiltration may be present but is often minimal. The intranuclear inclusion has been described in bile duct epithelium but is quite rare.

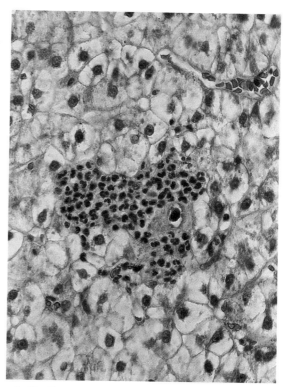

Figure 2–43. Cytomegalovirus infection in liver transplant. The liver cell in the center of the field contains a large basophilic nuclear inclusion and rather dense cytoplasm compared with the remaining hydropic hepatocytes. Although this photomicrograph shows a striking neutrophilic reaction adjacent to the infected liver cell, a lymphocytic reaction is usually more common (see Figure 10–35).

portal and interstitial fibrosis, giant cell transformation, and acute cholangitis may be seen in the neonate.

5. In transplanted livers, the early stage of the infection may be associated with small aggregates of neutrophils adjacent to or surrounding hepatocytes containing nuclear inclusions.

Differential Diagnosis

1. *Acute viral hepatitis* (A, B, non-A non-B [HCV]): Mild acute hepatitis caused by these hepatotropic viruses may be indistinguishable from CMV infection.
2. *Epstein-Barr (EBV) hepatitis:* Although the degree of lymphocytic response is more marked in EBV infection, the granulomatous response is minimal and intranuclear inclusions are not present.
4. *Drug-induced* (e.g., phenytoin): Morphologically, this may resemble CMV infection, although drugs tend to have less of a portal inflammatory response.
5. *Lymphocytic leukemia:* Portal and sinusoidal infiltration by lymphocytes is more prominent in leukemia, and granulomatous necrosis is not present.

Immunohistochemistry

1. *CMV antigen:* Nuclear and very rarely cytoplasmic staining may be identified in hepatocytes, bile ducts, and even Kupffer cells; demonstration of this antigen is usually limited to patients who are immunocompromised.

Clinical and Biologic Behavior

1. This virus is a member of the herpesvirus group, and infection may be acquired during birth in the majority of instances. The virus in these cases is not eradicated but becomes incorporated into the host's cells as a latent infection and reactivates during immunosuppressive therapy (e.g., following renal transplantation and chemotherapy for malignancy).
2. CMV may be acquired in adulthood from massive blood transfusions as occur during open-heart surgery.
3. CMV can be isolated from saliva, urine, blood, and tissues. The virus produces a focal cytopathic change on monolayer fibroblast cultures.
4. CMV-specific antibody by solid phase immunoassay is useful to detect primary infection; however, approximately 30% of immunosuppressed patients may produce IgM-specific antibody with recurrent infection.
5. The liver may be involved in congenital infection. Neonates present with hepatosplenomegaly, portal and interstitial hepatic fibrosis, jaundice, thrombocytopenia in association with microcephaly, periventricular calcification, chorioretinitis, and other signs of intrauterine infection. Brain damage is often permanent.
6. Clinically, CMV hepatitis is mild and self-limiting and accounts for approximately 8% of cases with an "infectious mononucleosis–like syndrome" with hepatic involvement. Liver tests reveal mild to moderate elevation of serum transaminases (200–300 IU/L) and alkaline phosphatase, and mild hyperbilirubinemia. Atypical lymphocytes may be seen on a peripheral smear.
7. Other associated conditions include Guillain-Barré syndrome, hemolytic anemia, meningoencephalitis, pneumonitis, and myocarditis
8. Rare cases of fatal massive hepatic necrosis have been reported, usually in immunocompromised patients.

References

Griffiths PD. Cytomegalovirus and the liver. Semin Liver Dis 1984;4:307–313.

Paya CV, Hermans PE, Wiesner RH, et al. Cytomegalovirus hepatitis in liver transplantation: Prospective analysis of 93 consecutive orthotopic liver transplantations. J Infect Dis 1989;160:752–758.

Snover DC, Horwitz CA. Liver disease in CMV mononucleosis: A light microscopic and immunoperoxidase study of six cases. Hepatology 1984;4:408–412.

Herpes Simplex Virus Infection

Major Morphologic Features

1. Coagulative necrosis involves large areas of parenchyma, with no zonal distribution.
2. Two types of intranuclear inclusions are seen in liver cells at edge of necrosis:
   a. Eosinophilic, with peripheral clear space or halo (Cowdry type A)
   b. Basophilic, filling up entire nucleus and giving ground-glass appearance (Cowdry type B)

Other Features

1. Cytoplasm of hepatocytes at edge of necrosis has a more eosinophilic appearance.
2. Inflammatory activity is variable, but generally sparse at edge of necrosis and in portal areas.
3. Hemorrhage surrounds and is within necrotic areas.
4. Giant cell transformation of hepatocytes, particularly in the neonate, occurs infrequently.
5. Massive hepatic necrosis has been described (undernourished children).
6. Inclusion bodies are *not* present in Kupffer cells or bile duct epithelium.

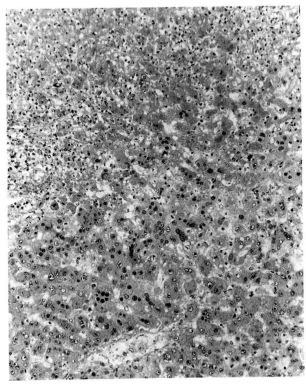

Figure 2–44. Herpes simplex virus infection. The parenchyma *(upper field)* has undergone extensive coagulative-type necrosis. Adjacent hepatocytes *(center)* exhibit dark-staining nuclei.

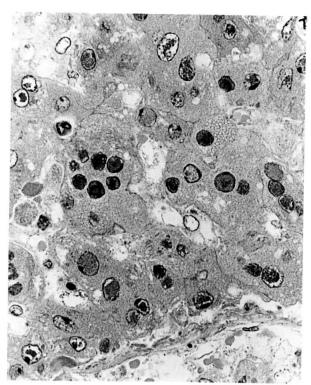

Figure 2–45. Herpes simplex virus infection. Higher power exhibits two types of nuclei: (1) dark-staining and basophilic, taking up the entire nucleus, often with a thin peripheral rim of chromatin material (Cowdry type B), and (2) clear with a central relatively large acidophilic mass (Cowdry type A). The type B inclusion is Feulgen positive and composed of virus particles. Eventually the virus enters the cytoplasm, leaving in its place the Feulgen-negative type A inclusion.

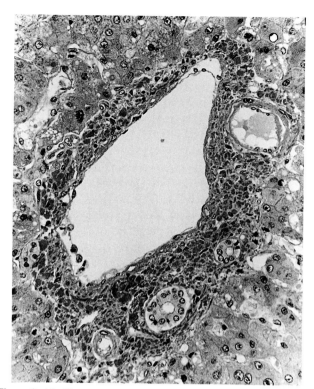

Figure 2–46. Herpes simplex virus infection. The portal tract in an area away from liver cell necrosis appears unremarkable, with no inflammatory infiltrate or bile duct change.

Differential Diagnosis

1. *Varicella-zoster:* Necrotic lesions and inclusion bodies may be identical with those of herpes simplex infection; however, unlike in herpes simplex, both granulomatous necrosis and viral inclusions within Kupffer cells and bile duct epithelium may be present in varicella infections.
2. *Vaccinia:* Necrosis is similar to that of herpes simplex but without inclusions (does not cause fatal liver disease).
3. *Eclampsia:* Coagulative necrosis tends to be periportal or midzonal, with prominent sinusoidal fibrin deposition; inclusions are not present.

Special Stains

1. *Feulgen reaction:* Nuclear staining is *positive* when the nucleus is filled with viral DNA (Cowdry type B) and *negative* when the virus has entered the cytoplasm (Cowdry type A).

Immunohistochemistry

1. *Herpesvirus type 1 and 2 antigens:* Intranuclear staining shows cells containing the ground-glass inclusions but is also occasionally positive in cytoplasm of hepatocytes in and around the necrotic lesions.

Clinical and Biologic Behavior

1. There are two variants of *Herpesvirus hominis:* Type 1 is common, is present in oral secretions in 50% of the general population, and is clinically manifested by ulceration of the lip and buccal mucosa; type 2 involves the genitalia and is spread by sexual contact. Both types may involve the liver.
2. Hepatic involvement is associated with disseminated infection and marked elevations of serum transaminase and bilirubin levels; disseminated intravascular coagulation is common.
3. Hepatic lesions are virtually never seen in normal humans but are found in immunocompromised patients (e.g., in patients on corticosteroids, during treatment for neoplastic disorders, and after transplantation), in malnourished children, and rarely in pregnant women.

Prognosis

1. In patients with symptomatic hepatic necrosis, death usually results in over 90% of patients 1 to 2 weeks after the beginning of symptoms.

References

Goodman ZD, Ishak KG, Sesterhenn IA. Herpes simplex hepatitis in apparently immunocompetent adults. Am J Clin Pathol 1986;85:694–699.

Marrie TJ, McDonald ATJ, Conen PE et al. Herpes simplex hepatitis: Use of immunoperoxidase to demonstrate the viral antigen in hepatocytes. Gastroenterology 1982;82:71–76.

Nahmias AJ, Roizman B. Infection with herpes-simplex viruses 1 and 2. N Engl J Med 1973;289:667–674, 719–725, 781–789.

Human Immunodeficiency Virus (HIV) Infection

Major Morphologic Features

1. Decreased or marked depletion of lymphocytes occurs within portal areas in more than 50% of cases.
2. Changes are secondary to opportunistic infections in up to 32% of cases (most commonly CMV, *Mycobacterium avium-intracellulare,* and *Cryptococcus neoformans*).

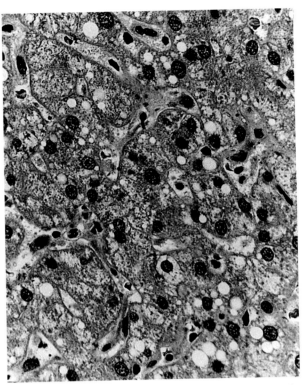

Figure 2–48. Human immunodeficiency virus infection. The parenchyma exhibits a variable degree of both macrovesicular and microvesicular fat. Kupffer cell hyperplasia is present. Although not seen in this photomicrograph, superinfection with various agents (e.g., *Mycobacterium avium-intracellulare*) is often present.

Other Features

1. Granulomas from infections are usually ill defined, and organisms, which may be present in Kupffer cells in the absence of granuloma formation, are often abundant.
2. Kupffer cell hyperplasia is variable.
3. Kupffer cells may exhibit erythrophagocytosis in approximately 10% of cases and have a foamy appearance when containing organisms.
4. Mild fatty change occurs in 25%, and variable degrees of cholestasis occur in 10% of cases.
5. Kaposi's sarcoma is present in up to 14% of cases.
6. Chronic co-infection with persistent hepatitis B has been reported in up to 32% of cases; however, chronic *active* hepatitis is rare.

Differential Diagnosis

1. *Disorders that may cause lymphocyte depletion include the following:*
   a. Hodgkin's disease with or without liver involvement
   b. Immunosuppression secondary to chemotherapy and renal dialysis

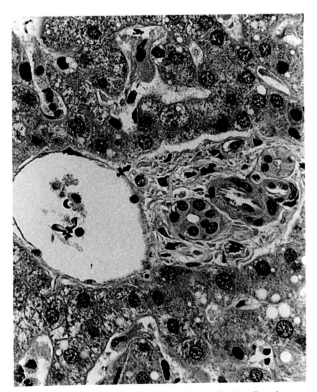

Figure 2–47. Human immunodeficiency virus infection. Portal tracts are normal in size with a relative paucity of inflammatory cells, especially lymphocytes.

c. Widespread carcinoma
d. Elderly population

Note: In any case in which opportunistic infections are identified in the liver, the acquired immunodeficiency syndrome should be in the differential diagnosis as the underlying immunodeficiency disorder.

Special Stains

1. Identification of co-infection is performed with the following:
   a. *Ziehl-Neelsen, Kinyoun's acid fast:* Acid-fast bacilli *(Mycobacterium tuberculosis* and *M. avium-intracellulare)*
   b. *Periodic acid–Schiff:* M. *avium-intracellulare* and fungi *(Cryptococcus neoformans)*
   c. *Methenamine silver:* Fungi, *Pneumocystis carinii*

Immunohistochemistry

1. *HBsAg, HBcAg:* These antigens identify co-infection with hepatitis B and may be positive in up to 32% and 5% of cases, respectively.

Clinical and Biologic Behavior

1. Acquired immunodeficiency syndrome (AIDS) and AIDS-related complex (ARC) are caused by infection with a group D retrovirus, previously named lymphadenopathy-associated virus (LAV), human T-cell lymphotropic virus type III (HTLV-III), and AIDS-associated retrovirus (ARV) and now officially recognized as the human immunodeficiency virus (HIV).
2. AIDS occurs in a group of previously healthy persons who have lost their immunity as a result of infection with HIV. Opportunistic infections and neoplasms develop in these patients.

Infectious Agents	Neoplasms
Cytomegalovirus	Kaposi's sarcoma
Epstein-Barr virus	Central nervous system
Herpesvirus hominis	lymphoma
Varicella-zoster	
Cryptosporidium	
Pneumocystis	
Toxoplasma	
Aspergillus	
Histoplasma	
Candida	
Cryptococcus	
Mycobacterium tuberculosis	
Mycobacterium avium-intracellulare	

3. The virus infects, replicates in, and eventually destroys T4 (helper) lymphocytes, with reversal of the helper/suppressor T-cell ratio and acquisition of anti-HIV.
4. Patient populations at high risk include intravenous drug users, homosexuals, patients receiving transfusion of blood products (especially hemophiliacs), and heterosexual contacts of the above patients as well as children of the above contacts.
5. Antibody can be found days to weeks after infection, with eventual development of AIDS (5 years average time period) and/or ARC (lymphadenopathy, fatigue, weight loss, diarrhea, night sweats, decreased T4 lymphocytes).
6. Liver disease is secondary to associated infections and neoplasms, not to the immunodeficiency disorder itself.
7. Chronic hepatitis from CMV can occur, but fibrosis is not a feature.

Prognosis

1. In patients with Kaposi's sarcoma, the median survival is 18 to 24 months; in patients with opportunistic infections, the survival is 6 to 8 months

References

Glasgow BJ, Anders K, Layfield LJ et al. Clinical and pathologic findings of the liver in the acquired immune deficiency syndrome (AIDS). Am J Clin Pathol 1985;83:582–588.
Lebovics E, Thung SN, Schaffner F et al. The liver in the acquired immunodeficiency syndrome: A clinical and histologic study. Hepatology 1985;5:293–298.
Nakanuma Y, Liew CT, Peters RL et al. Pathologic features of the liver in acquired immune deficiency syndrome (AIDS). Liver 1986;6:158–166.
Smith RD. The pathobiology of HIV infection: A review. Arch Pathol Lab Med 1990;114:235–239.

■ Rare Systemic Viral Infections With Hepatic Involvement: Lassa Fever and Yellow Fever

Major Morphologic Features

Lassa Fever
1. Coagulative hepatocellular necrosis and fragmentation of cytoplasm (apoptosis) are scattered throughout the lobule; although usually patchy, this occasionally produces confluent, bridging necrosis.

Yellow Fever
1. Coagulative type of midzonal necrosis with numerous acidophilic *(Councilman)* bodies is present.
2. Nuclei of surviving hepatocytes with enlarged eosinophilic nucleoli are present and in rare instances may contain distinct eosinophilic inclusions (Torres bodies).

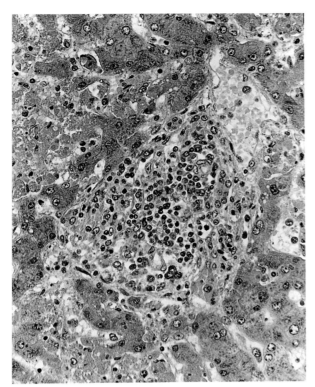

Figure 2–49. Lassa fever. The portal tract exhibits a moderate lymphocytic infiltration and hyperplasia. The periportal parenchyma *(upper left)* is undergoing a coagulative-type necrosis.

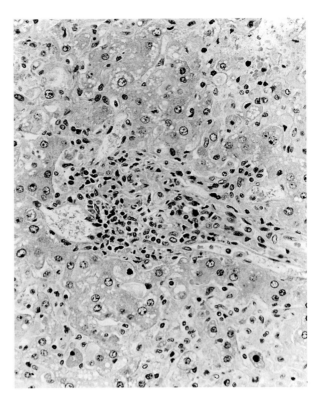

Figure 2–51. Yellow fever. The portal tract is normal in size with a moderate degree of lymphocytic infiltration and hyperplasia. The immediate surrounding periportal hepatocytes appear unremarkable; however, there is a suggestion of liver cell necrosis at the edges of the photomicrograph in the midzonal regions.

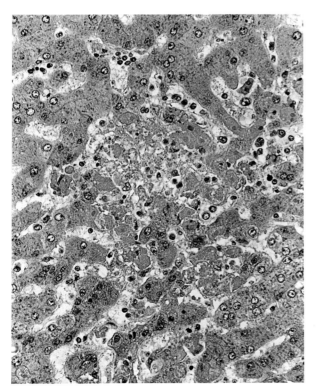

Figure 2–50. Lassa fever. The coagulative-type necrosis is rather poorly demarcated. Although an increase in circulating sinusoidal cells is apparent, infiltration into the necrotic hepatocytes is not seen. Inclusion bodies are not present on routine histologic examination, but abundant numbers of viral particles can be identified on electron microscopy.

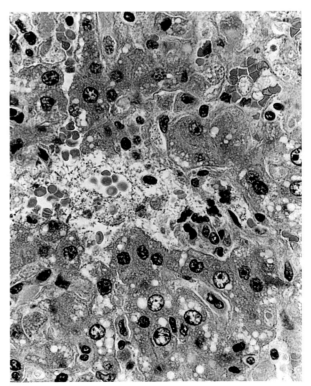

Figure 2–52. Yellow fever. The hepatocytes surrounding this terminal hepatic venule are intact, with only a mild degree of microvesicular fat. Moderate Kupffer cell hyperplasia is also present.

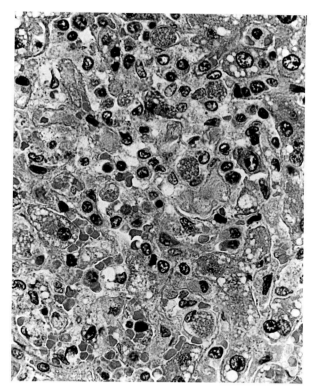

Figure 2–53. Yellow fever. This midzonal region exhibits a moderate infiltration by lymphocytes. Liver cell necrosis is apparent, with formation of numerous acidophil bodies.

Other Features (Both Entities)

1. Inflammatory activity in portal tracts is variable but usually minimal.
2. Kupffer cell hyperplasia is mild to moderate.
3. Mild fatty changes occur in yellow fever but are rare in Lassa fever.

Differential Diagnosis

1. *Acute viral hepatitis (A, B, non-A non-B [HCV]):* Both yellow fever and Lassa fever exhibit a coagulative type of necrosis, with accentuation of midzonal regions in yellow fever. The classic forms of viral hepatitis, however, may have a perivenular accentuation and are not associated with a coagulative type of necrosis.
2. *Other viral infections associated with acidophilic necrosis (Bolivian, Korean, and Argentinian hemorrhagic fever; Marburg virus infection, dengue fever):* These viral infections may morphologically resemble Lassa fever; epidemiology and isolation of the viruses are necessary for diagnosis.

Clinical and Biologic Behavior

Lassa Fever
1. Lassa fever is a multisystemic disease associated with fever, exudative pharyngitis, gastrointestinal and renal disturbances, and coagulation abnormalities.
2. The disease is caused by an arenavirus, a member of a group of RNA viruses responsible for hemorrhagic fevers and widely present in Western and Central Africa.
3. Infection is usually subclinical and transmitted by contact with rodent (reservoir) excrement.
4. Hepatomegaly, right upper quadrant pain, and tenderness are common; serum transaminase levels are elevated, but bilirubin level is usually normal.

Yellow Fever
1. Yellow fever is a multisystemic disease that presents with fever, renal dysfunction (acute tubular necrosis, hemoglobinuria), gastrointestinal hemorrhage, and coagulation abnormalities. Moderate to marked elevations in serum transaminases and bilirubin levels are usually present.
2. The disease is caused by an RNA group B arbovirus transmitted by the *Aedes aegypti* mosquito and is present in Africa, South America, and the Caribbean Islands.

Prognosis

Lassa Fever
1. The mortality is 5% to 14%; however, mortality in pregnant women is much higher.

Yellow Fever
1. Coma and death occur in 10% to 60%.

References

Howard CR, Ellis DS, Simpson DIH. Exotic viruses and the liver. Semin Liver Dis 1984;4:361–374.
Vieira W, Gayotto LC, De Lima CP et al. Histopathology of the human liver in yellow fever with special emphasis on the diagnostic role of the Councilman body. Histopathology 1983;7:195–208.
Walker DH, McCormick JB, Johnson KM et al. Pathologic and virologic study of fatal Lassa fever in man. Am J Pathol 1982;107:349–356.

General References

Edmondson HA, Peters RL. Liver. In: Kissane JM, Anderson WAD, eds. Pathology, 8th ed. St. Louis: C.V. Mosby, 1985:1111–1129.
Koff RS, Galambos JT. Viral hepatitis. In: Schiff L, Schiff ER, eds. Diseases of the Liver, 6th ed. Philadelphia: J.B. Lippincott, 1987:457–581.
Peters RL. Acute and chronic varieties of viral hepatitis. In: Oda T, ed. Hepatitis Viruses. Tokyo: University of Tokyo Press, 1978:197–233.
Peters RL. Viral hepatitis: A pathologic spectrum. Am J Med Sci 1975;270:17–31.
Scheuer PJ. Viral hepatitis. In: MacSween RNM, Anthony PP, Scheuer PJ, eds. Pathology of the Liver, 2nd ed. Edinburgh: Churchill Livingstone, 1987:202–223.

CHAPTER 3

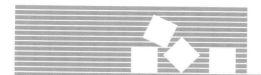

Cholestasis and Biliary Tract Disorders

■ Mechanical Duct Obstruction

Early Stages (First weeks after obstruction)

Major Morphologic Features

1. Proliferation and dilatation of interlobular ducts occur.
2. Periductal edema is present, and portal inflammatory infiltration consists predominantly of neutrophils.
3. *Acute cholangitis:* Neutrophils surround and invade the duct.
4. Perivenular cholestasis is evident within hepatocytes and dilated bile canaliculi.

Other Features

1. Cholangiolar proliferation occurs at periphery of portal tracts, with the cholangioles often containing bile and surrounded by neutrophils.
2. There are variable degrees of hepatocellular necrosis in cholestatic regions, with bile and periodic acid–Schiff-positive phagocytized material in macrophages and hyperplastic Kupffer cells.
3. *Microabscess formation:* Aggregates of neutrophils either involving destroyed interlobular bile ducts or formed within the parenchyma are seen in severe and usually untreated cases.
4. Portal inflammatory changes may be virtually absent in very early stages in spite of severe clinical presentation, occurring most often in instances of passed gallstones.
5. When obstruction has been present at least 1 month, one may see the following:

   a. *Bile lakes:* Accumulation of small pools of extracellular bile within portal or periportal regions is rare but virtually diagnostic of acute large duct obstruction.
   b. *Bile infarcts:* Aggregates of pale-staining, necrotic hepatocytes with intermixed fibrin and occasionally bile pigment are located predominantly in the periportal zone; they are rare but virtually diagnostic of acute large duct obstruction.
   c. *Feathery degeneration:* Hepatocytes with clear to foamy cytoplasm are found singly or in small groups.

Later Stages (Months to years after obstruction)

Major Morphologic Features

1. *Biliary fibrosis:* Portal fibrosis uniformly involves all portal tracts, with preservation of the basic lobular architecture (portal–terminal hepatic venule–portal).
2. *Secondary biliary cirrhosis:* Fibrous septa and irregular to round, small regenerative nodules are arranged in a "geographic" or "jigsaw puzzle" pattern, exhibiting periseptal lamellar fibrosis with a thin rim of edema around the periphery of the nodules.

Other Features

1. Periductal fibrosis is noted, with variable but often prominent bile duct reduplication; however, in cirrhotic stages bile ducts may be decreased in number or even absent.

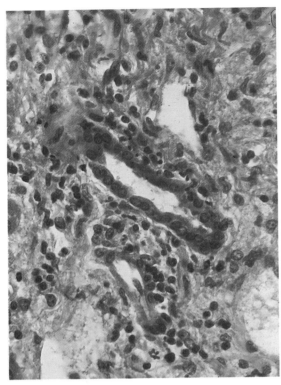

Figure 3–1. Mechanical duct obstruction. An interlobular bile duct within a portal tract exhibits slight dilatation. Periductal neutrophils are present but have not yet infiltrated into the duct wall in this early stage of obstruction.

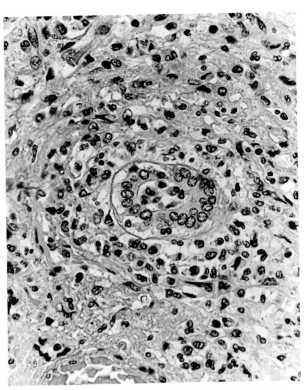

Figure 3–3. Mechanical duct obstruction. Acute cholangitis is illustrated by neutrophils invading the basement membrane and appearing within the duct wall and lumen. Slight dilatation of the lumen is also present.

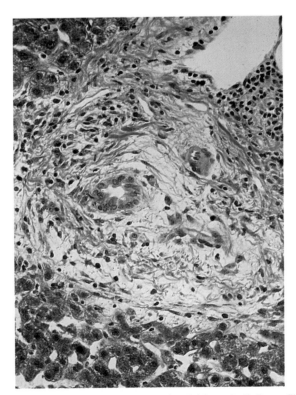

Figure 3–2. Mechanical duct obstruction (trichrome). Collagen fibers exhibit a loose staining pattern around the interlobular duct as a result of edema.

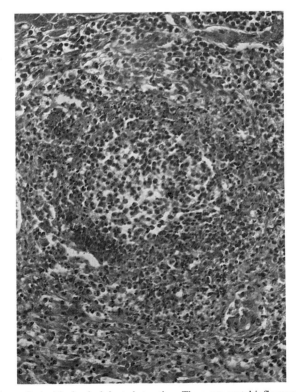

Figure 3–4. Mechanical duct obstruction. The acute portal inflammatory infiltration can progress in the untreated patient to form marked duct destruction and abscesses. At this stage microabscesses can often be seen in the parenchyma as well.

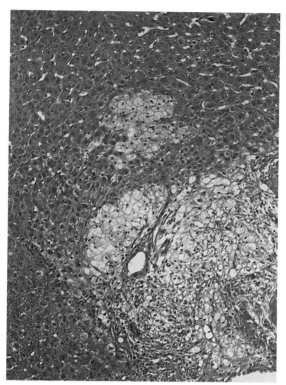

Figure 3–5. Mechanical duct obstruction. Aggregates of liver cells having a clear reticulated cytoplasm, appearing feathery in type, are often identified more commonly in periportal zones. With time these liver cells may undergo a lytic necrosis, forming bile infarcts.

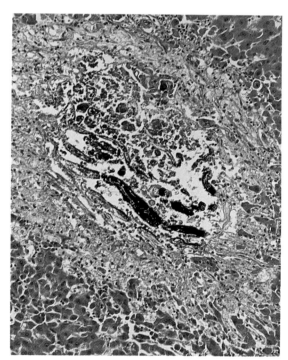

Figure 3–6. Mechanical duct obstruction. A toxic change of hepatocytes caused by accumulation of bile and bile salts is known as a *bile infarct* and is characterized by lytic necrosis of liver cells with the presence of bilirubin. Hepatocytes with foamy clear cytoplasm often having a feathery-type degeneration immediately surround the necrotic region. Bile infarcts, like bile lakes, are rare but pathognomonic for large duct obstruction.

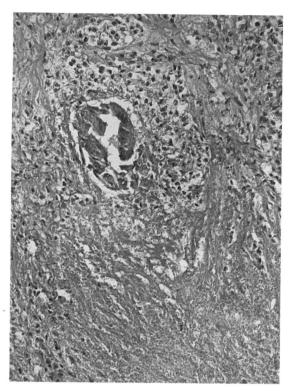

Figure 3–7. Mechanical duct obstruction. The interlobular duct is distorted and has undergrown individual cell necrosis. Bile has extravasated from the duct lumen, forming a *bile lake*. Neutrophils are also present surrounding the duct. Although bile lakes are believed to be pathognomonic for extrahepatic or intrahepatic large duct obstruction, this lesion is uncommonly found in liver biopsy specimens.

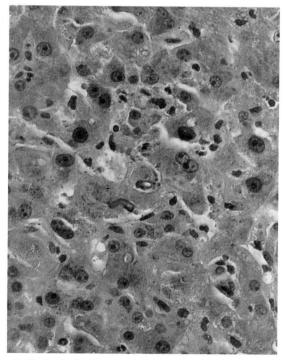

Figure 3–8. Mechanical duct obstruction. Perivenular hepatocytes exhibit dilated canaliculi filled with bile. Cholestasis can also be identified in liver cell cytoplasm and in Kupffer cells adjacent to hepatocytes that have undergone necrosis.

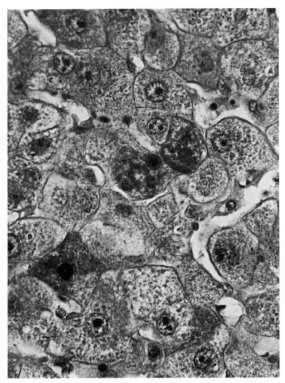

Figure 3–9. Mechanical duct obstruction. Alcoholic hyalin can be found in approximately 2% of patients with long-term obstruction. The hyalin is predominantly in periportal hepatocytes. Neutrophilic reaction to the hyalin, characteristic of acute alcoholic liver disease, is not typically noted.

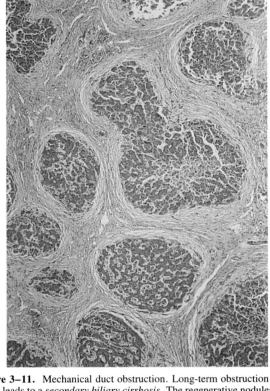

Figure 3–11. Mechanical duct obstruction. Long-term obstruction eventually leads to a *secondary biliary cirrhosis*. The regenerative nodules have a jigsaw puzzle appearance, and are surrounded by loose collagen laid down in a parallel fashion.

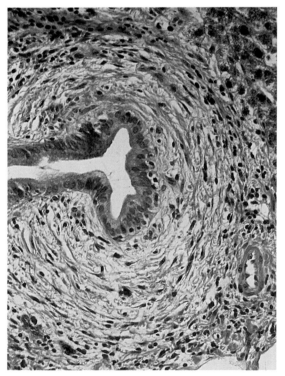

Figure 3–10. Mechanical duct obstruction (trichrome). As the liver disease progresses, periductal collagen is gradually laid down. Intermittent bouts of acute cholangitis, often subclinical, undoubtedly occur in these cases.

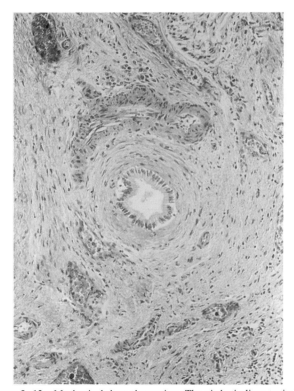

Figure 3–12. Mechanical duct obstruction. The cirrhotic liver typically exhibits periductal fibrosis involving the medium-sized interlobular ducts.

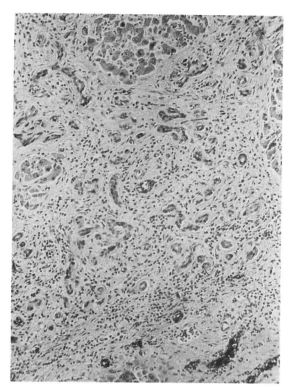

Figure 3–13. Mechanical duct obstruction. The fibrous septa in the cirrhotic stage often have proliferating interlobular ducts, as in this case; however, the septa rarely may be devoid of ducts. Variable degrees of lymphocytic infiltration are present.

2. Inflammatory mononuclear infiltrate occurs predominantly in fibrotic regions.
3. Thickening of hepatic arterioles is often present.
4. Bile ductules may rarely have an atypical appearance, with elliptical nuclei, absence of lumina, and a serpiginous growth pattern at the margins of the portal regions.
5. Periportal hepatocytes are often swollen and hydropic.
6. Mallory's hyalin is present in periportal hepatocytes

in 2% of cases; the hyalin is usually not associated with surrounding inflammatory cells.
7. Cholestasis is not as frequent as in acute obstruction and when present is perivenular or periportal.
8. Acute cholangitis, bile infarcts, bile lakes, and feathery degeneration may be seen, but not as frequently as in the earlier stages.
9. There is a moderate increase in copper and copper-binding protein (black intracytoplasmic granules on orcein stain) within periportal hepatocytes.
10. Extrahepatic bile ducts exhibit variable degrees of fibrosis and both acute and chronic inflammatory infiltration in instances of choledocholithiasis; this change is prominent at the site of obstruction or resultant stricture.

Differential Diagnosis

1. *Primary biliary cirrhosis*
2. *Primary sclerosing cholangitis*
   a. *Noncirrhotic stage* (refer to table below)
   b. *Severe fibrotic and cirrhotic stages:* It may be impossible to morphologically distinguish between the three entities on needle biopsy, since all three may show fibrous septa and decreased or absent ducts. Periductal fibrosis will rule out primary biliary cirrhosis, but ERCP, ultrasound, and/or serologic data are usually necessary for diagnosis.
3. *Impaired regeneration syndrome:* Dilated cholangioles may be filled with bile and surrounded by neutrophils; however, perivenular cholestasis is not present. Instead there is perivenular collapse of the reticulin framework from previous liver cell necrosis.
4. *Sepsis:* Acute portal inflammatory infiltration, cholestasis, and even acute cholangitis may be seen with sepsis. In these cases obstruction must be ruled out by ultrasound or ERCP.
5. *Toxic shock syndrome:* Portal changes of acute cho-

Feature	Mechanical Duct Obstruction	Primary Biliary Cirrhosis	Primary Sclerosing Cholangitis
Cholestasis	Perivenular	Periportal	Perivenular
Granuloma formation	Not present	Common	Not present
Predominant portal inflammatory cell	Neutrophil in acute; lymphocyte in chronic	Lymphocyte	Lymphocyte
Characteristic duct lesion	Acute cholangitis; periductal fibrosis and edema	Nonsuppurative destructive cholangitis	Periductal obliterative cholangitis
Atypical duct proliferation	Not present in acute; rare in chronic	Common	Rare
Mallory's hyalin	Rare (2%) in chronic	Common, especially in late stages (24%)	Rare
Radiologic changes: Endoscopic retrograde cholangiopancreatography (ERCP)	Dilatation proximal to obstruction (e.g., hilar, ampullary)	Normal	"Beaded" appearance of intrahepatic and extrahepatic ducts
Serologic: Antimitochondrial antibody	Absent	Present (95%)	Absent

langitis can be seen; the dramatic clinical features of fever, severe hypotension, diffuse myalgias/arthralgias, and diffuse erythroderma characterize this syndrome. Bile duct obstruction is excluded by ultrasound or ERCP.

6. *Acute alcoholic liver disease:* Neutrophilic infiltration is diffusely present within portal tracts in acute sclerosing hyaline necrosis but *not* oriented to the ducts as in acute cholangitis.

7. *Drug-induced* (e.g., chlorpropamide): Cholestasis with or without portal inflammatory changes may be present in certain drug reactions. Acute cholangitis is not typically seen.

8. *Pylephlebitis:* Acute portal inflammatory infiltration is oriented to the portal vein and not bile ducts; portal vein thrombosis may be present.

Special Stains

1. *Periodic acid–Schiff after diastase:* Hepatocytes and canaliculi containing bile, and Kupffer cells containing phagocytized material derived from necrotic liver cells often stain positively.

2. *Van Gieson:* Bile stains bright green.

3. In cases of chronic obstruction:
   a. *Orcein:* Copper-binding protein (*not* copper) presents as dark-brown to black intracytoplasmic granules in periportal hepatocytes.
   b. *Rubeanic acid:* Copper stains as black to black-green intracytoplasmic granules in periportal hepatocytes.

Clinical and Biologic Behavior

1. Common causes of mechanical duct obstruction are listed below:

Acute
   a. Choledocholithiasis
   b. Acute pancreatitis
   c. Early stages of common duct stricture (following biliary tract surgery, blunt abdominal trauma)
   d. Mass lesions either directly involving ducts (e.g., cholangiocarcinoma) or compressing extrahepatic ducts (e.g., lymph nodes from metastasis, lymphoma) or large intrahepatic bile ducts (e.g., hydatid cyst, abscess)

Chronic
   a. Benign long-term stricture secondary to surgical trauma, chronic pancreatitis, and rarely choledocholithiasis
   b. Extrahepatic biliary atresia
   c. Parasitic infections of biliary system (e.g., *Clonorchis sinensis*)
   d. Tumors of pancreas and extrahepatic ducts

2. Patients with acute obstruction typically present with jaundice, abdominal pain, and fever (Charcot triad) when cholangitis is present; serum bilirubin, GGTP,

5'-nucleotidase, and alkaline phosphatase levels are prominently elevated.

3. Bile lakes form secondary to leakage of bile directly from damaged interlobular ducts; bile infarcts are caused by direct toxic damage of bile to hepatocytes. Although these two changes are virtually diagnostic of large (intrahepatic or extrahepatic) duct obstruction, they are not commonly seen on liver biopsy specimens.

4. Cholestasis is predominantly perivenular, since bile is reabsorbed and recirculated in the periportal zone.

5. In *partial* duct obstruction, inflammation is usually associated with growth of bacteria in the biliary tree; if obstruction is not relieved, abscesses occur with eventual septicemia; in *total* obstruction, abscess formation and cholangitis are not as common.

6. Chronic obstruction leads to a periductal fibrosis from repeated bouts of cholangitis, most of which are subclinical or mild; resolution of the acute inflammatory change leaves scar formation encircling the involved ducts.

7. In patients with chronic pancreatitis, 8% develop strictures in the intrapancreatic segment of the common bile duct; although asymptomatic, 79% will demonstrate features of extrahepatic obstruction on liver biopsy specimens.

8. Length of time for development of biliary cirrhosis is as follows:
   a. Six months in neonates with extrahepatic biliary atresia; thus it is critical to diagnose these cases in less than 3 months after birth for successful surgical management.
   b. Common duct stricture, 7.1 years
   c. Choledocholithiasis, 4.6 years; this disorder develops less rapidly in those patients clinically symptomatic than in those who are asymptomatic.

9. Secondary biliary cirrhosis is associated less frequently with complications of cirrhosis (ascites, variceal bleeding) than in patients with cirrhosis of viral or alcoholic etiology.

Prognosis

Acute
1. When obstruction is subclinical, biliary fibrosis and eventual cirrhosis may develop.

Chronic
1. Relief of obstruction will lead to regression of portal and lobular changes in the noncirrhotic patient.
2. The patients with cirrhosis generally become asymptomatic.
3. Unlike the cirrhosis secondary to alcoholism or hepatitis B, hepatocellular carcinoma is not a complication.

References

Afroudakis A, Kaplowitz N. Liver histopathology in chronic bile duct stenosis due to chronic alcoholic pancreatitis. Hepatology 1981;1:65–72.

Desmet VJ. Cholestasis: Extrahepatic obstruction and secondary biliary cirrhosis. In: MacSween RNM, Anthony PP, Scheuer PJ, eds. Pathology of the Liver, 2nd ed. Edinburgh: Churchill Livingstone, 1987:388–401.

MacSween RNM. Mechanical duct obstruction. In: Peters RL, Craig JR, eds. Liver Pathology. New York: Churchill Livingstone, 1986:161–176.

Warshaw AL, Schapiro RH, Ferrucci JT Jr, et al. Persistent obstructive jaundice, cholangitis, and biliary cirrhosis due to common bile duct stenosis in chronic pancreatitis. Gastroenterology 1976;70:562–567.

■ Primary Biliary Cirrhosis

Major Morphologic Features (Four Stages)

1. Stage I: Florid nonsuppurative destructive cholangitis is present (64% cases):
   a. Interlobular bile ducts are damaged by prominent lymphocytic infiltration.
   b. Cytoplasmic vacuolization, nuclear pyknosis and karyorrhexis, and occasional epithelial hyperplasia of duct epithelium occur.
   c. Infiltration by plasma cells occurs around areas of duct destruction.
2. Stage II: Biliary fibrosis occurs with atypical duct proliferation:
   a. Lumina are scanty to absent.
   b. Epithelium is flattened and nuclei are hyperchromatic.
   c. Serpentine growth pattern is irregular.

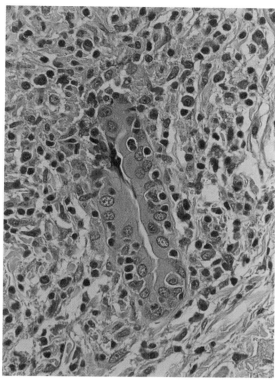

Figure 3–15. Primary biliary cirrhosis. A bile duct exhibits infiltration of its wall by lymphocytes, as well as focal necrosis of the epithelium. Both lymphocytes and plasma cells surround the duct.

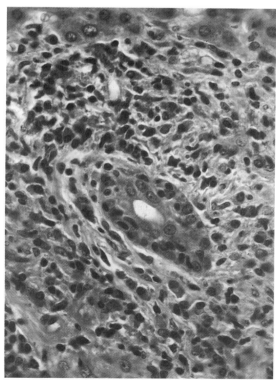

Figure 3–14. Primary biliary cirrhosis. A portal tract exhibits a hyperplastic interlobular bile duct with infiltration by lymphocytes. Macrophages, lymphocytes, and plasma cells are present surrounding the duct.

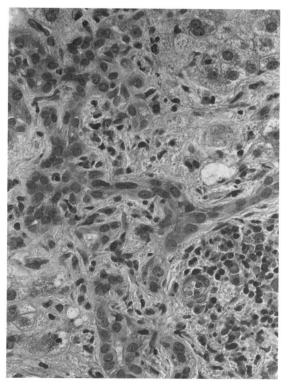

Figure 3–16. Primary biliary cirrhosis. Atypical duct structures are often seen in the precirrhotic stage. The ducts grow in a serpiginous fashion, often have flattened nuclei and no well-formed lumina.

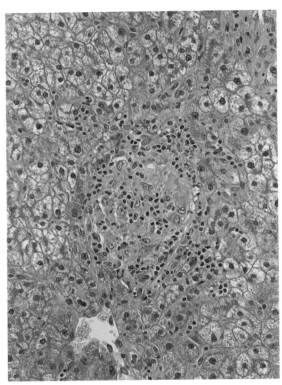

Figure 3–17. Primary biliary cirrhosis. Well-formed epithelioid granuloma may be found with the portal tract as well as the parenchyma. This photomicrograph exhibits a granuloma immediately adjacent to a terminal hepatic venule. The granulomas are often surrounded and infiltrated by lymphocytes. Although multinucleated giant cells may be present, they are unusual.

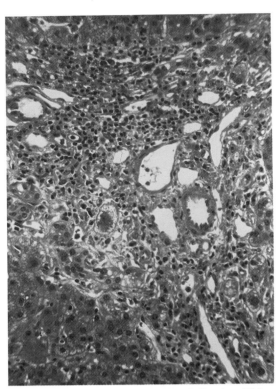

Figure 3–19. Primary biliary cirrhosis. Portal fibrosis exhibits marked proliferation and dilatation of vascular channels, consistent with portal hypertension in the precirrhotic stage. Bile ducts are usually decreased, as in this example.

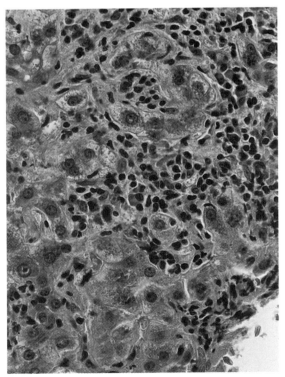

Figure 3–18. Primary biliary cirrhosis. In approximately 15% of cases, portal inflammatory cells may spill over into the parenchyma and surround individual hepatocytes, resembling chronic active hepatitis.

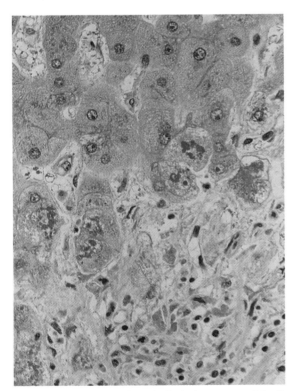

Figure 3–20. Primary biliary cirrhosis. In the latter stages of the disease, approximately one fourth of the cases may exhibit periportal or periseptal hepatocytes containing alcoholic hyalin, which is sometimes quite abundant. Neutrophilic infiltration adjacent to the hyalin is unusual.

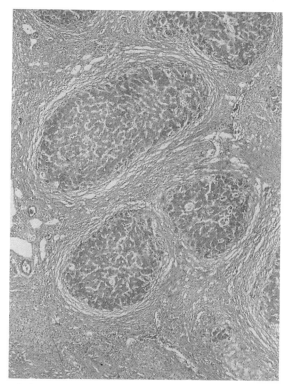

Figure 3–21. Primary biliary cirrhosis. The regenerative nodules in the cirrhotic stage are usually small and surrounded by loose collagen bundles arranged in a parallel fashion.

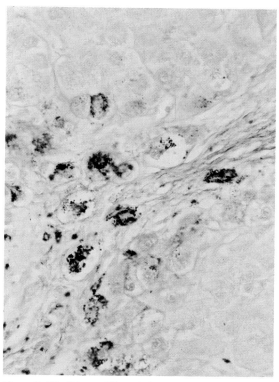

Figure 3–23. Primary biliary cirrhosis (orcein). Copper-binding protein is abundantly present in periportal hepatocytes. This is a characteristic feature of chronic biliary tract disease (e.g., primary biliary cirrhosis, primary sclerosing cholangitis).

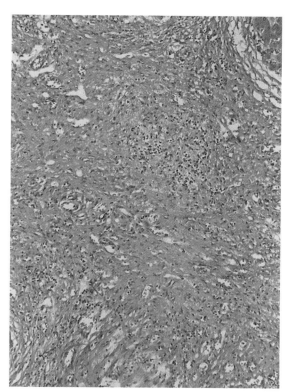

Figure 3–22. Primary biliary cirrhosis. The fibrous septa in the cirrhotic liver typically are devoid of ducts. Mild mononuclear inflammatory infiltration is present.

3. Stage III: Biliary fibrosis progresses with decrease in ducts.
4. Stage IV: Biliary cirrhosis (irregular, "geographic," or "jigsaw puzzle" pattern; periseptal lamellar fibrosis; edema surrounding nodules) is evident with marked decrease to absence of small to medium-sized ducts. Although inflammatory changes to some degree may still involve larger interlobular ducts and large ducts toward the hilum, those ducts generally remain intact (hence ERCP is normal).

Other Features

1. Portal areas show increase in lymphocytic infiltration and hyperplasia and mild increase in plasma cells; disruption of limiting plate with spillover of inflammatory cells into parenchyma (resembling "piecemeal" necrosis) is often present.
2. Neutrophils are sometimes present within portal tracts and scattered among atypical ducts; very rarely, morphologic destructive duct changes may resemble acute cholangitis, similar to that seen with large duct obstruction.
3. Thickening of hepatic arterioles is often present.
4. Focal hepatocytolysis and variable degrees of Kupffer cell hyperplasia and mononuclear inflammatory change are present within the lobule, with no

distinct zonal distribution or variation; however, in up to 15% of cases portal and parenchymal inflammatory reaction may resemble chronic active hepatitis.

5. Noncaseating epithelioid granulomas are adjacent to damaged ducts in early stages (up to 38% cases); granulomas are less commonly present in the parenchyma.

6. Mallory's hyalin is noted within periportal hepatocytes in latter stages of the disease (24%); these cells are generally not associated with a neutrophilic infiltration.

7. Cholestasis is evident in later stages, with zonal distribution usually periportal or periseptal.

8. Copper and copper-binding protein in periportal or periseptal hepatocytes (15%–37%) is found in early stages, becoming more common (90%) and abundant as the disease progresses.

9. Although there are characteristic changes for the different stages (I and II: large duct lesion, granulomas; III and IV: decreased ducts, presence of Mallory's hyalin), it is important to note that a crossover of major features occurs, such as the presence of large duct lesions with extensive fibrosis (23%) or even cirrhosis (9%).

Differential Diagnosis

1. *Mechanical duct obstruction*
2. *Primary sclerosing cholangitis:* See table on page 39.
3. *Chronic active hepatitis:* Ten to 15% of cases of primary biliary cirrhosis and chronic active hepatitis have similar inflammatory changes in portal and lobular regions. Differential features favoring primary biliary cirrhosis are the typical destructive duct lesions, granuloma formation, increase in copper-binding protein, and decrease in ducts as fibrosis advances. In addition, although chronic active non-A, non-B hepatitis may exhibit atypical duct lesions, the sinusoidal collagen and fatty change seen in that condition is not a feature of primary biliary cirrhosis.
4. *Drug-induced reaction* (e.g., chlorpromazine): Although changes of decreased or atypical ducts may rarely be present, antimitochondrial antibody testing is always negative with drugs.

Special Stains

1. *Orcein:* Copper-binding protein (*not* copper) presents as dark brown to black intracytoplasmic granules in periportal hepatocytes.
2. *Rubeanic acid:* Copper stains as black to black-green intracytoplasmic granules in periportal hepatocytes.

Clinical and Biologic Behavior

1. Primary biliary cirrhosis is a chronic progressive cholestatic liver disease typically found in middle-aged women (90%) and is responsible for 0.6% to 2.0% of deaths from cirrhosis worldwide.

2. The onset is insidious, with pruritus preceding jaundice; other clinical features include xanthomas, osteopenia, steatorrhea, hepatosplenomegaly, and, in advanced disease, manifestations of portal hypertension (ascites, esophageal varices, and portal systemic encephalopathy).

3. Laboratory data include elevated serum IgM, alkaline phosphatase, 5'-nucleotidase, gamma-glutamyl transpeptidase, and cholesterol levels. The serum bilirubin becomes elevated in advanced disease (severe fibrosis or cirrhosis) and consequently is used as a prognostic indicator.

4. Antimitochondrial antibody is present in 95% of patients, and circulating immune complexes occur 60% to 90% of the time; other autoantibodies include antinuclear, antithyroid, lymphocytotoxic, and platelet-bound antibodies.

5. Autoimmune disorders are present in 84% of cases and include Sjögren's syndrome, scleroderma and CREST syndrome, rheumatoid arthritis, lymphocytic interstitial pneumonia, systemic lupus erythematosus, and autoimmune thyroiditis.

6. A subgroup of patients may be entirely asymptomatic and diagnosed incidentally by increased serum alkaline phosphatase levels; biopsy shows characteristic morphologic features. It is not certain if these patients have a normal life span since recent evidence suggests decreased survival in these cases.

7. An additional subgroup of patients fulfill all criteria for primary biliary cirrhosis but have a normal or only slightly elevated alkaline phosphatase level.

8. Liver biopsy may show features of chronic active hepatitis, but response to corticosteroids is unlike that seen in autoimmune chronic active hepatitis. Subsequent clinical course is that of primary biliary cirrhosis.

9. Autopsy studies have shown that a normal liver contains a mean of 1.3 to 1.5 bile ducts per portal tract; in the fibrotic stages of primary biliary cirrhosis the ducts are decreased to 0.3 per portal tract.

10. Increased hepatic copper is due to bile retention (normal 2.7 mg copper/100 g dry weight of liver; mechanical duct obstruction, 12.8 mg; primary biliary cirrhosis, 44.1 mg)

11. Initial injury may be secondary to activated cytotoxic lymphocytes directed against bile ducts expressing histocompatibility antigens (Class I HLA-A, B and C, and Class II HLA-DR) in primary biliary cirrhosis but not in normal bile ducts.

Prognosis

1. The mean survival after onset of symptoms is approximately 11 years; it is uncertain whether survival in asymptomatic patients is the same as in the control population.
2. Presence of granulomas is found to be a good prognostic indicator.
3. Hepatic transplantation should be considered when hepatic failure develops; however, graft-versus-host reaction, a disease with similar morphologic features, has been reported in liver allografts.

References

Kaplan MM. Primary biliary cirrhosis. N Engl J Med 1987;316:521–528.

Kaplan MM. Medical treatment of primary biliary cirrhosis. Semin Liver Dis 1989;9:138–143.

Ludwig J, Czaja AJ, Dickson ER, et al. Manifestations of nonsuppurative cholangitis in chronic hepatobiliary diseases: Morphologic spectrum, clinical correlations and terminology. Liver 1984;4:105–116.

Mackay IR, Gershwin ME. Primary biliary cirrhosis: Current knowledge, perspectives, and future directions. Semin Liver Dis 1989;9:149–157.

MacSween RNM. Primary biliary cirrhosis. In: Peters RL, Craig JR, eds. Liver Pathology. New York: Churchill Livingstone, 1986:177–191.

Portmann B, Popper H, Neuberger J, et al. Sequential and diagnostic features in primary biliary cirrhosis based on serial histologic study in 209 patients. Gastroenterology 1985;88:1777–1790.

■ Primary Sclerosing Cholangitis

The term *pericholangitis* refers to inflammation and fibrosis surrounding the small to medium-sized bile ducts. It has recently been suggested that this condition is part of a spectrum of primary sclerosing cholangitis and therefore will not be considered as a separate entity.

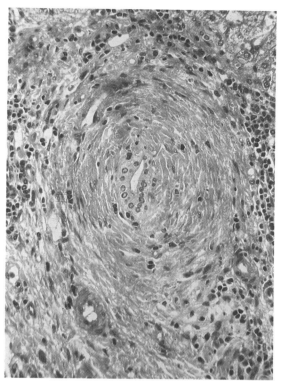

Figure 3–25. Primary sclerosing cholangitis. The bile duct shows extensive periductal *onion skin* fibrosis. The duct epithelium in areas is thin.

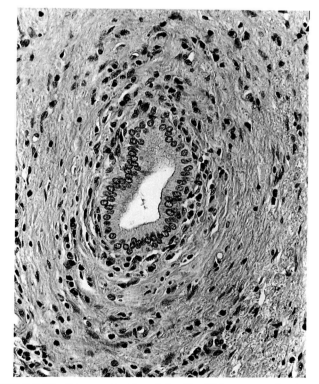

Figure 3–26. Primary sclerosing cholangitis. Higher power of an interlobular bile duct shows extensive periductal fibrosis and a moderate mononuclear inflammatory infiltrate surrounding, but in this case not infiltrating, the duct wall.

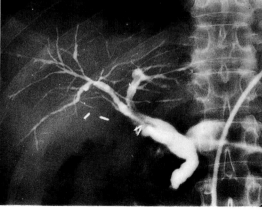

Figure 3–24. Primary sclerosing cholangitis (endoscopic retrograde cholangiopancreatography). The interlobular bile ducts are thinned throughout and show focal beading, characteristic of this disorder. This change can be diffuse or localized.

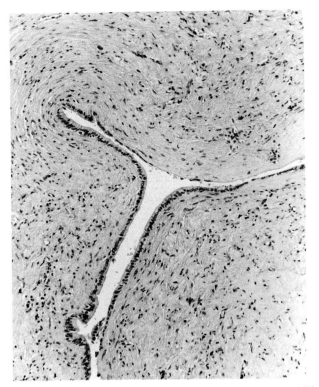

Figure 3–27. Primary sclerosing cholangitis. This large duct exhibits compression by collagen, with extensive thinning and focal dropout of epithelial cells. The collagen contains a mild infiltrate by mononuclear cells.

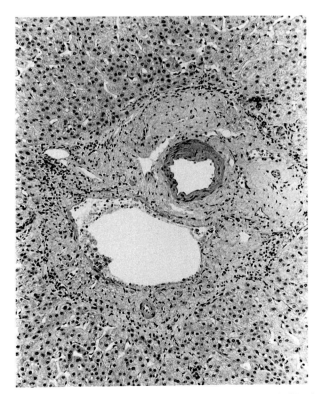

Figure 3–28. Primary sclerosing cholangitis. The portal tract is fibrotic, with a mild mononuclear inflammatory infiltrate. Interlobular duct structures and cholangioles are entirely absent.

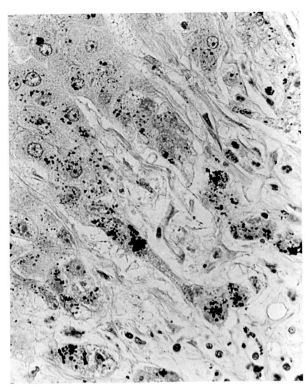

Figure 3–29. Primary sclerosing cholangitis (orcein). Copper-binding protein is abundantly present in periseptal hepatocytes.

Major Morphologic Features

1. Destructive sclerosing interlobular duct lesion is seen:
   a. Prominent periductal fibrosis, focal necrosis of duct epithelium, and significant narrowing and eventual obliteration of duct wall and lumen are present.
   b. Lymphocytic infiltration surround and often infiltrate the duct wall.
2. Ducts decrease or become absent as disease advances, with biliary fibrosis and eventual biliary cirrhosis (irregular "geographic", or "jigsaw puzzle" pattern, periseptal lamellar fibrosis, and edema).

Other Features

1. Lymphocytic infiltration and hyperplasia occur in portal areas, with occasional spillover of cells into adjacent parenchyma.
2. Proliferation of interlobular ducts alongside sclerosing lesions may occur.
3. Cholestasis is usually perivenular in early stages, although not common; periseptal bile may be seen in severely fibrotic or cirrhotic lesions.
4. There are variable degrees of macrovesicular fatty change, more commonly seen when associated with ulcerative colitis.

5. Focal hepatocytolysis is present but usually minimal.
6. As the disease segmentally involves the ducts, changes of mechanical duct obstruction are often identified in portal tracts and parenchyma distal to the fibrous duct lesion.
7. Copper and copper-binding protein in periportal hepatocytes can be seen in early stages and becomes more common and abundant as the disease progresses.
8. Alcoholic hyalin, although rare, can occasionally be identified in periportal hepatocytes.
9. Fibrosis and variable degrees of chronic inflammatory infiltration are present in the involved extrahepatic bile ducts. The gallbladder exhibits fibrosis and chronic inflammation resembling chronic cholecystitis.

Differential Diagnosis

1. *Mechanical duct obstruction*
2. *Primary biliary cirrhosis:* See table on page 39.
3. *Chronic active hepatitis:* Although the portal and parenchymal inflammatory changes may resemble chronic hepatitis, most notably of the non-A, non-B type with atypical ducts, the characteristic periductal sclerosing lesion and/or absence of ducts are characteristic for primary sclerosing cholangitis.

Special Stains

1. *Orcein:* Copper-binding protein (*not* copper) presents as dark brown to black intracytoplasmic granules in periportal hepatocytes.
2. *Rubeanic acid:* Copper stains as black to black-green intracytoplasmic granules in periportal hepatocytes.

Clinical and Biologic Behavior

1. Primary sclerosing cholangitis occurs in middle-aged men 70% of the time.
2. The disorder presents with bile duct obstruction, fever, abdominal pain, intermittent fluctuating jaundice, marked elevation of alkaline phosphatase activity, and modest elevation of serum transaminase levels.
3. Chronic ulcerative colitis is associated in 30% to 75% of cases, either before or after the colitis manifests itself; 1% to 4% of all patients with ulcerative colitis will develop primary sclerosing cholangitis; in addition, 7% of patients with both primary sclerosing cholangitis and ulcerative colitis will develop cholangiocarcinoma.
4. The characteristic radiologic appearance on ERCP of the ''beaded'' appearance of the intrahepatic and extrahepatic bile ducts, with segmental strictures and saccular dilatation, is virtually diagnostic of the disease.
5. Other associated diseases include retroperitoneal and mediastinal fibrosis, Riedel's thyroiditis, vasculitis, orbital pseudotumor, Sjögren's syndrome, and chronic pancreatitis.
6. Generally there is involvement of the entire biliary tract, including the gallbladder; however, pure intrahepatic primary sclerosing cholangitis with segmental involvement can occur, with the main hepatic and common ducts free of the disease.
7. The entity previously titled ''pericholangitis'' is a form of liver disease associated with ulcerative colitis, consisting predominantly of portal lymphocytic infiltration and hyperplasia surrounding bile ducts; on review, many of these cases are in fact primary sclerosing cholangitis involving the small interlobular ducts.
8. The majority of the time, results of a liver biopsy are consistent with or suggestive of the disorder; unfortunately, the classic and virtually diagnostic fibrous obliterative duct lesion is seen in less than one-third of biopsy specimens, with ERCP almost always necessary for diagnosis.
9. As the disease progresses, complications of portal hypertension develop, eventually leading to hepatic failure. In patients with ulcerative colitis and prior colectomy, varices may develop with bleeding at the ileostomy site.

Prognosis

1. Biliary cirrhosis develops 3 to 5 years after initial presentation, although this time period can be considerably variable.

References

Chapman RW. Primary sclerosing cholangitis. J Hepatol 1985;1:179–186.
LaRusso NF, Wiesner RH, Ludwig J, et al. Primary sclerosing cholangitis. N Engl J Med 1984;310:899–903.
Ludwig J, Czaja AJ, Dickson ER, et al. Manifestations of nonsuppurative cholangitis in chronic hepatobiliary diseases: Morphologic spectrum, clinical correlations and terminology. Liver 1984;4:105–116.
Ludwig J, LaRusso NF, Wiesner RH. Primary sclerosing cholangitis. In: Peters RL, Craig JR, eds. Liver Pathology. New York: Churchill Livingstone, 1986:193–213.
Nakanuma Y, Hirai N, Kono N, et al. Histological and ultrastructural examination of the intrahepatic biliary tree in primary sclerosing cholangitis. Liver 1986;6:317–325.
Wiesner RH, LaRusso NF. Clinicopathologic features of the syndrome of primary sclerosing cholangitis. Gastroenterology 1980;79:200–206.

■ Recurrent Pyogenic Cholangiohepatitis

Major Morphologic Features

1. Dilatation of large intrahepatic ducts occurs, with acute inflammatory infiltration focally surrounding and invading duct walls.
2. Abscess formation is present in 85% of cases.

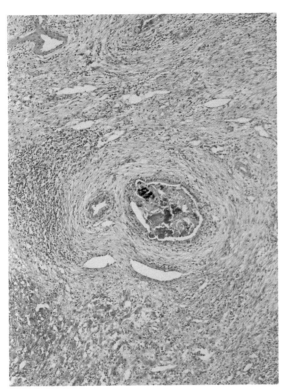

Figure 3–30. Recurrent pyogenic cholangiohepatitis. On low power the large bile duct is dilated and filled with calculi and eosinophilic sludge. Inflammatory cells, predominantly neutrophils, surround and infiltrate the duct wall.

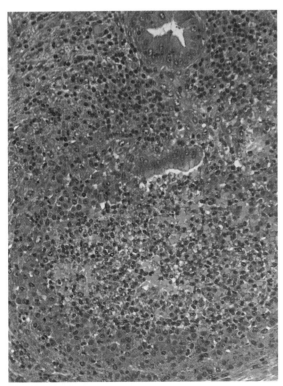

Figure 3–31. Recurrent pyogenic cholangiohepatitis. The bile duct is partially destroyed and replaced by neutrophils. A residual focus of duct epithelium can still be identified.

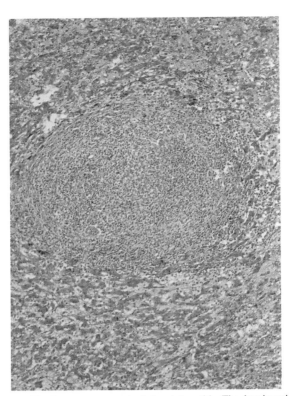

Figure 3–32. Recurrent pyogenic cholangiohepatitis. The duct is entirely destroyed and replaced by a large aggregate of neutrophils, forming an abscess.

Other Features

1. Perivenular cholestasis is often present.
2. Smaller portal areas distal to large duct lesions show signs of acute and chronic obstruction, most notably periductal fibrosis and occasionally acute cholangitis.
3. Liver distal to sites of duct involvement may undergo atrophy.
4. There is a predilection for left lobe involvement, with right lobe often showing minimal changes.
5. In more advanced cases, biliary fibrosis and arteriolar thickening are common.
6. *Pylephlebitis:* Inflammation of portal veins may be present; infarction of parenchyma may be seen but is not common.
7. Intrahepatic calculi and biliary sludge are present in virtually all cases.
8. Extrahepatic bile ducts may show variable degrees of dilatation, fibrosis, and both acute and chronic inflammatory change.

Differential Diagnosis

1. *Extrahepatic obstruction:* Various causes of acute cholangitis, such as choledocholithiasis, must be considered, but these entities are usually not present

with *intrahepatic* calculi and changes of pylephlebitis.

2. *Primary sclerosing cholangitis:* Periductal fibrosis is present in both entities, but destructive fibrosing duct lesions, with prominent mononuclear inflammatory infiltration, and eventual decrease in ducts *without* abscess formation, characteristic of primary sclerosing cholangitis, are not present in recurrent pyogenic cholangiohepatitis.

3. *Caroli's disease:* This disorder most often uniformly involves the entire intrahepatic biliary tree without predilection for the left lobe. In addition, Caroli's disease affects large and small ducts while recurrent pyogenic cholangiohepatitis tends to involve the larger ducts near the hilum.

Clinical and Biologic Behavior

1. Also known as Oriental cholangiohepatitis, recurrent pyogenic cholangiohepatitis is seen most frequently in Southeast Asia and is the third most common cause of acute abdominal emergency in Hong Kong.

2. The disorder is found with equal frequency in both sexes; the onset of symptoms is in the second to fourth decades, with right upper quadrant pain, fever, and jaundice that recurs with increasing frequency and severity.

3. Biliary calculi and sludge are characteristically brown-black (bilirubin), with cultures positive for enteric organisms (principally *Escherichia coli*) over 90% of the time; the gallbladder is involved in only 25% of the cases.

4. ERCP shows characteristic features of a dilated biliary tree containing both intrahepatic and extrahepatic calculi; for unclear reasons the majority of the intrahepatic stones (occurring in 25% of cases) are confined to the left hepatic ductal system.

5. *Clonorchis sinensis* infestation of the biliary tree is present in approximately 50% of the patients; *Ascaris lumbricoides* may also be present.

6. The frequency of cholangiocarcinoma is increased in these patients.

7. The pathogenesis is uncertain; although *Clonorchis* is present in only 50% of the cases, the etiology is speculated to be in part due to the deposition of eggs and intraductular parasite fragments provoking inflammatory change, increased goblet cell secretion, and resultant stone formation.

8. Acute pancreatitis is a common accompaniment (12%), and complications of recurrent pyogenic cholangiohepatitis include liver abscess, biliary enteric fistula, gram-negative sepsis, and portal vein thrombosis.

Prognosis

1. Intrahepatic calculi involving the left lobe of the liver are difficult to manage and may lead to left hepatic lobectomy.

References

Chou S-T, Chan CW. Recurrent pyogenic cholangitis: A necropsy study. Pathology 1980;12:415–428.

Craig JR. Recurrent pyogenic cholangiohepatitis. In: Peters RL, Craig JR, eds. Liver Pathology. New York: Churchill Livingstone, 1986:215–219.

Seel DJ, Park YK. Oriental infestational cholangitis. Am J Surg 1983;146:366–370.

■ **Intrahepatic Cholestasis**

Postoperative Cholestasis

Intrahepatic Cholestasis of Pregnancy

Benign Recurrent Intrahepatic Cholestasis

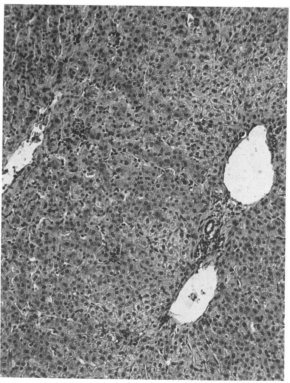

Figure 3–33. Intrahepatic cholestasis. The portal tract is normal in size with a minimal mononuclear inflammatory infiltrate. The perivenular hepatocytes exhibit an increase in pigment. Rare foci of hepatocytolysis are present.

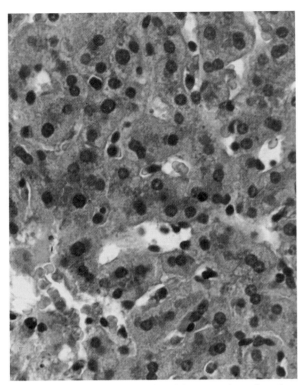

Figure 3–34. Intrahepatic cholestasis. High power of a perivenular zone exhibits bile within both dilated canaliculi and liver cell cytoplasm. Mild Kupffer cell hyperplasia is present.

Major Morphologic Feature

1. Cholestasis occurs within perivenular hepatocytes and dilated canaliculi.

Other Features

1. Portal tract shows minimal to absent mononuclear inflammatory infiltration.
2. Bile ducts are normal to only slightly increased in number.
3. Kupffer cell hyperplasia is slight.
4. Phagocytized red blood cells are occasionally present within Kupffer cells in postoperative cholestasis.
5. Giant cell transformation has been identified in cholestasis of pregnancy.
6. Portal and sinusoidal fibrosis does *not* occur.

Differential Diagnosis

1. *All three conditions:* These three types of cholestasis morphologically resemble each other; the clinical setting is essential for diagnosis.
2. *Drug-induced reaction* (e.g., oral contraceptives): Cholestasis resolves with subsidence of the drug.

3. *Early acute duct obstruction:* Typical portal tract changes, such as edema, duct dilatation and proliferation, that are usually present in obstruction may in fact be absent in its very early stages and resemble these benign cholestatic disorders.
4. *Sepsis:* Perivenular cholestasis with little portal reaction may occur in some instances of septicemia; blood culture and history are necessary for diagnosis.

Special Stains

1. *Van Gieson:* Bile stains bright green.

Clinical and Biologic Behavior

Postoperative Cholestasis
1. Frequency of postoperative cholestasis is low (2/1000 elective surgical procedures) and more common after cardiac surgery.
2. The disorder presents usually within 1 to 2 days after a prolonged surgical procedure, with pruritus and hyperbilirubinemia (as high as 40 mg/dL) but only minimally elevated alanine aminotransferase and aspartate aminotransferase activities.
3. Postoperative cholestasis is secondary to a combination of bilirubin overload (hemolysis from transfusions, stress of patients with hemolytic disorder), and decrease in secretory function of the liver cells.

Intrahepatic Cholestasis of Pregnancy
1. Intrahepatic cholestasis occurs in 2% to 6% of uncomplicated pregnancies and manifests in the third trimester, with pruritus and only slight bilirubin elevation (1–2 mg/dL), resolving within a few hours to days after delivery.
2. Although there are generally no obstetric complications, there is a slight increase in the incidence of stillborn and premature births.
3. Scandinavian, Polish, and Chilean women appear most susceptible.
4. There is an increased incidence of gallstone formation.
5. Etiology may be related to liver cell dysfunction from gonadal and placental hormones.

Benign Recurrent Intrahepatic Cholestasis
1. Benign recurrent intrahepatic cholestasis usually begins in childhood, with repeated bouts of pruritus and jaundice throughout life.
2. There is a slight male predominance.
3. Attacks are separated by months to years, during which time clinical, biochemical, and liver biopsy features are completely normal.
4. Although the pathogenesis is not known, hypersensitivity to environmental agents and possible alteration of bile acid metabolism have been postulated.

Prognosis

1. Mortality that occurs in postoperative cholestasis is related to surgical complications (e.g., sepsis) and *not* to hepatic dysfunction.

References

Collins JD, Bassendine MF, Ferner R, et al. Incidence and prognostic importance of jaundice after cardiopulmonary bypass surgery. Lancet 1983;2:1119–1129.

Minuk GY, Shaffer EA. Benign recurrent intrahepatic cholestasis. Gastroenterology 1987;93:1187–1193.

Rolfes DB, Ishak KG. Liver disease in pregnancy. Histopathology 1986;10:555–570.

Schmid M, Heft ML, Gattiker R, et al. Benign postoperative intrahepatic cholestasis. N Engl J Med 1965;272:545–550.

General References

Desmet VJ. Cholestasis: Extrahepatic obstruction and secondary biliary cirrhosis. In: MacSween RNM, Anthony PP, Scheuer PJ, eds. Pathology of the liver, 2nd ed. Edinburgh: Churchill Livingstone, 1987:364–423.

Portmann B, MacSween RNM. Diseases of the intrahepatic bile ducts. In: MacSween RNM, Anthony PP, Scheuer PJ, eds. Pathology of the Liver, 2nd ed. Edinburgh: Churchill Livingstone, 1987:424–453.

Review by International Group (Baptista A, Bianchi L, de Groote J, et al.). Histopathology of the intrahepatic biliary tree. Liver 1983;3:161–175.

Scheuer PJ. Biliary disease and cholestasis. In: Scheuer PJ, ed. Liver Biopsy Interpretation, 3rd ed. London: Baillière Tindall, 1980:36–59.

White TT. Obstructive biliary tract disease. West J Med 1982; 136:484–504.

CHAPTER 4

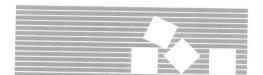

Alcoholic Liver Disease

■ Fatty Liver

Major Morphologic Feature

1. Macrovesicular fat is present within hepatocytes; accentuation often occurs in the perivenular (zone 3) region.

Other Features

1. Small numbers of microvesicular fat droplets are occasionally present.
2. Focal hepatocytolysis is present but scanty.
3. *Lipogranuloma:* Coalescence of fat droplets elicits a mild mononuclear inflammatory and rarely giant cell reaction because of extracellular fat.
4. Kupffer cell hyperplasia is minimal to absent.
5. Portal tracts are unremarkable in simple fatty liver; underlying chronic alcoholic liver disease exhibits varying degrees of both portal and sinusoidal collagen deposition.

Differential Diagnosis

1. *Obesity/adult-onset diabetes mellitus:* The macrovesicular fat in both these conditions does not typically have a zonal distribution; in addition, diabetes usually exhibits glycogen nuclei in periportal hepatocytes.
2. *Malnutrition:* Macrovesicular fat in severe malnutrition, and occasionally in chronic debilitating infections such as tuberculosis, is predominantly periportal.
3. *Status post jejunoileal bypass surgery for morbid obesity:* Within the first few months after surgery, almost all the hepatocytes exhibit a macrovesicular fatty change, with this degree lessening in latter months to years after surgery.
4. *Drugs* (e.g., corticosteroids, sulfasalazine): A drug-induced fatty liver does not tend to have a zonal distribution pattern.

Special Stain

1. *Masson trichrome:* The presence of sinusoidal collagen is indicative of not simply a fatty liver induced by alcohol but of some degree of alcoholic liver disease.

Clinical and Biologic Behavior

1. Fatty change is the most common morphologic change in the liver of an alcoholic and is seen in 90% of biopsied and autopsied cases.
2. Alcohol is predominantly metabolized by alcohol dehydrogenase to form acetaldehyde, a substance toxic to mitochondrial structure and function. Fatty change results to some extent by an increase in synthesis of triglycerides and by decreased oxidation of fatty acids. In addition, mobilization of triglycerides from peripheral stores occurs in the chronic alcoholic.
3. A minor metabolic pathway is the microsomal ethanol oxidizing system, also involved in drug metabolism; induction of this system by ethanol may enhance the hepatic metabolism of certain drugs.
4. The degree of fat approximately varies with the amount of alcohol intake and to some extent the quantity of protein in the diet.
5. Alcohol stimulates collagen formation; although stains for collagen may not demonstrate sinusoidal

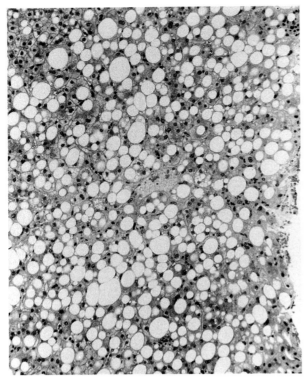

Figure 4–1. Fatty liver, alcoholic etiology. In any person who drinks modest quantities of alcohol there is almost always some degree of fatty change whether alcoholic liver disease is present or not. The most common feature is a macrovesicular fatty change, most prominent in the perivenular zone (note terminal hepatic venule at *center*).

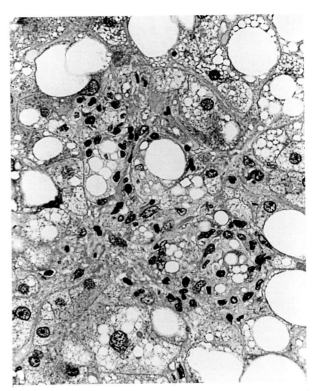

Figure 4–2. Fatty liver, alcoholic etiology. Distended hepatocytes that have ruptured are often present in alcoholic fatty livers. The extravasated fat elicits a chronic inflammatory infiltrate, forming a *lipogranuloma*. These structures are more prominent in the perivenular zone.

collagen in simple fatty change, chemical analysis of these livers shows moderate increases in hydroxyproline, a major amino acid found in collagen fibers.

6. Fat is generally graded as 1+, involving up to 25% of hepatocytes; 2+, 25% to 50% of hepatocytes; 3+, 50% to 75% of hepatocytes, and 4+, greater than 75% of hepatocytes.
7. Hepatomegaly may be the only abnormality on physical examination, and no stigmata of chronic liver disease is present. Mild elevations in serum transaminase levels may occur.
8. Increased fat in the liver is seen on computed tomography, evidenced by low density areas in the liver, and may be focal in nature.

Prognosis

1. Simple fatty change is asymptomatic; the fat will disappear in a severe fatty liver within 8 weeks of abstinence of alcohol.

References

Edmondson HA, Peters RL. Liver. In: Kissane JM, Anderson WAD, eds. Pathology, 8th ed. St. Louis: C.V. Mosby, 1985:1135–1137.
Horn T, Junge J, Christoffersen P. Early alcoholic liver injury. Activation of lipocytes in acinar zone 3 and correlation to degree of collagen formation in the Disse space. J Hepatol 1986;3:333–340.

Lieber CS, Davidson CS. Some metabolic effects of ethyl alcohol. Am J Med 1962;33:319–327.
Lieber CS, Schmid R. Stimulation of hepatic fatty acid synthesis by ethanol. Am J Clin Nutr 1961;9:436–438.
Rubin E, Lieber CS. Alcohol-induced hepatic injury in nonalcoholic volunteers. N Engl J Med 1968;278:869–876.

■ Acute Alcoholic Liver Disease

Acute Fatty Liver With or Without Cholestasis

Major Morphologic Features

1. Prominent macrovesicular fatty change occurs; although there may be perivenular (zone 3) accentuation, more often all zones of the lobule are equally involved.
2. Cholestasis may be present.

Other Features

1. Minimal sinusoidal collagen deposition occurs within the space of Disse.
2. Focal hepatocytolysis is usually mild; lipogranuloma may be present.
3. Microvesicular fat is usually present, but minimal.

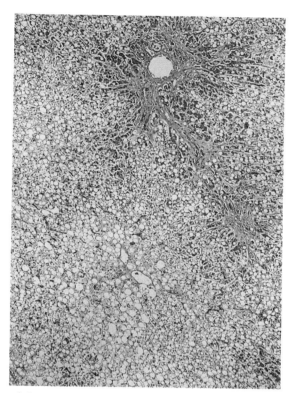

Figure 4–3. Acute fatty liver. This photomicrograph on low power exhibits fatty change involving virtually all of the hepatocytes, with slight sparing of the liver cells immediately adjacent to a portal tract (*top*).

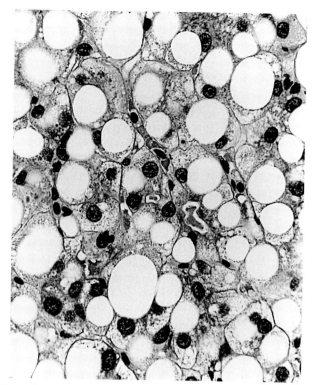

Figure 4–5. Acute fatty liver. Cholestasis may be present, shown here as bile within dilated canaliculi. The fatty change is macrovesicular.

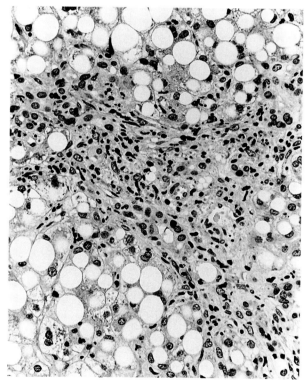

Figure 4–4. Acute fatty liver. The portal tract is fibrotic. Bile ducts are present, with slight dilatation involving a duct at the bottom of the portal region. Inflammatory cells consist predominantly of neutrophils, with no distinct orientation of these cells to any specific portal structure.

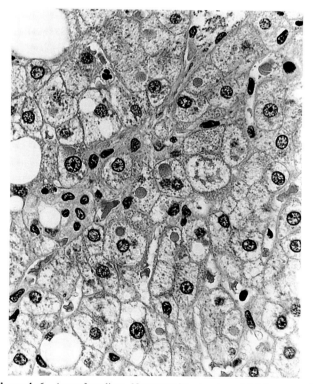

Figure 4–6. Acute fatty liver. Numerous hepatocytes exhibit large round eosinophilic inclusions within the cytoplasm. Electron microscopy demonstrates these inclusions to be enlarged mitochondria (*megamitochondria*), which are infrequent in nonalcoholic liver disease.

4. *Megamitochondria:* Enlarged mitochondria, often identified in hydropic hepatocytes, are of two types:
   a. *Round:* Single or small numbers of eosinophilic cytoplasmic inclusions may approach the size of the nucleus and are characteristic of alcoholic liver disease.
   b. *Spindle shaped:* Multiple long thin crystalline-type eosinophilic inclusions are seen in both alcoholic and nonalcoholic liver diseases.
5. Mild mononuclear inflammatory infiltrate is seen in the portal tracts; in addition, scattered neutrophils are usually present but not oriented to any portal structure.

Differential Diagnosis

1. *Obesity/adult-onset diabetes mellitus:* Generally these conditions do not have the same degree of fat as acute alcoholic fatty liver and do not exhibit cholestasis. In diabetes, glycogen nuclei in periportal hepatocytes are seen.
2. *Status post jejunoileal bypass surgery for morbid obesity:* Condition may be indistinguishable from acute fatty liver in the early months after surgery.
3. *Drug-induced* (e.g., corticosteroids, sulfasalazine): Usually drug-induced fatty change is not as severe as acute alcoholic fatty liver, and zonal distribution is not typically present with drugs.

Special Stains

1. *Periodic acid–Schiff after diastase:* This stain is useful in examination of cytoplasmic inclusions, since alpha-1-antitrypsin, *not* megamitochondria, stains positively.
2. *Masson trichrome:* Thin blue strands of sinusoidal collagen are more readily identifiable. In addition, megamitochondria usually stain bright red.

Clinical and Biologic Behavior

1. The patient usually presents with nonspecific complaints of nausea, vomiting, and malaise; associated features of alcohol withdrawal and occasionally jaundice may be present.
2. Marked hepatomegaly is present, with liver weights at autopsy exceeding 3000 g.
3. Laboratory tests show mildly elevated aspartate aminotransferase levels, with alanine aminotransferase levels often normal; serum bilirubin may be normal or slightly elevated.
4. Fat will disappear 6 to 12 weeks after cessation of drinking.
5. Heavy drinking (>80 g of alcohol per day) must occur for at least 3 to 5 years before acute alcoholic liver disease will present.

6. Patients with "acute portal fibrosis" may have a markedly elevated alkaline phosphatase level; the clinical features and other laboratory data are similar to those in acute fatty liver.

Treatment and Prognosis

1. Cessation of drinking is mandatory.
2. Complications of acute alcoholic liver disease, such as infections and acute and/or chronic pancreatitis, may affect outcome.

References

Edmondson HA. Alcoholic liver disease. In: Peters RL, Craig JR, eds. Liver Pathology. New York: Churchill Livingstone, 1986:257–259.

Randall B. Fatty liver and sudden death: A review. Hum Pathol 1980;11:147–153.

Randall B. Sudden death and hepatic fatty metamorphosis. JAMA 1980;243:1723–1725.

Acute Sclerosing Hyaline Necrosis

Major Morphologic Features

1. Extensive perivenular sinusoidal fibrosis (sclerosis) occurs, with partial or total obliteration of the terminal hepatic venules.

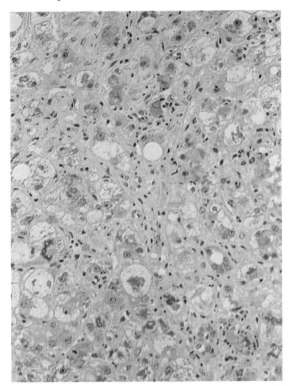

Figure 4–7. Acute sclerosing hyaline necrosis. The terminal hepatic venule is totally sclerosed and surrounded by abundant collagen. The hydropic hepatocytes contain variable degrees of fat and alcoholic hyalin and are infiltrated by neutrophils.

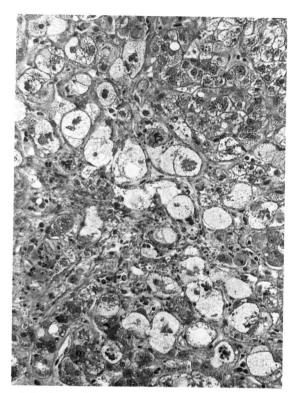

Figure 4–8. Acute sclerosing hyaline necrosis (trichrome). The terminal hepatic venule (*center*) is heavily surrounded by sinusoidal collagen extending into the midzonal region. Hepatocytes are hydropic, some containing scanty cytoplasmic material that most likely represents alcoholic hyalin.

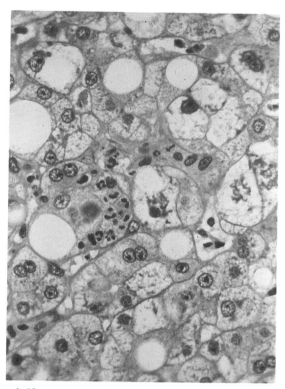

Figure 4–10. Acute sclerosing hyaline necrosis. Alcoholic hyalin is present in numerous hydropic hepatocytes. One hepatocyte containing both fat and hyalin is partially surrounded by neutrophils.

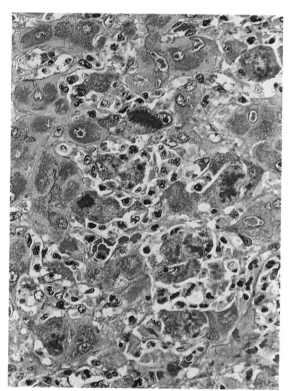

Figure 4–9. Acute sclerosing hyaline necrosis (trichrome). Many of the hepatocytes are surrounded by neutrophils. The alcoholic hyalin stains both red and blue.

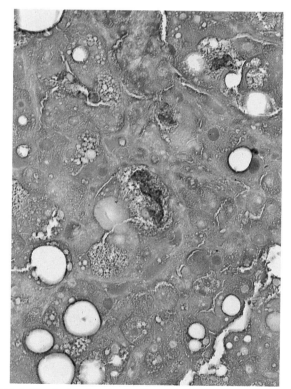

Figure 4–11. Acute sclerosing hyaline necrosis, alcoholic hyalin (immunoperoxidase). This special stain demonstrates alcoholic hyalin in a liver cell (*center*). The stain is helpful when hyalin, on hematoxylin and eosin staining, appears atypical or questionable.

2. Hydropic change of hepatocytes, most prominent in the perivenular zone, is evident, with many of these cells containing an amorphous, clumped eosinophilic cytoplasmic material (*alcoholic hyalin, Mallory bodies*).
3. Cells with hyalin are often surrounded and invaded by neutrophils.

Other Features

1. Portal tracts with variable degrees of arachnoid fibrosis and mild to moderate neutrophilic infiltration are present, the neutrophils not oriented to any particular structure.
2. Variable degrees of bile duct and cholangiolar proliferation occur; neutrophils may surround slightly dilated cholangioles.
3. Variable degrees of macrovesicular fatty change, usually with perivenular accentuation, occur; occasionally, a small number of cells may exhibit microvesicular fat.
4. Perivenular cholestasis may be present.
5. Megamitochondria are often seen in swollen hepatocytes.
6. Focal hepatocytolysis with a mixture of both mononuclear and neutrophilic inflammatory infiltrates is also identified in midzonal and periportal regions.

Differential Diagnosis

1. *Obesity/adult-onset diabetes mellitus:* Hyaline necrosis and sinusoidal collagen may rarely be identified in obese and/or diabetic patients. The degree of change is not as severe as in acute sclerosing hyaline necrosis; in addition, glycogen nuclei are usually present in periportal hepatocytes of the diabetic.
2. *Status post jejunoileal bypass surgery for morbid obesity:* Two to 7% of these patients may develop hepatic failure 2 to 9 months after surgery, with the morphologic features being identical to acute sclerosing hyaline necrosis.
3. *Other conditions in which alcoholic hyalin may be present:* Wilson's disease, Indian childhood cirrhosis, chronic cholestatic disorders (primary biliary cirrhosis, chronic biliary outflow obstruction), ingestion of certain drugs (amiodarone, griseofulvin, corticosteroids), and hepatocellular carcinoma (see table on page 239) may exhibit alcoholic hyalin, although in most cases other morphologic features and clinical history easily exclude acute sclerosing hyaline necrosis.

Special Stains

1. *Masson trichrome:* Sinusoidal collagen fibers are accentuated by their blue staining pattern; alcoholic hyalin stains bright red or blue, and megamitochondria stain red.
2. *Mallory's phloxine:* Alcoholic hyalin stains intensely red; older hyalin is pink to colorless.

Immunohistochemistry

1. *Cytokeratin:* Antibodies to this protein strongly stain alcoholic hyalin; cells without hyalin on hematoxylin and eosin may also exhibit membrane or cytoplasmic staining.
2. *Alcoholic hyalin:* Antibodies to alcoholic hyalin itself will distinguish cytoplasmic clumping from hyalin.
3. *Horseradish peroxidase:* This stain nonspecifically binds alcoholic hyalin.

Clinical and Biologic Behavior

1. There is a broad range of clinical abnormalities in acute alcoholic hepatitis. In mild disease, patients are asymptomatic, but in severe cases, jaundice, ascites, and hepatic encephalopathy are present, leading to increased mortality. Hepatomegaly, hepatic pain and tenderness, leukocytosis (rarely as high as $100,000/cm^3$), fever, and hepatic systolic bruit are frequently present.
2. Serum total and direct bilirubin levels are elevated, and serum albumin and prothrombin activity are depressed, markedly so in severe cases. Alkaline phosphatase elevation is variable. Aspartate aminotransferase levels are elevated, usually in the 100 to 300 IU/1 range, but alanine aminotransferase levels are substantially lower and in some cases normal. Technetium liver spleen scan demonstrates marked redistribution of isotope to the spleen and bone marrow; isotope flow scan shows increased arterial flow in a large proportion of cases.
3. For unclear reasons a worsening of the clinical and laboratory parameters 2 to 4 weeks after cessation of alcohol may occur.
4. *Alcoholic hyalin* is a principal feature; although present in over 20 liver disorders, it is seen most abundantly in acute sclerosing hyaline necrosis.
5. Alcoholic hyalin consists of bundles and aggregates of *intermediate filaments*, microtubular structures that are part of the cytoskeleton of the hepatocyte; ultrastructurally it has been separated into three categories: I—irregular, connecting filaments; II—branching, randomly arranged tubular filaments (most common type); III—granular, with filaments at periphery.
6. Different staining patterns of hyalin are seen on trichrome stain (red or blue) and may be related to different subtypes or age of the hyalin.
7. The dense deposition of collagen fibers (predominantly type III) most marked in the perivenular si-

nusoids causes partial or complete obliteration of the terminal hepatic venules, with obstruction to hepatic venous outflow and consequent post-sinusoidal portal hypertension.

8. With abstinence, the new collagen fibers may be broken down by collagenase and ultimately resorbed; however, continuous deposition of periportal and perivenular collagen leads to bridging of portal-portal and portal-perivenular regions. Regeneration of hepatocytes next to this fibrous tissue leads to nodule formation, eventually resulting in *cirrhosis*.

9. In acute sclerosing hyaline necrosis significant fibrosis is usually present. At initial presentation, the vast majority of patients will have significant underlying chronic liver disease, with established portal and perivenular fibrosis; 40% of cases are cirrhotic at initial presentation, demonstrable at biopsy.

10. Thirty-five per cent of all patients dying of alcoholic liver disease will have considerable hyaline necrosis at autopsy.

Treatment and Prognosis

1. General measures include abstinence, nutritive support, and treatment of vitamin deficiencies, ascites, and hepatic encephalopathy. Bacterial infections of ascites and the respiratory and urinary tracts are treated with appropriate antibiotics.

2. Since the precise mechanism of hepatic damage is not certain, a number of empiric treatments have been tried. In controlled trials with corticosteroids, short-term morbidity and mortality were unaffected, although it was suggested that a subgroup of severely ill patients with encephalopathy may benefit.

3. The development of renal failure (hepatorenal syndrome), encephalopathy nonresponsive to therapy, or progressive decrease in prothrombin activity is associated with a poor outcome (80% mortality).

References

Edmondson HA, Peters RL, Reynolds TB, et al. Sclerosing hyaline necrosis of the liver in the chronic alcoholic. Ann Intern Med 1963;59:646–673.

Gerber MA, Popper H. Relation between central canals and portal tracts in alcoholic hepatitis: A contribution to the pathogenesis of cirrhosis in alcoholics. Hum Pathol 1972;3:199–207.

Maddrey WC. Alcoholic hepatitis: Clinicopathologic features and therapy. Semin Liver Dis 1988;8:91–102.

Pares A, Caballeria J, Bruguera M, et al. Histological course of alcoholic hepatitis: Influence of abstinence, sex, and extent of hepatic damage. J Hepatol 1986;2:33–42.

Reynolds TB, Benhamou JP, Blake T, et al. Treatment of acute alcoholic hepatitis. Gastroenterology Int 1989;2:208–216.

Reynolds TB, Hidemura R, Michel H, et al. Portal hypertension without cirrhosis in alcoholic liver disease. Ann Intern Med 1969;70:497–506.

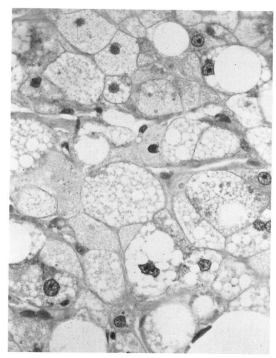

Figure 4–12. Alcoholic foamy degeneration. Hepatocytes surrounding the terminal hepatic venule are distended by fatty change, the predominant type being microvesicular. In some of the hepatocytes the size of the individual fat globules is exceptionally small and can be confirmed with fat stains (frozen sections) and electron microscopy. Liver cell nuclei are often present toward the center of the cell and are slightly smaller than normal.

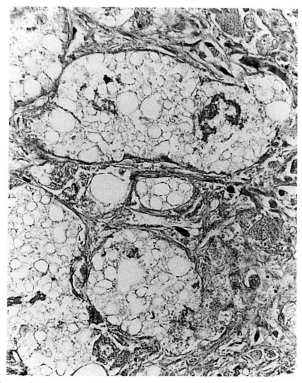

Figure 4–13. Alcoholic foamy degeneration. These hepatocytes have merged as a result of severe swelling and lysis of cytoplasmic membranes (*lytic change*). All liver cells are filled with microvesicular fat. Alcoholic hyalin is also present in a lytic hepatocyte (*upper right*).

Alcoholic Foamy Degeneration

Major Morphologic Features

1. Perivenular hepatocytes contain microvesicular fat; the cytoplasm has a granular to "foamy" appearance.
2. Thin strands of sinusoidal collagen occur predominantly within the perivenular zone.

Other Features

1. Portal tracts with variable degrees of arachnoid fibrosis and mild neutrophilic infiltration are present but not oriented to any particular structure.
2. There are variable degrees of bile duct proliferation.
3. Macrovesicular fat is almost always present in perivenular and midzonal regions; many perivenular cells exhibit both macrovesicular and foamy fatty changes.
4. Nuclei of foamy hepatocytes are centrally located and slightly smaller than normal.
5. Megamitochondria are often found in foamy hepatocytes.
6. Some degree of cholestasis may be present.
7. Focal hepatocytolysis is present but mild.
8. Alcoholic hyalin and sclerosis of terminal hepatic venules is absent in *pure* form; however, *mixed* forms of alcoholic foamy degeneration and acute sclerosing hyaline necrosis often occur in which sinusoidal collagen, hyaline necrosis, and foamy cells are all present.

Differential Diagnosis

1. *Conditions producing microvesicular fatty change:*
   a. *Fatty liver of pregnancy:* This condition usually resolves after delivery.
   b. *Reye's syndrome:* This syndrome is rare in adults.
   c. *Drugs and toxins:* Morphologic features of valproic acid, mushroom toxins, and intravenously administered tetracycline are similar. (On frozen sections of fresh or formalin fixed tissue, tetracycline can be demonstrated as a golden-brown autofluorescent material within the cytoplasm of hepatocytes.)
   d. *Diabetes mellitus:* Glycogen nuclei are also prominent.

NOTE: Among the diseases listed, portal and sinusoidal collagen deposition is seen only in diabetes.

Special Stains

1. *Oil red O:* Foamy cells may not appear to contain fat on hematoxylin and eosin stain of routinely processed tissue; if fresh or formalin fixed wet tissue is available, oil red O stains the fat bright red on frozen section.
2. *Periodic acid–Schiff:* This stain is often helpful in outlining microvesicular fat by staining glycogen located immediately adjacent to fat globules.

Clinical and Biologic Behavior

1. Patients present with acute onset of hepatomegaly (90%), jaundice (90%), and abdominal pain (59%); ascites is usually absent.
2. In laboratory tests serum alanine aminotransferase levels range between 100 and 300 IU/L, although rarely they may be as high as 700 IU/L at initial presentation; aspartate aminotransferase levels of 100 IU/L are usually noted. Hyperbilirubinemia, sometimes as high as 20 mg/dL, occurs, with serum albumin levels and prothrombin activity mildly abnormal. White blood cell count is usually normal. The transaminase pattern may suggest viral hepatitis or mechanical bile duct obstruction.
3. Ultrastructural features of foamy cells show striking damage and loss of organelles, with diffuse distribution of fine fat droplets.
4. Microvesicular fat may resolve shortly after hospitalization; liver biopsy may reveal only macrovesicular fatty change with the diagnosis of alcoholic foamy degeneration being missed.
5. In very severe cases, seen almost only at autopsy, adjacent cell membranes may rupture, termed *lytic necrosis;* these cases often have variable degrees of hyaline necrosis but without neutrophilic infiltration.
6. Microvesicular foamy hepatocytes and changes of acute sclerosing hyaline necrosis may be prominent morphologic features in the same biopsy specimen, representative of the wide spectrum of changes seen in acute alcoholic liver disease.
7. Four per cent of all patients dying of alcoholic liver disease will exhibit foamy degeneration of hepatocytes.

Prognosis

1. Patients quickly improve after cessation from alcohol, with falling serum bilirubin levels; however, hepatomegaly may persist for months.
2. Prognosis appears to be significantly better than that of acute sclerosing hyaline necrosis.

References

Koyama K, Kanayama M, Uchida T, et al. Serial liver biopsies of two patients with alcoholic foamy degeneration. Jpn J Hepatol 1984;25:657–665.

Montull S, Pares A, Bruguera M, et al. Alcoholic foamy degeneration in Spain: Prevalence and clinicopathological features. Liver 1989;9:79–85.

Uchida T, Kao H, Quispe-Sjogren M, et al. Acute foamy degeneration: A pattern of acute alcoholic injury of the liver. Gastroenterology 1983;84:683–692.

■ Chronic Alcoholic Liver Disease

Alcoholic Cirrhosis

Major Morphologic Features

Precirrhotic Stage
1. Increased portal and perivenular fibrosis occurs in an arachnoid pattern, usually in a liver with varying degrees of fatty change.
2. Bridging of fibrous regions is evident between portal-perivenular zones, and between perivenular regions of adjacent lobules, with regeneration of hepatocytes forming small nodules.

Cirrhotic Stage
1. Fibrous septa formation is present, with development of complete, although often ill-defined small regenerative nodules.

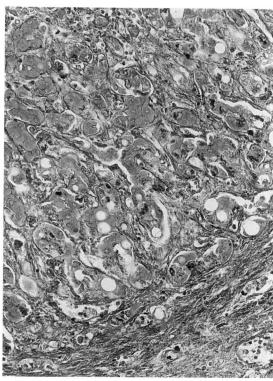

Figure 4–15. Alcoholic cirrhosis (trichrome). Sinusoidal collagen is present in the periseptal regions, surrounding individual and small groups of liver cells.

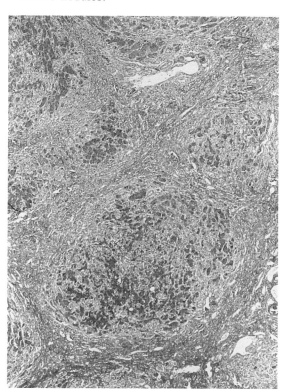

Figure 4–14. Alcoholic cirrhosis (trichrome). The architecture is distorted by fibrosis and regenerative nodule formation. Even on low power sinusoidal collagen can be appreciated within the nodules.

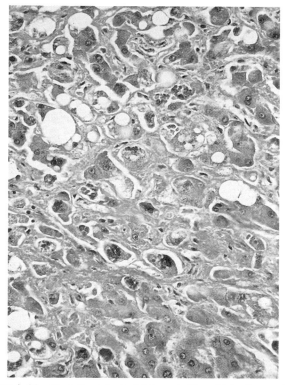

Figure 4–16. Alcoholic cirrhosis (trichrome). Sinusoidal collagen within this nodule is abundant, with no regenerative activity of individual liver cells. Occasional hepatocytes contain alcoholic hyalin that stains red.

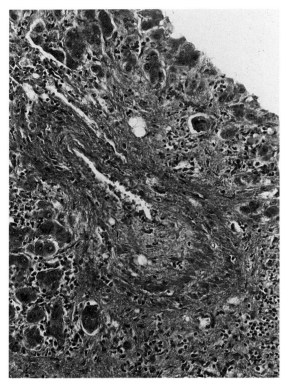

Figure 4–17. Alcoholic cirrhosis (trichrome). A sublobular vein is almost totally sclerosed and occluded.

2. Arachnoid sinusoidal fibrosis is present, extending from fibrous septa into nodules.
3. Fibrous septa are widened by formation of dense collagen as the cirrhosis progresses.

Other Features

1. There are variable degrees of both mononuclear and occasionally neutrophilic infiltration of the septa.
2. There are variable degrees of bile duct proliferation.
3. Vascular channels in septa (response of altered blood flow and portal hypertension) are increased.
4. Macrovesicular fat is usually present, less often in advanced stages of cirrhosis.
5. Sublobular hepatic veins have variable degrees of sclerosis.
6. Cholestasis may be present.
7. *Diffuse interstitial fibrosis:* A small percentage of cases may exhibit a prominent sinusoidal fibrosis in both precirrhotic and cirrhotic stages, uniformly involving the entire lobule or nodule.
8. Nuclear anisocytosis and dysplasia of hepatocytes are not a prominent feature in the alcoholic who is actively drinking.
9. In larger nodules in the alcoholic who has stopped drinking, small portal structures and the cord–sinusoid pattern may be reestablished.

10. Septa are somewhat thinner in patients who have undergone portacaval anastomosis.
11. Focal hyaline necrosis *without* neutrophilic infiltration may be present.

Differential Diagnosis

1. *Cirrhosis secondary to obesity/adult-onset diabetes mellitus:* Patients with diabetes exhibit increased numbers of glycogen nuclei; however, many alcoholics develop a diabetic state.
2. *Post jejunoileal bypass surgery:* Cirrhosis may occur in a small percentage of these patients 2 or more years after surgery. The nodules, although often containing fat, are fairly well demarcated, and the septa are thin, with little sinusoidal collagen.
3. *Wilson's disease:* Fat, sinusoidal collagen, and alcoholic hyalin may be seen. Copper (rubeanic acid stain) and copper-binding protein (orcein stain) are greatly increased in Wilson's disease, and sinusoidal collagen is usually mild.
4. *Chronic active hepatitis with cirrhosis:*
   a. *Non-A, non-B (HCV) etiology:* Mild fatty change and sinusoidal collagen are often present. Differentiation from alcoholic cirrhosis can be difficult on morphologic grounds alone if dealing with an inactive cirrhosis, especially since approximately 10% of alcoholic cirrhotics may have coexisting chronic non-A, non-B hepatitis.
   b. *Inactive chronic hepatitis B:* The alcoholic cirrhotic who has stopped drinking may develop dysplasia of periseptal hepatocytes, a feature often noted in chronic active hepatitis B. Ground-glass cells are present in more than half of the cases of chronic hepatitis B. A subtle morphologic feature is the nature of regenerative change: in chronic active hepatitis, regeneration is *irregular,* even within the same nodule, while in alcoholic cirrhosis, although regeneration can vary from one lobe of the liver to another, it is usually *regular* within single and groups of nodules present in surgical biopsy specimens.

Special Stain

1. *Masson trichrome:* Sinusoidal collagen is present as well as denseness of the fibrous septa.

Immunohistochemistry

1. *HBsAg, HBcAg, alpha-1-antitrypsin:* These antigens are useful in eliminating other possible etiologies in instances in which the cirrhosis is relatively inactive.

Clinical and Biologic Behavior

1. Common clinical presentation in decompensated state, with or without concomitant acute sclerosing hyaline necrosis, includes jaundice, ascites, debilitation, impotence/amenorrhea, loss of skeletal muscle mass, and other features related to alcohol itself (i.e., delirium tremens, pancreatitis, polyneuritis, gastritis with hemorrhage).
2. Splenomegaly occurs in only 30% of patients with alcoholic cirrhosis.
3. Patients often present with signs of chronic liver disease such as vascular spiders and palmar erythema. Visible collateral veins on the abdominal wall indicate portal hypertension. Ankle edema occurs when hypoalbuminemia develops.
4. Unless there is superimposed acute sclerosing hyaline necrosis, laboratory tests reveal mild to moderate elevations of serum aspartate aminotransferase, generally below 100 IU/L, with normal levels of alanine aminotransferase; serum IgA (polymeric IgA) is usually elevated in alcoholic cirrhosis but not in cirrhosis of other etiologies.
5. In early stages of cirrhosis, the liver is almost always enlarged, sometimes achieving weights of up to 5000 g; in advanced stages, the liver is of normal size or is slightly atrophic (900 g).
6. Dense sclerosis is typically seen in areas between the gallbladder bed and the hepatic vein outflow to the inferior vena cava, an area demarcating the vascular boundary between the true median portions of the right and left lobes.
7. Regenerative changes present as proliferating hydropic hepatocytes with sharp, distinct nuclear and cytoplasmic membranes. Mitoses are not typically seen. Sinusoidal borders appear to be poorly defined or absent, and inflammatory changes and Kupffer cell hyperplasia are not present. These regenerative changes in the cirrhotic liver can be variable and are more prominent away from the dense sclerotic regions.
8. The nodules in the active drinker are generally between 1 and 4 mm in diameter; in the patient who abstains from alcohol for months to years, the nodules can become larger (1.5 cm or more), grossly mimicking cirrhosis from chronic viral hepatitis.
9. If drinking continues, the nodules are always small, since there is constant subdivision of enlarging regenerative nodules by sinusoidal fibrogenesis; in addition, there is inhibition, to varying degrees, of regeneration of liver cells by alcohol itself.
10. Alcohol can induce fibrogenesis without overt episodes of acute liver disease, since approximately 40% of cases first present clinically in the cirrhotic stage.
11. In 30% of patients, the biopsy specimen shows appreciable amounts of fat, while in 20% there is some degree of hyaline necrosis.
12. Hepatic arteries and the arterial bed are increased in size in cirrhotics, with an increase in communication between the hepatic arterial and portal venous systems.
13. Decompensation is precipitated by heavy drinking (superimposed acute liver disease), as well as by gastrointestinal hemorrhage, infection, injury, or other causes of stress to the liver.
14. Hepatocellular carcinoma occurs in approximately 6% of all alcoholic cirrhotics and is more common in those who have abstained from drinking for a number of years; the average age of the alcoholic who has stopped drinking and develops hepatocellular carcinoma is 60 years, 10 years older than the alcoholic who continues to drink and dies of the consequences of cirrhosis without hepatocellular carcinoma.

Fine-Needle Aspiration

Although this technique is not used for diagnosis of alcoholic liver disease, the incidence of hepatocellular carcinoma is approximately 6% in patients with alcoholic cirrhosis. Aspiration may therefore be performed in the workup of mass lesions in these patients, where tumor cells may be demonstrated.

Treatment and Prognosis

1. Once the patient has reached the cirrhotic stage, abstinence from drinking does not significantly decrease complications from the consequences of portal hypertension.
2. Management of complications is similar regardless of the cause of the cirrhosis (see Chapter 1).
3. Controlled trials of propylthiouracil in ambulatory cirrhotics showed a benefit in survival in those who received therapy despite continued drinking.
4. One-year survival after onset of ascites was 35% and after onset of gastrointestinal hemorrhage was 28% to 55%.
5. Five-year survival after portacaval shunt was 50% at 2 years and 25% at 5 years.

References

Anthony PP, Ishak KG, Nayak NC, et al. The morphology of cirrhosis. J Clin Pathol 1978;31:395–414.

Glund C, Christoffersen P, Eriksen J, et al. Influence of ethanol on development of hyperplastic nodules in alcoholic men with micronodular cirrhosis. Gastroenterology 1987;93:256–260.

Popper H. Pathologic aspects of cirrhosis: A review. J Pathol 1977;87:228–264.

Ruebner BH. Collagen formation and cirrhosis. Semin Liver Dis 1986;6:212–220.

Progressive Perivenular Alcoholic Fibrosis

Major Morphologic Changes

1. Extensive dense sclerosis of the terminal hepatic venule and zone 3 is present.
2. Portal tract shows minimal fibrosis.
3. There is minimal to absent regenerative activity of hepatocytes; in the "pure" form of the disease, cirrhosis does *not* occur.

Other Features

1. Portal tract shows mild mononuclear inflammatory infiltrate and occasional scattered neutrophils.
2. Sinusoidal collagen in periportal and midzonal regions is present but minimal.
3. Bile duct proliferation is mild.
4. There are variable but mild degrees of macrovesicular fatty change.

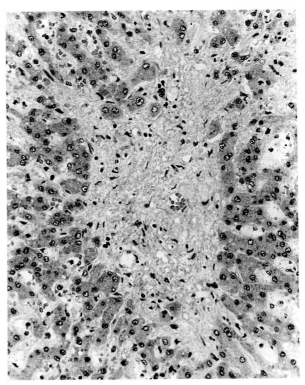

Figure 4–19. Progressive perivenular alcoholic fibrosis. High power of the terminal hepatic venule shows dense collagen containing numerous small vascular structures.

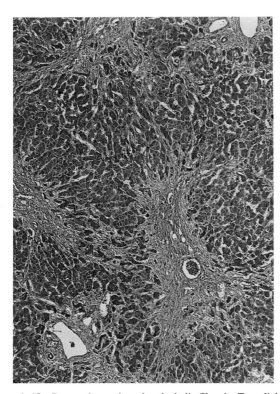

Figure 4–18. Progressive perivenular alcoholic fibrosis. Two slightly fibrotic portal tracts are present (*corners of the field*). The three terminal hepatic venules are extensively surrounded by dense sinusoidal collagen. Numerous reconstituted small vascular structures are present in these areas. The midzonal and periportal hepatocytes form an intact cord–sinusoid pattern, with little regenerative activity. This photomicrograph in some ways resembles the impaired regeneration syndrome of viral hepatitis (see Figure 2–12); however, the perivenular areas are densely fibrotic in progressive perivenular alcoholic fibrosis and not collapsed as in impaired regeneration.

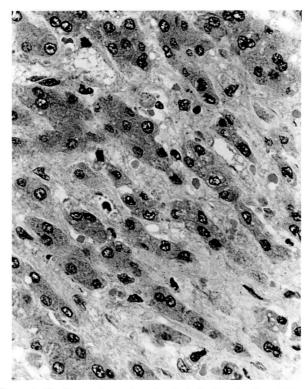

Figure 4–20. Progressive perivenular alcoholic fibrosis. Sinusoidal collagen is present adjacent to individual thin hepatic cords, with little regenerative activity.

5. Cholestasis is rarely present.
6. Scanty amounts of alcoholic hyalin may be present in liver cells adjacent to the sclerotic regions.
7. Cord–sinusoid pattern is usually distinct owing to absence of regeneration.
8. "Mixed" forms (i.e., with regenerative nodules) may be present in the same liver; although this change is common in autopsy specimens, it is rarely found in the same liver biopsy specimen.

Differential Diagnosis

1. *Portal and perivenular fibrosis (precirrhotic stage) of chronic alcoholic liver disease:* This condition may be quite similar to progressive perivenular alcoholic fibrosis except that the perivenular fibrosis is more extensive and denser in progressive perivenular alcoholic fibrosis. Typical precirrhotic portal and perivenular fibrosis also exhibits some degree of parenchymal regenerative activity.

Special Stain

1. *Masson trichrome:* Collagen in the perivenular zone stains intensely blue.

Clinical and Biologic Behavior

1. Progressive perivenular alcoholic fibrosis uniformly involving the liver is a relatively uncommon morphologic subtype of chronic alcoholic liver disease in which the main pathophysiologic changes revolve around the dense sclerosis in the perivenular zone, causing severe venous outflow obstruction and resulting portal hypertension; in the past the lesion was termed *chronic sclerosing hyaline disease.*
2. The major distinction between progressive perivenular alcoholic fibrosis and the typical perivenular fibrosis seen in most cases of alcoholic liver disease is its denseness and extensive involvement of zone 3, without regenerative nodule formation but with concomitant clinical features of advanced cirrhosis.
3. Patients first present with jaundice, ascites, and other signs of chronic liver disease; ascites is usually resistant to diuretic therapy.
4. Laboratory data are similar to the data seen in alcoholic cirrhosis, with hypoalbuminemia, mild increase in aspartate aminotransferase and normal alanine aminotransferase, hyperbilirubinemia, decreased prothrombin activity, and occasionally leukocytosis.
5. Peritoneoscopy reveals a liver with a smooth to slightly granular surface, without nodule formation.
6. The incidence of progressive perivenular alcoholic fibrosis, derived from a series of 517 consecutive autopsies from patients with any form of alcoholic liver disease, is 5%; a "mixed" form with cirrhosis is more common (17%).
7. A clinical distinction between progressive perivenular alcoholic fibrosis and alcoholic cirrhosis is the incidence of hepatocellular carcinoma: the latter has *not* been shown to develop in the former either in pure or mixed form (71 consecutive cases studied), while the incidence in alcoholic cirrhosis is from 6% to 12% in various large series.

Treatment and Prognosis

1. Management is directed to the consequences of portal hypertension outlined in Chapter 1.
2. Survival of patients is the same as those with alcoholic cirrhosis (age of death 48 years vs. 51 years for cirrhosis).

References

Edmondson HA. Alcoholic liver disease. In: Peters RL, Craig JR, eds. Liver Pathology. New York: Churchill Livingstone, 1986:268–272.
Edmondson HA, Peters RL. Liver. In: Kissane JM, Anderson WAD, eds. Pathology, 8th ed. St. Louis: C.V. Mosby, 1985:1140–1141.
Reynolds TB, Kanel GC. Alcoholic liver disease. In: Stein JH, ed. Internal Medicine, 2nd ed. Boston: Little, Brown and Co, 1987:223.

General References

Edmondson HA. Pathology of alcoholism. Am J Clin Pathol 1980;74:725–742.
Edmondson HE, Peters RL. Liver. In: Kissane JM, Anderson WAD, eds. Pathology, 8th ed. St. Louis: C.V. Mosby, 1985:1135–1148.
Edmondson HA. Alcoholic liver disease. In: Peters RL, Craig JR, eds. Liver Pathology. New York: Churchill Livingstone, 1986:255–283.
de la Hall P. Alcoholic liver disease. In: MacSween RNM, Anthony PP, Scheuer PJ, eds. Pathology of the Liver, 2nd ed. Edinburgh: Churchill Livingstone, 1987:281–309.
Lieber CS. Biochemical and molecular basis of alcohol-induced injury to liver and other tissues. N Engl J Med 1988;319:1639–1650.
MacSween RNM, Burt AD. Histologic spectrum of alcoholic liver disease. Semin Liver Dis 1986;6:221–232.
Reynolds TB, Kanel GC. Alcoholic liver disease. In: Stein JH, ed. Internal Medicine, 2nd ed. Boston: Little, Brown and Co, 1987:218–224.
Scheuer PJ. Liver disease in the alcoholic. In: Scheuer PJ, ed. Liver Biopsy Interpretation, 3rd ed. London: Baillière Tindall, 1980:75–87.

CHAPTER 5

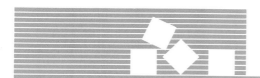

Drugs and Toxins

■ Classification

Basic Mechanisms of Disease

Feature	Direct	Intrinsic Injury Indirect (Toxic Metabolic Byproducts)	Idiosyncratic Injury
Reproducible in animals	+	+	−
Dose relationship	+	+	−
Temporal relationship	+	+	−
Specific morphologic changes	+	+	−
Hypersensitivity	−	−	+
Examples	Carbon tetrachloride Phosphorus	Acetaminophen Cocaine	Phenytoin Methyldopa

Predominant Morphologic Features

Feature	Examples
1. Hepatocellular necrosis without inflammatory reaction	Acetaminophen Cocaine
2. Hepatitis-like reaction a. Acute	Isoniazid Halothane (later stage)
b. Chronic (persistent, active)	Phenytoin Nitrofurantoin
3. Cholestasis a. Pure	Oral contraceptives
b. Mixed (with hepatitis)	Erythromycin
c. Chronic (with bile duct injury)	Chlorpromazine
4. Fibrosis	Methotrexate Vitamin A Alcohol
5. Fatty change	Prednisone Tetracycline
6. Vascular abnormalities	Anabolic steroids *Senecio* alkaloids
7. Granuloma formation	Phenylbutazone Sulfasalazine
8. Neoplasms a. Benign	Oral contraceptives
b. Malignant	Polyvinyl chloride
9. Miscellaneous (e.g., inclusions)	Procainamide

■ Hepatocellular Necrosis Without Significant Inflammatory Reaction

Perivenular (Zone 3)

Acetaminophen
Aflatoxin B1
Carbon tetrachloride
Chloroform
Halothane (early stage) and other halogenated
    hydrocarbons (methoxyflurane, enflurane)
Phalloidin
Pyrrolizidine alkaloids
Urethane

Midzonal (Zone 2)

Beryllium
Dioxane

Periportal (Zone 1)

Allyl formate
Endotoxin from *Proteus vulgaris*
Ferrous sulfate
Phosphorus

Perivenular or Peripor

Cocaine

Diffuse

Galactosamine
Tetrachlorethane
Trinitrotoluene

Acetaminophen

Major Morphologic Features

1. Coagulative-type of liver cell necrosis involves perivenular zone 3; this change is most prominent 4 to 6 days after ingestion of drug.
2. Collapse of perivenular reticulin framework occurs 6 to 10 days after ingestion, with marked midzonal and periportal hepatocellular regenerative activity.

Other Features

1. Portal tracts show no significant changes; portal fibrosis does *not* occur.

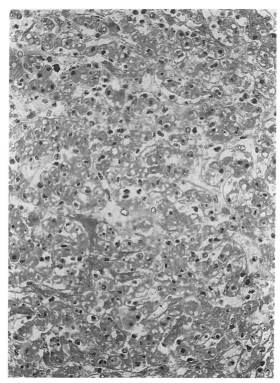

Figure 5–1. Acetaminophen toxicity. The hepatocytes in the perivenular zone in the early stage (4 to 6 days after drug exposure) exhibit a coagulative-type necrosis. Most of the nuclei have become pyknotic. A mild inflammatory infiltrate adjacent to necrotic liver cells is present.

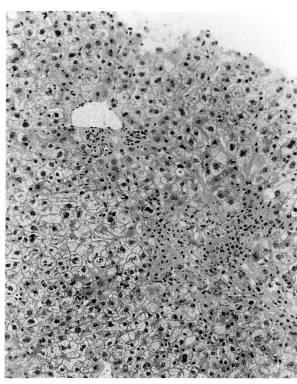

Figure 5–2. Acetaminophen toxicity. The portal tract (*upper left*) is of normal size, with no inflammatory infiltration. The perivenular zone (*lower right*) exhibits changes seen 6 to 10 days after exposure, with drop-out of hepatocytes and their replacement by Kupffer cells and macrophages. This area of cell necrosis is well demarcated from the adjacent hydropic hepatocytes.

2. Phagocytosis of necrotic hepatocytes by mononuclear and Kupffer cells is prominent in collapsed perivenular regions.
3. Inflammatory infiltration and Kupffer cell hyperplasia are absent in midzonal and periportal zones.
4. Necrosis extends into midzonal regions in more severe cases.
5. Cholestasis is quite rare.
6. All lobules throughout the liver are uniformly involved.

Differential Diagnosis

1. *Ischemic necrosis:* Eosinophilic coagulative necrosis, occurring in perivenular regions in severe hypoxia, resembles acetaminophen toxicity. Predisposing factors for ischemia, and plasma acetaminophen levels are helpful in confirming the diagnosis.
2. *Acute viral hepatitis:* Clinically the two entities may present in a similar manner, and plasma drug levels are not helpful unless the test is performed within the first 16 hours after ingestion. Serum aminotransferase activities are markedly elevated in acetaminophen toxicity, sometimes reaching levels greater than 10,000 IU/L. Serum lactate dehydrogenase levels are generally much higher in drug- and ischemic-

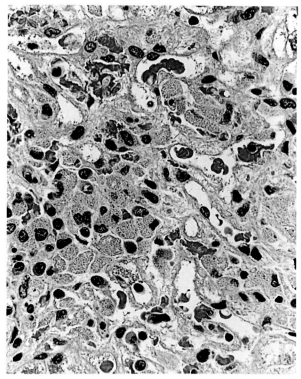

Figure 5–3. Acetaminophen toxicity. High power of the perivenular zone exhibits absence of hepatocytes and their replacement by Kupffer cells and macrophages. Occasional lymphocytes are present. Many of the macrophages contain an abundant granular cytoplasmic pigment representing phagocytized lipochrome.

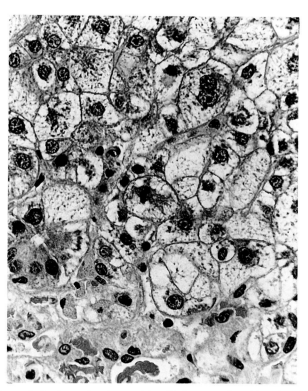

Figure 5–4. Acetaminophen toxicity. High power of a midzonal region (perivenular necrosis at the bottom of the field) shows hydropic hepatocytes representing areas of regeneration.

related injury. Biopsy is usually not necessary for diagnosis unless the possibility of viral hepatitis and the risk of chronic hepatitis need exclusion, since acetaminophen liver injury does not lead to chronic disease. Features of morphologic differentiation are described below:

Feature	Acute Viral Hepatitis	Acetaminophen Toxicity
Inflammation	Diffuse with spotty necrosis	Minimal, only in areas of perivenular necrosis
Kupffer cell hyperplasia	Prominent	Absent
Portal lymphoid hyperplasia	Prominent	Absent

Special Stain

1. *Periodic acid–Schiff after diastase:* Positive lysosomal granules in perivenular mononuclear and Kupffer cells are prominent owing to phagocytosis of necrotic hepatocytes.

Clinical and Biologic Behavior

1. *Metabolism:* Acetaminophen is rapidly absorbed, with peak levels attained 30 to 60 minutes after ingestion (therapeutic: 9 μg/mL); it is metabolized in liver, with a half-life of 2 hours.
2. With ingestion of a large dose of the drug (e.g., 10 g), saturation of glucuronic acid and sulfate conjugates leads to generation of toxic metabolites by the mixed function oxidases. When capacity of glutathione conjugation is exceeded, covalent binding and liver cell necrosis result.
3. Nausea and vomiting occur within a few hours of ingestion. Between 24 and 72 hours, abdominal pain and jaundice develop, associated with marked elevations in serum aminotransferase levels. Decreased prothrombin activity occurs early and precedes aminotransferase elevation. Renal failure develops in 10% to 40% of patients; in severe injury, renal tubular necrosis, myocardial damage, coma, and death may result.
4. Metabolic half-life (normally 2 hours) increases twofold to threefold with hepatotoxicity; mortality is increased if metabolic half-life is prolonged to 10 hours.

5. The risk of liver injury can be estimated from a semi-log plot of plasma concentration (μg/mL) versus time after ingestion; liver damage with necrosis is expected if the patient's level falls *above* a line connecting 200 μg/mL at 4 hours and 50 μg/mL at 12 hours.
6. The single toxic dose of acetaminophen necessary to produce significant liver cell damage is 10 g or more, although small doses (5–8 g) over weeks may also cause liver injury; in patients whose mixed function oxidase system is enhanced (e.g., by alcohol or barbiturates), liver injury may develop with lower doses (3–5 g) of acetaminophen.
7. Chronic administration to rats has induced cirrhosis, and rare cases of acute hepatic necrosis and chronic active hepatitis-like features in humans associated with long-term low-dose (4–6 g/d) therapy have been reported.

Treatment and Prognosis

1. The objective of therapy is to prevent liver injury by repleting glutathione in persons confirmed to have ingested a toxic dose, or those at risk, by administering N-acetylcysteine (Mucomyst), preferably orally or intravenously.
2. Recovery is excellent if the patient is treated before 10 hours following ingestion. Therapy is usually not effective after the onset of liver injury.
3. Factors affecting mortality include advanced age, severity of liver injury, delayed therapy, concomitant use of alcohol and other drugs, and pre-existing disease in other organ systems.
4. Death from fulminant hepatic failure can be avoided by hepatic transplantation.

References

Black M. Acetaminophen hepatotoxicity. Gastroenterology 1980;78:382–392.
Davis M. Protective agents for acetaminophen overdose. Semin Liver Dis 1986;6:138–147.
Portmann B, Talbot IC, Day DW et al. Histopathological changes in the liver following a paracetamol overdose: Correlation with clinical and biochemical parameters. J Pathol 1975;117:169–181.
Smilkstein MJ, Knapp GL, Kulig KW et al. Efficacy of oral N-acetylcysteine in the treatment of acetaminophen overdose: Analysis of the National Multicenter study (1976–1985). N Engl J Med 1988;319:1557–1562.

■ **Hepatocellular Necrosis With Acute Hepatitis-like Features**

Alpha-methyldopa
Dapsone
Halothane (latter stage) and other halogenated hydrocarbons (methoxyflurane, enflurane)
Indomethacin
Isoniazid
Nitrofurantoin
Oxyphenisatin

Phenylbutazone
Phenytoin
Rifampin
Sulfasalazine

Isoniazid

Major Morphologic Features

1. Hydropic hepatocytes involve all zones, with focal necrosis and Kupffer cell hyperplasia.
2. Lymphocytic exudation occurs within portal tracts and parenchyma.

Other Features

1. Slight periportal accentuation of inflammation and necrosis may be present in early stages.
2. Cholestasis is infrequent.
3. Submassive and massive hepatic necrosis is rare.
4. Endophlebitis may be present around terminal hepatic venules.
5. Irregular inflammatory activity and "piecemeal" necrosis resembling features of chronic active hepatitis have been reported.

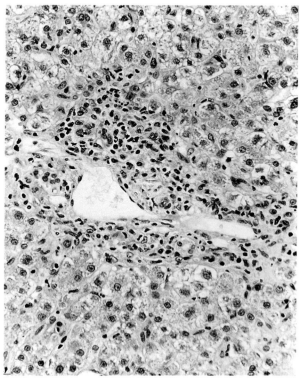

Figure 5–5. Isoniazid toxicity. The portal tract is normal in size and exhibits a moderate lymphocytic infiltration and hyperplasia. Bile ducts are present and normal in number.

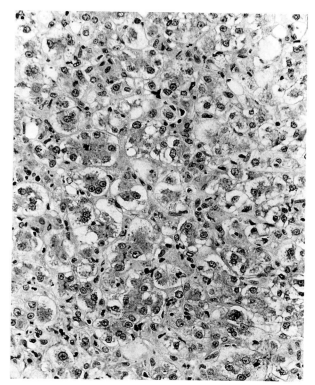

Figure 5–6. Isoniazid toxicity. The parenchyma exhibits a distorted cord–sinusoid pattern with hydropic hepatocytes, focal necrosis, and prominent Kupffer cell hyperplasia.

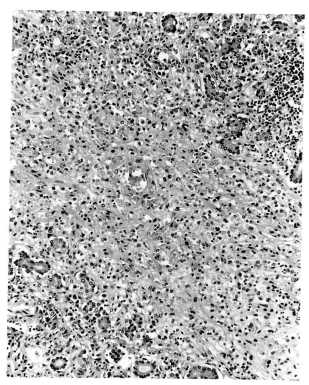

Figure 5–8. Isoniazid toxicity. This severe case shows total dropout of liver cells in all zones. Lymphocytes and hyperplastic Kupffer cells remain within the lobule. Two portal tracts (*upper right, lower left*) exhibit prominent numbers of bile ductules. The portal tracts are closer together because of the marked dropout of hepatocytes and resultant collapse of the reticulin framework.

Differential Diagnosis

1. *Acute viral hepatitis:* Prominent parenchymal inflammatory exudates seen in viral hepatitis are not as severe in isoniazid hepatitis. Periportal accentuation of the inflammatory change that may be seen with isoniazid hepatitis is not noted in viral hepatitis.

Clinical and Biologic Behavior

1. The incidence of acute hepatitis is 0.1% to 1.0% of all patients receiving isoniazid, but in those older than 35 years of age the incidence is 2% to 3%. Approximately 10% who develop clinically apparent hepatotoxicity die of fulminant hepatic failure, with estimated overall mortality of 0.1%.

2. Isoniazid hepatotoxicity occurs in two patterns: (1) *subacute hepatic injury* in 12% to 20% of recipients, occurring at an average of 3 months of drug use with asymptomatic elevation (threefold to fourfold) of serum aminotransferase levels, which resolve when the medication is continued; and (2) *overt hepatic injury,* which resembles viral hepatitis with onset 2 to 11 months after continued ingestion.

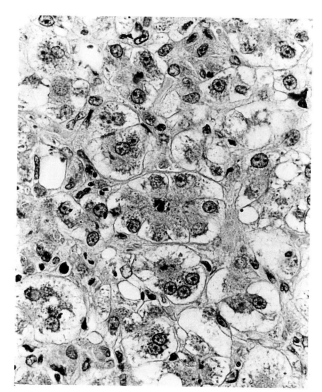

Figure 5–7. Isoniazid toxicity. High power of the parenchyma exhibits hydropic hepatocytes, focal necrosis, and Kupffer cell hyperplasia. A dilated canaliculus containing dark-staining bile (*center*) is present.

Prompt recognition of toxicity and withdrawal of drug results in resolution in 60% to 80% of cases. In older patients and with continued therapy despite symptoms the risk of severe hepatitis and hepatic failure is increased.

3. Isoniazid is metabolized through the cytochrome P-450 pathway as *fast acetylators,* in which 94% of the administered dose is acetylated and excreted, and as *slow acetylators,* in which 63% is acetylated and 37% free isoniazid is excreted. It is not clear if isoniacid hepatoxicity is related to fast acetylator status. The metabolic byproduct acetylhydrazine appears to be the toxic metabolite.

4. Phenobarbital and other enzyme inducers of the cytochrome P-450 system may favor hepatotoxicity.

5. Plasma levels of isoniazid or metabolites do not correlate with liver cell necrosis.

6. There is little documented evidence for cirrhosis developing as a sequel to isoniazid-induced liver injury.

Treatment and Prognosis

1. Treatment is supportive and necessitates early drug withdrawal. Mortality is increased in women older than 35 years of age and when delay in recognition and continued ingestion of the drug occur despite early liver injury.

2. Although approximately 10% of patients who are symptomatic will die of submassive necrosis, the availability of hepatic transplantation will reduce this mortality.

References

Black M, Mitchell JR, Zimmerman HJ et al. Isoniazid-associated hepatitis in 114 patients. Gastroenterology 1975;69:289–302.

Garibaldi RA, Drusin RE, Ferebee SH, et al. Isoniazid-associated hepatitis: Report of an outbreak. Am Rev Respir Dis 1972;106:357–365.

Maddrey WC, Boitnott JK. Isoniazid hepatitis. Ann Intern Med 1973;79:1–12.

Mitchell JR, Zimmerman HJ, Ishak KG, et al. Isoniazid liver injury: Clinical spectrum, pathology and probable pathogenesis. Ann Intern Med 1976;84:181–192.

Moulding TS, Redeker A, Kanel GC. Twenty isoniazid-associated deaths in one state. Am Rev Respir Dis 1989;140:700–705.

Phenytoin

Major Morphologic Features

1. Viral hepatitis–like features:
   a. Hepatocytolysis, hydropic change, acidophilic necrosis, and Kupffer cell hyperplasia occur.
   b. Portal inflammatory infiltrate consists of lymphocytes, neutrophils, and eosinophils.
2. Mononucleosis-like features:
   a. Intact cord–sinusoid pattern, focal necrosis,

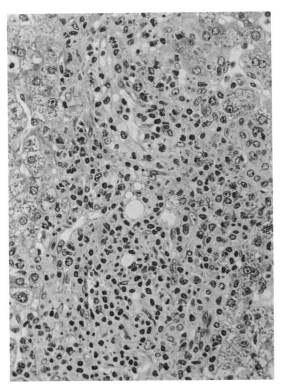

Figure 5–9. Phenytoin toxicity. The portal tract is slightly enlarged by infiltration with both lymphocytes and numerous eosinophils.

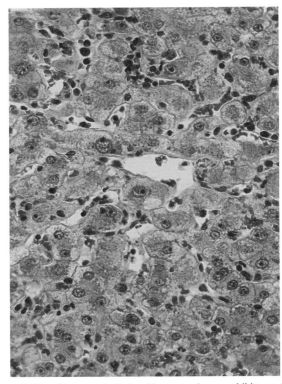

Figure 5–10. Phenytoin toxicity. The parenchyma exhibits an intact cord–sinusoid pattern. Hepatocytes are normal in size to slightly hydropic. Kupffer cell hyperplasia and a slight increase in circulating lymphocytes are present. Liver cell necrosis is not evident in this field.

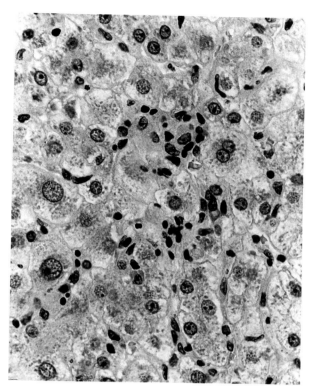

Figure 5–11. Phenytoin toxicity. Focal necrosis, hepatocytolysis, and Kupffer cell hyperplasia are present. Hepatocytes are slightly hydropic.

Kupffer cell hyperplasia and hypertrophy are evident.
  b. Increased numbers of lymphocytes in sinusoids exhibit a beaded or "Indian file" pattern.
  c. Portal inflammatory infiltrate consists of lymphocytes, neutrophils, and eosinophils.

Other Features

1. Portal and parenchymal inflammatory infiltrate may be minimal, with ground-glass type cells resembling those seen in persistent hepatitis type B.
2. Occasional poorly defined noncaseating granulomas sometimes exhibiting multinucleated giant cells are seen.
3. Cholestasis is rare.
4. Submassive and massive hepatic necrosis with prominent portal inflammatory infiltrate is uncommon.

Differential Diagnosis

1. *Acute viral hepatitis:* Eosinophils and granulomatous necrosis are not features of acute viral hepatitis.
2. *Acute hepatitis secondary to infectious mononucleosis:* Eosinophils are not a feature of infectious mononucleosis.
3. *Persistent hepatitis B:* The ground-glass type cells

seen in chronic hepatitis B are positive on orcein and immunoperoxidase stains for HBsAg but negative in phenytoin hypersensitivity.

Special Stains

1. *Orcein, aldehyde fuchsin:* These stains differentiate ground-glass type cells in drug-induced injury (negative) versus chronic hepatitis B (positive).

Immunohistochemistry

1. *HBsAg:* This antigen differentiates ground-glass type cells in drug-induced injury (negative) versus chronic hepatitis B (positive).

Clinical and Biologic Behavior

1. The overall incidence of phenytoin hepatotoxicity is less than 1%, rarer in the pediatric age group, and slightly increased in blacks.
2. Acute injury presents somewhat similar to acute viral hepatitis, occurring 1 to 8 weeks after ingestion of the drug, but fever (75%), rash (63%), hepatomegaly (12%), lymphadenopathy, and splenomegaly (60%) are associated.
3. On laboratory tests, leukocytosis is noted in almost all cases (eosinophilia in 89%), with elevations of serum aminotransferase levels (ranging from 300 to 800 IU/L, rarely as high as 3500 IU/L) and serum bilirubin level (usually <10 mg/dL) and mild elevation of alkaline phosphatase activity.
4. Less common features include pharyngitis, malaise, myalgia, pruritus, thrombocytopenia, interstitial nephritis, and megaloblastoid change in the blood and bone marrow. In some, lymphadenopathy and atypical lymphocytes resemble infectious mononucleosis.
5. The hepatotoxicity is considered to be caused by hypersensitivity, based on clinical presentation of fever, rash, and eosinophilia; prompt reproducibility on rechallenge; circulating antibodies to the drug; and lack of relationship to dose.

Treatment and Prognosis

1. Prompt resolution of symptoms occurs with withdrawal of the drug. Corticosteroids ameliorate more severe features of hypersensitivity, such as exfoliation.

References

Harinasuta U, Zimmerman HJ. Diphenylhydantoin sodium hepatitis. JAMA 1968;203:1015–1018.

Lee TJ, Carney CN, Lapid J, et al. Diphenylhydantoin-induced hepatic necrosis: A case study. Gastroenterology 1976;70:422–424.

Mullick FG, Ishak KG. Hepatic injury associated with diphenylhydantoin therapy: A clinicopathologic study of 20 cases. Am J Clin Pathol 1980;74:442–452.

Halothane

Major Morphologic Features

Early Stage (First Week)
1. Coagulative-type necrosis occurs in perivenular zone.
2. Minimal mononuclear inflammatory infiltration is evident within the parenchyma and portal tracts.

Later Stage (Second to Third Weeks)
1. Resorption of necrotic cells occurs, with perivenular stromal collapse.
2. Focal hepatocytolysis, ballooning degeneration of liver cells, Kupffer cell hyperplasia, and mild to moderate predominantly lymphocytic infiltration are present within the remaining zones of the parenchyma.
3. Portal tracts show moderate lymphocytic infiltration and hyperplasia.

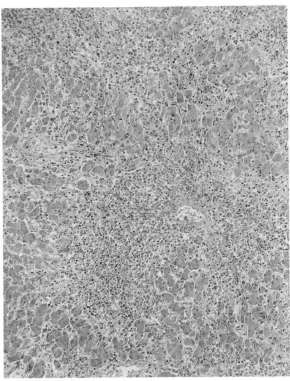

Figure 5–13. Halothane toxicity. The perivenular and midzonal regions in this early stage (first week after exposure) exhibit coagulative-type necrosis of hepatocytes. Kupffer cell hyperplasia is present next to adjacent viable hepatocytes.

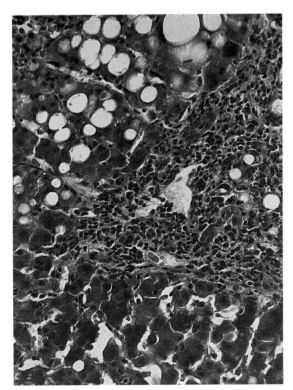

Figure 5–12. Halothane toxicity. The portal tract (*right*) exhibits a moderate lymphocytic infiltration and hyperplasia. The periportal hepatocytes exhibit variable macrovesicular fatty change. Kupffer cell hyperplasia is present, but liver cell necrosis is minimal.

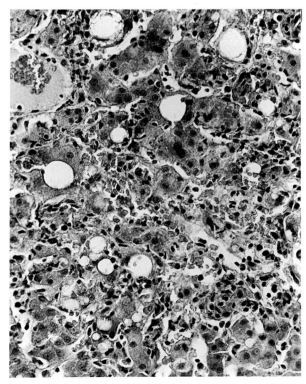

Figure 5–14. Halothane toxicity. The perivenular zone in later stages (second to third week) exhibits prominent lymphocytic infiltration, focal necrosis, and Kupffer cell hyperplasia and resembles acute viral hepatitis. Mild macrovesicular fatty change is also present.

Other Features

Early Stage
1. There is fairly sharp demarcation between necrotic region and viable hepatocytes.
2. Macrovesicular fatty change is mild.

Later Stage
1. Acidophil bodies are often present.
2. Cholestasis is usually mild but is prominent in cases of significant necrosis and collapse.
3. In severe cases confluent, submassive, or massive hepatic necrosis is observed.
4. Cholangiolar proliferation is often prominent.
5. Mild to moderate increase in eosinophils may be present within the portal tract and parenchyma.

Differential Diagnosis

1. *Drug reactions that elicit a coagulative-type necrosis* (e.g., acetaminophen): In halothane toxicity a more prominent diffuse inflammatory response is seen within the lobules if the biopsy is performed *after* the first week and may resemble acute viral hepatitis, whereas in acetaminophen toxicity inflammation is seen *only* in sites of perivenular necrosis.
2. *Acute viral hepatitis:* Biopsy findings during the second to third weeks after clinical onset of hepatotoxicity may be morphologically indistinguishable from those of acute viral hepatitis, although in halothane hepatotoxicity the inflammatory infiltrate is less prominent. A well-defined margin of perivenular necrosis is more often noted with halothane liver injury.

Clinical and Biologic Behavior

1. Hepatic injury occurs in approximately 1/9,000 exposed individuals, with fatal illness in 1/40,000 exposures.
2. Adults and women have an increased susceptibility when compared with children and males. Older and obese persons appear at increased risk of hepatotoxicity.
3. Clinical features develop 1 to 14 days (mean, 6 days) after initial exposure; with multiple exposures, the interval decreases (mean, 3 days).
4. Onset is abrupt (60%–80%), and fever and chills are common; other features include rash (10%), myalgia (20%), and anorexia and nausea (50%); jaundice occurs 3 to 4 days later.
5. Marked elevation of serum aminotransferase levels (3000–4000 IU/L) occurs, with hyperbilirubinemia, decreased prothrombin activity, and mildly elevated alkaline phosphatase activity; leukocytosis is usually present, with eosinophilia in 50% of these cases.
6. Most symptomatic patients have had prior exposure (75% of cases).
7. Mechanism of toxicity is not clear. Both toxic and hypersensitivity mechanisms may be operative. Hypoxia potentiates toxicity and is postulated to form toxic-free radicals by cytochrome P-450, which then leads to lipid peroxidation and cell necrosis.
8. Hepatotoxic changes may vary from mild and subclinical to fulminant massive hepatic necrosis.
9. Other halogenated hydrocarbons, such as enflurane and methoxyflurane, may also produce hepatotoxicity.
10. Halothane must be distinguished from post-transfusion viral hepatitis since viral hepatitis may become chronic while halothane-related injury does not; it is necessary to ensure that subsequent reexposure to halogenated hydrocarbons is avoided.

Treatment and Prognosis

1. Treatment is supportive. Mortality is 20% to 60% in jaundiced patients. Hepatic transplantation should be offered to patients with fulminant hepatic failure.
2. There is no evidence for a causal relationship between halothane liver injury and development of cirrhosis.

References

Benjamin SB, Goodman ZD, Ishak KG, et al. The morphologic spectrum of halothane-induced hepatic injury: Analysis of 77 cases. Hepatology 1985;5:1163–1171.

Carney FM, Van Dyke RA. Halothane hepatitis: A critical review. Anesth Analg Curr Res 1972;51:135–160.

DeGroot H, Noll T. Halothane hepatotoxicity: Relation between metabolic activation, hypoxia, covalent binding, lipid peroxidation and liver cell damage. Hepatology 1983;3:601–606.

Morgenstern L, Sacks HJ, Marmer MJ. Postoperative jaundice associated with halothane anesthesia. Surg Gynecol Obstet 1965;121:728–732.

Peters RL, Edmondson HA, Reynolds TB, et al. Hepatic necrosis associated with halothane anesthesia. Am J Med 1969;47:748–764.

Trey C, Lipworth L, Chalmer T, et al. Fulminant hepatic failure: Presumable contribution to halothane. N Engl J Med 1968;279:798–801.

■ Hepatocellular Necrosis With Chronic Hepatitis-like Features

Alpha-methyldopa
Aspirin
Chlorpromazine
Dantrolene
Disulfiram
Ethanol
Isoniazid
Methotrexate
Nitrofurantoin
Oxyphenisatin
Perhexilene maleate

Propylthiouracil
Sulfonamides
Tricrynafen

Nitrofurantoin

Major Morphologic Changes

1. Portal fibrosis with mononuclear inflammatory infiltrate is present.
2. Spillover of inflammatory cells into adjacent parenchyma occurs, surrounding individual and small groups of liver cells ("piecemeal" necrosis).
3. Focal liver cell necrosis and mononuclear inflammatory infiltration are *irregularly* distributed within the lobules.

Other Features

1. Hepatocytes exhibit variable degrees of hydropic change.
2. Cholestasis is sometimes a prominent feature.
3. Kupffer cell hyperplasia is mild to moderate.
4. Macrovesicular fatty change is occasionally present.
5. Lobular inflammatory changes may sometimes be uniform rather than irregular, resembling a mild acute viral hepatitis.

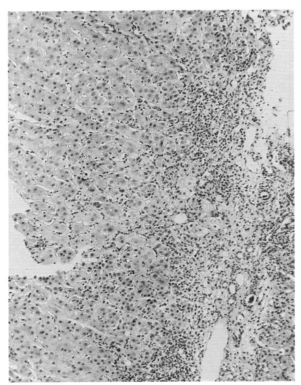

Figure 5–15. Nitrofurantoin toxicity. The portal tract is fibrotic. A moderate number of mononuclear inflammatory cells have infiltrated into the periportal region, surrounding hepatocytes.

6. Submassive necrosis is rare.
7. Severe fibrosis and even cirrhosis have been reported with chronic administration of the drug.

Differential Diagnosis

1. Chronic active hepatitis:
   a. *Viral etiology:* Presence of ground-glass cells confirms chronic hepatitis B.
   b. *Autoimmune:* Increased numbers of plasma cells in portal tracts and parenchyma are typical of this disease.

Clinical and Biologic Behavior

1. In patients with chronic active hepatitis confirmed by biopsy, the latent period from initial exposure to presentation is usually more than 6 months (range 30 days to 3 years).
2. The disorder occurs more often in women.
3. Jaundice is usually present, and the serum bilirubin level rarely exceeds 10 mg/dL; serum aminotransferase levels are moderately elevated and occasionally reported to be approximately 1000 IU/L.
4. An autoimmune etiology is suggested by positive immune serologic tests such as antinuclear antibody (82%) and smooth muscle antibody (73%).
5. Approximately two thirds of the patients with clinical symptoms have had prior exposure to the drug.
6. Patients may occasionally present with an acute illness after a latent period ranging from 2 days to 5 months, with fever (51%), eosinophilia (75%), rash (33%), fatigue, arthralgias, and myalgias; biopsy specimens show features of acute hepatitis.
7. Cirrhosis has been reported after long-term use.
8. Pathogenesis of hepatic injury is probably hypersensitivity, evidenced by fever, rash, eosinophilia, and prompt recurrence of symptoms and laboratory abnormalities after re-exposure.

Treatment and Prognosis

1. Termination of the drug leads to prompt resolution of symptoms in most patients; however, rare patients have continued to exhibit morphologic features of chronic active hepatitis a few months later.
2. Fulminant hepatitis related to nitrofurantoin has not been observed; rare cases of cirrhosis have been reported.

References

Klemola H, Penttila O, Runeberg L et al. Anicteric liver damage during nitrofurantoin medication. Scand J Gastroenterol 1975;10:501–505.

Selroos O, Edgran J. Lupus-like syndrome associated with pulmonary reaction to nitrofurantoin: Report of three cases. Acta Med Scand 1975;197:125–129.

Sharp JR, Ishak KG, Zimmerman HJ. Chronic active hepatitis and severe hepatic necrosis associated with nitrofurantoin. Ann Intern Med 1980;92:14–19.

Stricker BHC, Blok APR, Class FHJ, et al. Hepatic injury associated with the use of nitrofurans: A clinicopathological study of 52 reported cases. Hepatology 1988;8:599–606.

■ Cholestasis and Duct Injury

Cholestasis Without Inflammatory Change

Anabolic steroids (fluoxymesterone, oxymetholone, methyltestosterone)

Oral contraceptives (ethinyl estradiol, norethindrone acetate)

Cholestasis With Inflammatory Change

Acetohexamide
Azathioprine
Chlorpromazine
Chlorpropamide
Cimetidine
Erythromycin
6-Mercaptopurine
Naproxen
Nitrofurantoin
Oxyphenisatin
Penicillin
Sulfonamides
Tamoxifen
Total parenteral nutrition
Verapamil

Bile Duct Degeneration

4,4'- Diaminoidiphenylmethane
Paraquat

Acute Cholangitis

Allopurinol
Chlorpromazine
Chlorpropamide
Hydralazine

Chronic Primary Biliary Cirrhosis–like Features

Ajmaline
Arsenicals
Chlorpromazine
Methyl testosterone
Sulfonylurea agents
Tolbutamide

Oral Contraceptives

Major Morphologic Feature

1. Cholestasis is evident in hepatocytes, and dilated canaliculi are most prominent in the perivenular zone.

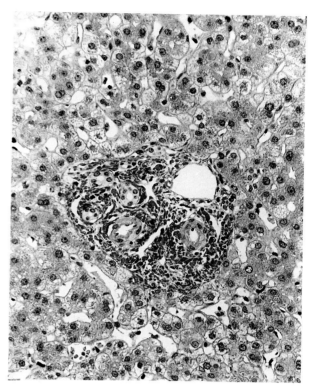

Figure 5–16. Oral contraceptive toxicity. The portal tract is well defined, with only a slight increase in duct structures and no significant inflammatory infiltrate. The surrounding parenchyma exhibits a normal cord–sinusoid pattern, with minimal Kupffer cell hyperplasia and no liver cell necrosis.

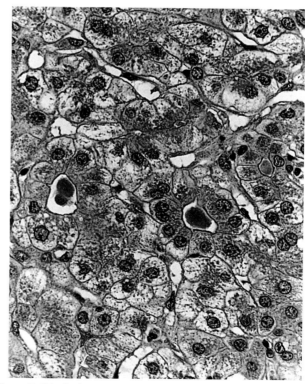

Figure 5–17. Oral contraceptive toxicity. Bile is present within dilated canaliculi. Hepatocytes are only slightly hydropic.

Other Features

1. Portal tracts exhibit no significant inflammatory or bile duct changes.
2. Hepatocytes may be slightly hydropic.
3. Focal necrosis is usually scanty and more often in a perivenular location.
4. Hepatocytes may form acinar-like structures around dilated canaliculi.
5. Kupffer cells are normal to slightly hyperplastic.
6. Cholestasis may be severe and involve all three zones.
7. Chronic use may rarely be associated with hepatic vein thrombosis, peliosis hepatis, liver cell adenoma, and hepatocellular carcinoma.

Differential Diagnosis

1. *Extrahepatic biliary obstruction:* Duct proliferation and dilatation, portal edema, and acute cholangitis, which are typical of large duct obstruction, are not present with oral contraceptives; however, in cases of rapid passage of common duct stones, the biopsy may only show minimal portal changes with cholestasis, and may be difficult to distinguish from drug-induced cholestasis.

Special Stains

1. *Van Gieson:* Bile stains bright green.

Clinical and Biologic Behavior

1. The clinical features develop within 1 to 6 months after drug ingestion, with nausea, pruritus, malaise, and anorexia, followed by jaundice; fever, arthralgias, and rash are not present.
2. Laboratory tests show hyperbilirubinemia (3–13 mg/dL) with mild elevations of serum aminotransferase and alkaline phosphatase levels.
3. The overall incidence is approximately 1/10,000 users, but the disorder has been reported more frequently in natives of Scandinavia (1/4,000), Argentina, and Chile.
4. Cholestasis caused by oral contraceptives is more likely to develop in women with benign recurrent cholestasis; a history of jaundice or pruritus during pregnancy is present in 50% of women who also develop jaundice while on oral contraceptives.
5. An increased frequency of cholelithiasis is noted owing to increased cholesterol saturation of the bile.
6. Jaundice is most likely caused by decreased uptake of bile acids from the blood and resultant interference of normal bile excretion.

Treatment and Prognosis

1. Cessation of medication leads to remission within a few weeks, although rarely liver test abnormalities can persist for months.

References

Edmondson HA, Henderson B, Benton B. Liver-cell adenomas associated with use of oral contraceptives. N Engl J Med 1976;294:470–472.
Ishak KG. Hepatic lesions caused by anabolic and contraceptive steroids. Semin Liver Dis 1981;1:116–128.
Ockner RK, Davidson CS. Hepatic effects of oral contraceptives. N Engl J Med 1967;276:331–334.
Schaffner F. The effect of oral contraceptives on the liver. JAMA 1966;198:155–157.

Chlorpromazine

Major Morphologic Features

1. Cholestasis is evident in hepatocytes, and dilated canaliculi are most prominent in the perivenular regions.
2. Portal tract shows mild to moderate infiltration by lymphocytes and eosinophils (early stages).

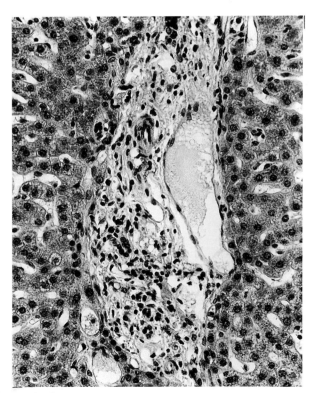

Figure 5–18. Chlorpromazine toxicity. The portal tract is slightly enlarged and contains lymphocytes, eosinophils, neutrophils, and rare plasma cells. Bile ducts are present but not directly involved by this infiltrate.

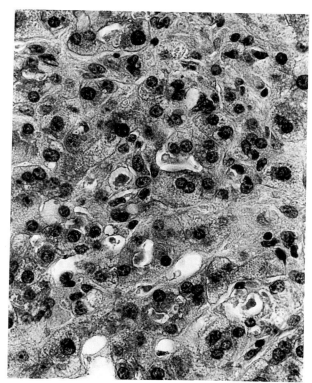

Figure 5–19. Chlorpromazine toxicity. Dilated canaliculi contain bile. Kupffer cell hyperplasia and occasional hepatocytolysis are present.

Other Features

1. Bile duct proliferation is minimal.
2. Liver cells may have variable degrees of cytoplasmic swelling.
3. Acidophil bodies are rare.
4. Hepatocytolysis is present but minimal.
5. Kupffer cell hyperplasia is mild.
6. Bile pigment in some cases is dark green-black.
7. Nonsuppurative destructive changes of interlobular bile ducts by lymphocytes with decrease in number of ducts, resembling primary biliary cirrhosis, has rarely been reported in patients on long-term therapy.

Differential Diagnosis

1. *Extrahepatic biliary obstruction:* Bile duct proliferation and dilatation, portal tract edema, and often acute cholangitis typically seen in large duct obstruction are not present in chlorpromazine-induced liver injury, where eosinophils are a predominant portal inflammatory feature.
2. *Primary biliary cirrhosis:* The rare case of destructive duct lesions associated with chlorpromazine morphologically resembles primary biliary cirrhosis. Cessation of the drug leads to eventual remission of the lesion, although it may persist for months. A positive antimitochondrial antibody, seen in 95% of cases of primary biliary cirrhosis, is not present in chlorpromazine-related primary biliary cirrhosis–like lesions.

Special Stains

1. *Van Gieson:* Bile stains bright green.
2. *Rubeanic acid:* In some instances there is an increase in intracytoplasmic black to black-green granules (copper) in periportal hepatocytes.

Clinical and Biologic Behavior

1. Twenty to fifty percent of all patients on chlorpromazine therapy have mild elevations of serum aminotransferase levels but are asymptomatic; however, 1% to 2% develop jaundice.
2. One third of these patients present with an acute illness 1 to 5 weeks after administration of the drug, with chills, fever, and malaise, followed by pruritus and jaundice 1 week later; abdominal tenderness (50%) and hepatomegaly (40%) may also occur.
3. Laboratory data reveal hyperbilirubinemia (mean 12 mg/dL), with serum aminotransferase levels five times normal and alkaline phosphatase three to four times normal.
4. Age range of susceptibility to drug toxicity is variable (20–80 years), with men more frequently affected.
5. Readministration of the drug leads to prompt recurrence of symptoms in approximately half of the patients.
6. Because almost half of all patients taking chlorpromazine exhibit mild enzyme elevations, it is believed that the drug or metabolic byproducts may be mildly hepatotoxic, with 1% to 2% of the patients additionally experiencing an idiosyncratic reaction (increased numbers of eosinophils in portal areas).

Treatment and Prognosis

1. After the drug is stopped there is total resolution of the illness within 10 weeks in 75% of cases (range, 2–12 months); in 17% recovery may be prolonged (up to 16 months) and primary biliary cirrhosis–like features lasting for several years have been rarely reported.

References

Ishak KG, Irey NS. Hepatic injury associated with the phenothiazines: Clinicopathologic and follow-up study of 36 patients. Arch Pathol 1972;93:283–304.

Levine RA, Briggs GW, Lowell DM. Chronic chlorpromazine cholangiolitic hepatitis: Report of a case with immunofluorescent studies. Gastroenterology 1966;50:665–670.

Popper H, Rubin E, Gardiol D et al. Drug-induced liver disease. Arch Intern Med 1965;115:128–136.

■ Fibrosis

Aflatoxin
Arsenicals
Chlorpromazine
Copper sulfate
Dantrolene
Disulfiram
Drugs associated with chronic active hepatitis
    Alpha-methyldopa
    Nitrofurantoin
    Oxyphenisatin
Ethanol
Iproniazid
Isoniazid
Methotrexate
Perhexilene maleate
Pyrrolizidine alkaloids
Thorotrast
Total parenteral nutrition
Vinyl chloride
Vitamin A

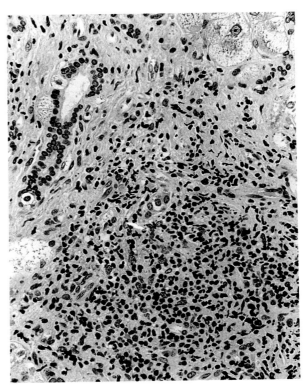

Figure 5–20. Methotrexate toxicity. The portal tract is enlarged by fibrosis and a moderate lymphocytic infiltration and hyperplasia.

Methotrexate

Major Morphologic Features

1. Portal arachnoid fibrosis and sinusoidal collagen deposition are present.
2. Moderate to marked nuclear anisocytosis and dysplasia of hepatocytes, prominent in all zones, are seen.

Other Features

1. Portal lymphocytic infiltration and hyperplasia are mild to moderate.
2. Cord–sinusoid pattern is distorted owing to irregularity and enlargement of hepatocytes.
3. Liver cells may be hydropic or have an eosinophilic, mosaic "plant-like" appearance.
4. Hyperchromatic liver cell nuclei often have cytoplasmic invagination; binucleate cells are common.
5. Glycogen nuclei are often present.
6. There are variable degrees of fatty change, predominantly macrovesicular, with no zonal distribution.
7. Features from one lobule to another are fairly uniform.
8. Focal necrosis and mononuclear inflammatory infiltration in the parenchyma may occur, with features resembling chronic active hepatitis.
9. Cirrhosis may occur; however, no well-defined regenerative nodules are present while the patient is

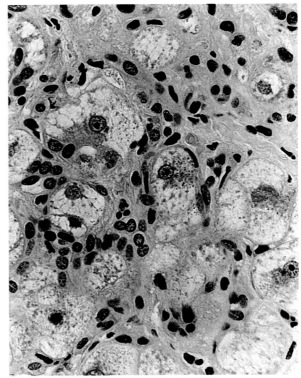

Figure 5–21. Methotrexate toxicity. Small groups of hydropic hepatocytes are surrounded by lymphocytes. Kupffer cell hyperplasia is present. Sinusoidal collagen surrounds most of the liver cells.

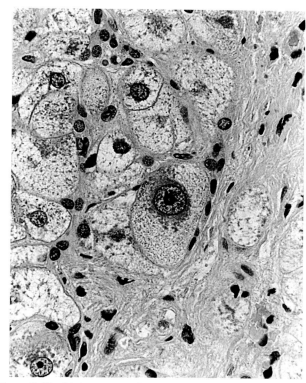

Figure 5–22. Methotrexate toxicity. Many of the hepatocytes show significant dysplastic change. The liver cell (*center*) shows a markedly enlarged nucleus with abundant cytoplasm. Adjacent hepatocytes, in contrast, exhibit much smaller features. Sinusoidal collagen is present and prominent.

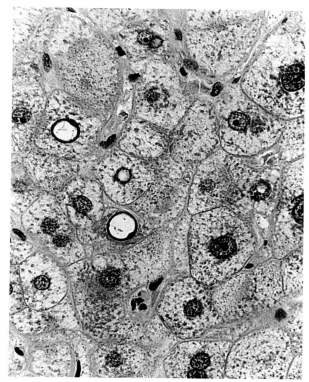

Figure 5–23. Methotrexate toxicity. Occasional hepatocytes are enlarged, with two exhibiting glycogen nuclei.

still on medication. Nodularity becomes more prominent after the drug therapy is stopped.

Differential Diagnosis

Feature	Methotrexate	Alcoholic Liver Disease	Chronic Active Hepatitis	
			B	Non-A/Non-B
Dysplasia	+ +	−	+ +	+
"Plant-like" cells	+ +	−	−	−
Sinusoidal collagen	+	+ +	−	+
Alcoholic hyalin	−	+ +	−	−
Ground-glass cells	−	−	+ +	−
Variability of changes in different lobules	−	+	+ +	+

Clinical and Biologic Behavior

1. Methotrexate, a folate antagonist, inhibits the S-phase of the mitotic cycle, halting DNA synthesis and cell division. Liver cell injury is most likely intrinsic, since the effect is dose related and to a large degree predictable.
2. Typically there is an insidious onset of liver cell damage, with hepatomegaly (50%), splenomegaly (15%), and ascites (10%) present before diagnosis.
3. On laboratory tests, only mild, often transient elevation of serum aminotransferase levels is noted; hyperbilirubinemia, when present, is mild.
4. Liver cell injury is directly proportional to the duration of therapy and amount ingested. Fibrosis is usually observed as the cumulative dose becomes greater than 2 to 4 g.
5. The likelihood of injury is inversely proportional to the interval between doses, with small daily doses more likely to cause fibrosis than larger weekly doses.
6. Potentiating factors to fibrogenesis include obesity and alcoholism; children are unusually susceptible.

Treatment and Prognosis

1. Liver biopsy should be performed as baseline study prior to methotrexate therapy, with follow-up biopsy at 6 to 12-month intervals or at stage when the cumulative dose is 1.5 to 2 g; if fibrosis is seen at that time, the drug should be discontinued.
2. The fibrosis and cirrhosis that develops with methotrexate is considered "less aggressive" and may become quiescent with withdrawal of the drug.

References

Almeyda J, Barnardo D, Baker H. Drug reactions: XV. Methotrexate, psoriasis and the liver. Br J Dermatol 1971;85:302–305.

Dahl MGC, Gregory MM, Scheuer PJ. Liver damage due to methotrexate in patients with psoriasis. Br Med J 1971;1:625–630.

Evans WE, Christensen ML. Drug interactions with methotrexate. J Rheumatol 1985;12(suppl):15–20.

Tolman KG, Clegg DO, Lee RG, et al. Methotrexate and the liver. J Rheumatol 1985;12(suppl):29–34.

Tugwell P, Bennett K, Gent M. Methotrexate in rheumatoid arthritis: Indications, contraindications, efficacy and safety. Ann Intern Med 1987;107:358–366.

■ Fatty Change

Macrovesicular

Bleomycin
Borates
Dichloroethylene
Ethanol
Ethyl chloride
Hydrazine
L-Asparaginase
Methotrexate
Methyl bromide
Microcycline
Perhexilene maleate
Phosphorus
Steroids
Sulfasalazine
Total parenteral nutrition
Warfarin

Microvesicular

Aflatoxin
Aspirin
Camphor
Ethanol
Hypoglycin A
Phalloidin
Tetracycline
Valproic acid

Tetracycline

Major Morphologic Features

1. Microvesicular fat is evident within the cytoplasm of virtually all hepatocytes; some cases may exhibit a perivenular accentuation.

Other Features

1. Focal hepatocytolysis and mononuclear inflammatory infiltration are present but minimal.
2. Variable degrees of macrovesicular fat may also be present, most often in the recovery phase.

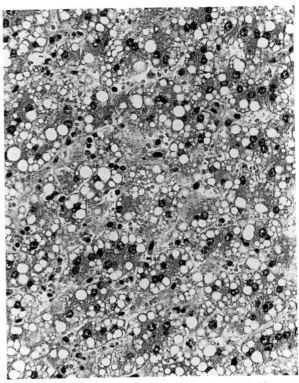

Figure 5–24. Tetracycline toxicity. The basic cord–sinusoid pattern is preserved. Every hepatocyte contains multiple fat globules. Although macrovesicular fat (greater than the size of the liver cell nucleus) is present, the predominant fat globules are microvesicular.

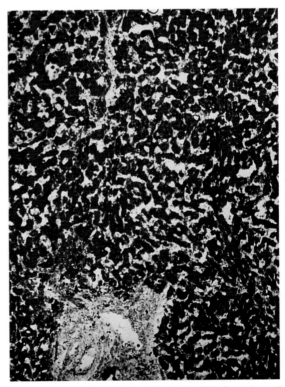

Figure 5–25. Tetracycline toxicity (oil red O). This fat stain on frozen section shows on low power that all hepatocytes contain abundant fat. The portal tract (*bottom*) is devoid of fat.

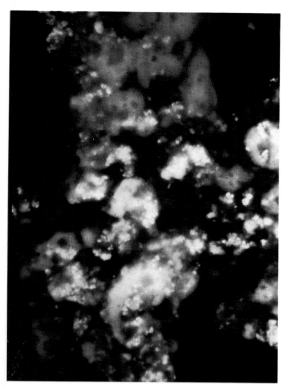

Figure 5–26. Tetracycline toxicity (autofluorescence). The abundant golden-brown fluorescent pigment represents tetracycline within the cytoplasm of the hepatocytes.

3. Hepatocytes containing microvesicular fat tend to have slightly small nuclei located in the center of the cytoplasm; macrovesicular fat pushes nucleus toward the periphery.
4. Cholestasis is minimal to absent.
5. Portal tract shows no significant changes.

Differential Diagnosis

1. *Other conditions associated with microvesicular fatty change include:*
   a. *Reye's syndrome:* This syndrome is rare in adults.
   b. *Acute foamy degeneration of alcoholic liver disease:* Sinusoidal collagen and occasionally alcoholic hyalin may also be present.
   c. *Fatty liver of pregnancy:* This condition usually resolves following delivery.
   d. *Drugs and toxins:* Morphologic features of valproic acid and mushroom toxins characteristically exhibit microvesicular fat.
   e. *Adult-onset diabetes mellitus:* Glycogen nuclei are prominent.

Special Stains

1. *Oil red O:* Hepatocytes may not appear to contain microvesicular fat on hematoxylin and eosin stain of routinely processed tissue; if fresh or formalin fixed wet tissue is available, oil red O stains the fat bright red on frozen section.
2. *Periodic acid–Schiff:* This stain is often helpful in outlining microvesicular fat by staining glycogen located immediately adjacent to fat globules.

Autofluorescence

1. Tetracycline within hepatocytes is intensely golden brown on examination of frozen section.

Clinical and Biologic Behavior

1. Patients present with nausea, vomiting, and abdominal pain, followed by jaundice.
2. Laboratory data show aminotransferase elevations up to 200 IU/L and rarely 500 IU/L; bilirubin is less than 10 mg/dL, and prothrombin activity is markedly decreased.
3. Tetracycline toxicity is more common in women; pregnancy appears to enhance susceptibility to injury.
4. Toxicity usually follows administration of at least 1 g/d or more intravenously, with signs beginning 4 to 6 days after initiation of therapy; it is very unlikely to occur with oral tetracycline use.
5. Pancreatitis is present in approximately 50% of cases; other features include acute tubular necrosis, fat accumulation in renal tubular cells, and gastrointestinal ulceration.
6. Mechanism of liver cell damage is most likely secondary to indirect hepatotoxicity, since hepatocellular damage is reproducible in animals and is dose related.

Treatment and Prognosis

1. Prompt recognition and discontinuation of the drug usually leads to resolution of hepatic injury.
2. Mortality is quite high in patients who are symptomatic.
3. With the availability of many broad-spectrum antibiotics, intravenous tetracycline is rarely used and consequently this disorder is now virtually nonexistent.

References

Kunelis CT, Peters RL, Edmondson HA. Fatty liver of pregnancy and its relationship to tetracycline therapy. Am J Med 1965;38:359–377.

Peters RL, Edmondson HA, Mikkelsen WP, et al. Tetracycline-induced fatty liver in nonpregnant patients. Am J Surg 1967;113:622–632.

Schenker S, Breen KJ, Heimberg M. Pathogenesis of tetracycline induced fatty liver. In: Gerok W, Sickinger K, eds. Drugs and the Liver. Stuttgart: F.K. Schattauer-Verlag, 1975:269–280.

■ Vascular Abnormalities

Peliosis-like Lesions

Androgenic/anabolic steroids
Diethylstilbestrol
Estrone sulfate
Phalloidin
Vitamin A

Sinusoidal Dilatation

Oral contraceptives

Hepatic Venous Outflow Obstruction (Veno-occlusive Disease)

Aflatoxin
Arsenicals
Azathioprine
Danazol
Decarbazine
Dimethyl busulfan
Ethanol
Mitomycin C
Oral contraceptives
Pyrrolizidine alkaloids
Tamoxifen
Thorotrast
Thioguanine
Urethane
Vinyl chloride
Vitamin A

Vasculitis

Allopurinol
Chlorpropamide
Chlorthiazide
Penicillin
Phenylbutazone
Phenytoin
Sulfonamides

Hepatoportal Sclerosis (Noncirrhotic Portal Fibrosis)

Arsenicals
Copper sulphate
Vinyl chloride

Vitamin A

Major Morphologic Features

1. Hypertrophy and hyperplasia of Ito cells containing fat, predominantly microvesicular in type, occur.
2. Sinusoidal collagen deposition, with some lobules exhibiting perivenular accentuation, is present.

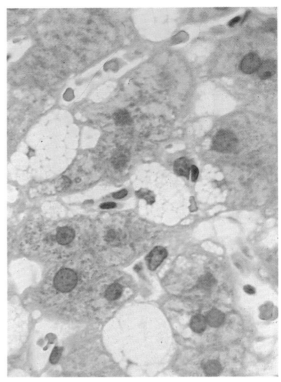

Figure 5–27. Vitamin A toxicity. Ito cells are distended and contain abundant small fat droplets. The Ito cell at the bottom of the field also contains larger fat vesicles. The nuclei of these cells are small and slightly stellate. The hepatocytes do not contain fat.

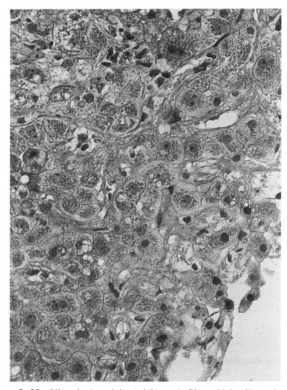

Figure 5–28. Vitamin A toxicity (trichrome). Sinusoidal collagen is present. Ito cells are also present but less abundant than in Figure 5-27.

Other Features

1. There are variable degrees of focal hepatocytolysis, with macrophages and Kupffer cells often filled with lipid.
2. Hepatocytes are generally normal in size with occasional but slight hydropic change; variable degrees of atrophic change may also be present adjacent to sinusoids containing abundant collagen.
3. Acidophil bodies are infrequent.
4. Macrovesicular fat in hepatocytes is minimal to absent.
5. Slight sinusoidal dilatation may be present; peliosis-like lesions have been described.
6. Glycogen nuclei are occasionally present.
7. Portal tract shows minimal to absent mononuclear inflammatory infiltrate.
8. Alcoholic hyalin-like material has been described in hydropic hepatocytes.
9. In rare instances erythrocytes have been identified within the space of Disse.

Differential Diagnosis

1. *Alcoholic liver disease:* The presence of fat, sinusoidal collagen, and alcoholic hyalin is typical of alcoholic liver disease. Ito cells are not increased in the alcoholic; in addition, neutrophilic infiltration within the lobule as well as an arachnoid portal fibrosis noted in acute and chronic alcoholic liver disease are not features of vitamin A toxicity.
2. *Chronic non-A, non-B (HCV) hepatitis:* Although sinusoidal collagen and fat within hepatocytes are often seen in chronic non-A, non-B hepatitis, Ito cells are not hyperplastic.

Special Stains

1. *Oil Red O:* Ito cells stain red on frozen section of fresh or formalin-fixed tissue.
2. *Masson trichrome:* Sinusoidal collagen is accentuated.

Autofluorescence

1. Vitamin A within the Ito cells is intensely green on frozen sections.

Clinical and Biologic Behavior

1. Chronic hypervitaminosis A presents as fatigue and weakness, anorexia, constipation, brittle nails and scaly dry rough skin, loss of hair, and cortical bone thickness.
2. Patients present with features of portal hypertension such as ascites, splenomegaly, and esophageal varices. Hepatomegaly is usually present, presumably caused by an increase in size and number of Ito cells.
3. Laboratory data show normal to slightly elevated aminotransferase, alkaline phosphatase, and bilirubin levels, with normal prothrombin activity.
4. Serum levels of retinol and retinol-binding protein are unreliable, since malnutrition, liver disease, and alcoholism may result in spurious findings. Hepatic vitamin A levels are markedly elevated (~10 times normal).
5. Most cases of hepatotoxicity occur in patients who admit to prolonged ingestion of vitamin A in doses of 20,000 to 40,000 IU daily for years (7–10 years) and usually in the setting of nutritional faddism. (The recommended daily requirement of vitamin A is 5000 IU.)
6. Ito cells may be precursors of fibroblasts, since transitional cells have been identified; excessive vitamin A, stored in Ito cells as inactive retinyl palmitate ester, causes Ito cell hyperplasia, hypertrophy, and possible fibrogenesis, with resultant collagen deposition in sinusoids, resulting in venous outflow obstruction and portal hypertension.

Treatment and Prognosis

1. Cessation of vitamin A intake results in gradual resolution of signs and symptoms. In patients with portal hypertension and ascites, resolution may not follow withdrawal of the drug despite return of vitamin A levels to the normal range. Therapy is directed to management of complications.

References

Hendricks FJ, Brouwer A, Knook DL. The role of hepatic fat-storing (stellate) cells in retinoid metabolism. Hepatology 1987;6:1368–1371.
Jacques EA, Buschmann RJ, Layden TJ. The histopathologic progression of vitamin A-induced hepatic injury. Gastroenterology 1979;76:599–602.
Leo MA, Lieber CS. Hypervitaminosis A: A liver lover's lament. Hepatology 1988;8:412–417.
Russell RM, Boyer JL, Bagheri SA, et al. Hepatic injury from chronic hypervitaminosis A resulting in portal hypertension and ascites. N Engl J Med 1974;291:435–440.
Zafrani ES, Bernuan B, Feldmann G. Peliosis-like ultrastructural changes of the hepatic sinusoids in human hypervitaminosis A: Report of three cases. Hum Pathol 1984;15:1166–1170.

■ Granulomas

Allopurinol
Alpha-methyldopa
Carbamazepine
Hydralazine
Oxyphenbutazone
Penicillin

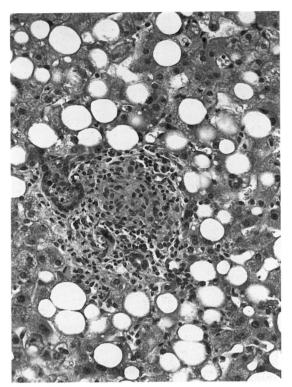

Figure 5–29. Granuloma (trichrome). A well-defined epithelioid granuloma is present within the portal tract and is secondary to the drug sulfasalazine in a patient with ulcerative colitis. The portal tract is slightly expanded but not fibrotic.

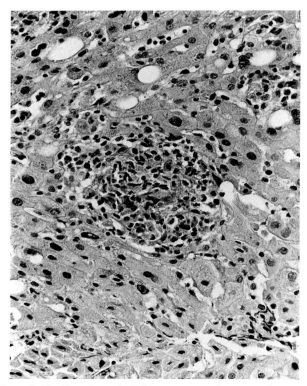

Figure 5–30. Granuloma. An inflammatory granuloma secondary to sulfonamide is present within the parenchyma and consists of lymphocytes, macrophages, and occasional plasma cells and neutrophils.

Phenylbutazone
Phenytoin
Quinidine
Sulfasalazine
Sulfonamides
Sulfonylurea agents

1. Granulomas are both noncaseating *epithelioid* (e.g., phenytoin) and *inflammatory* (lymphocytes, plasma cells, neutrophils; e.g., sulfasalazine) types.
2. They are located within portal areas as well as the parenchyma, with no zonal distribution.
3. Granulomas are usually associated with mild nonspecific inflammatory changes in portal areas and lobules.

References

Ishak KG, Mullick FG. Drug-induced and toxic liver injury. In: Peters RL, Craig JR, eds. Liver Pathology. New York: Churchill Livingstone, 1986:236–237.
McMaster KR, Hennigar GR. Drug-induced granulomatous hepatitis. Lab Invest 1981;44:61–73.
Zimmerman HJ, Ishak KG. Hepatic injury due to drugs and toxins. In: MacSween RNM, Anthony PP, Scheuer PJ, eds. Pathology of the Liver, 2nd ed. Edinburgh: Churchill Livingstone, 1987:518.

■ Neoplasms

Benign
Liver Cell Adenoma

Anabolic steroids
Oral contraceptives

Malignant
Hepatocellular

Aflatoxin
Anabolic steroids
Arsenicals
Mycotoxins
Oral contraceptives
Thorotrast
Vinyl chloride

Cholangiocarcinoma

Thorotrast
Vinyl chloride

Angiosarcoma

Anabolic steroids
Arsenicals
Copper sulphate
Diethylstilbestrol
Phenelzine
Thorotrast
Vinyl chloride

(See Chapter 9 for morphologic features of various neoplasms.)

1. Thorotrast and polyvinyl chloride are linked with numerous primary hepatic neoplasms, most notably angiosarcoma (see page 199).

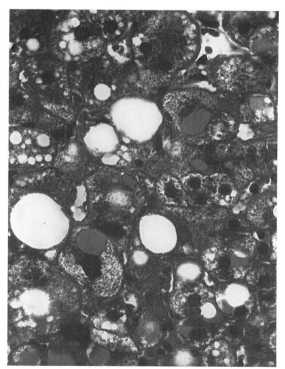

Figure 5–31. Thorotrast injury. This radiopaque solution contains 20% thorium dioxide, an emitter of alpha, beta, and gamma radiation. Not in present use by radiologists because of its association with angiosarcoma and noncirrhotic portal fibrosis, thorotrast can be identified years after administration, owing to its biologic half-life of approximately 400 years, and is seen within macrophages and Kupffer cells, appearing as a dull green, coarse and refractile pigment.

Figure 5–32. Procainamide toxicity. Single large round eosinophilic cytoplasmic inclusions are evident in many liver cells. The inclusions, which rapidly disappear on discontinuance of the medication, resemble those seen in perivenular hepatocytes secondary to anoxia.

2. Thorotrast can be distinctly identified as a gray-green refractile pigment within Kupffer cells and portal macrophages.
3. Association between oral contraceptives and benign liver cell adenoma is well established with only a very rare case exhibiting malignant transformation to hepatocellular carcinoma.

References

Edmondson HA, Henderson B, Benton B. Liver-cell adenomas associated with use of oral contraceptives. N Engl J Med 1976;294:470–472.

Farber E. On the pathogenesis of experimental hepatocellular carcinoma. In: Okuda K, Peters RL eds. Hepatocellular carcinoma. New York: John Wiley and sons, 1976:1–22.

Heath CW Jr, Falk H, Creech JL Jr. Characteristics of cases of angiosarcoma of the liver among vinyl chloride workers in the United States. Ann NY Acad Sci 1975;246:231–236.

■ Miscellaneous Drug-induced Lesions

Situation	Example
1. Discrete cytoplasmic inclusions	Procainamide
2. Ground-glass–like hepatocytes	Phenobarbital
	Phenytoin
3. Increase in pigment:	
a. Lipochrome	Phenacetin
b. Iron	Ethanol
c. Radiopaque	Thorotrast
4. Alcoholic hyalin	Amiodarone
	Diethylaminoethoxyhexestrol
	Estrogens
	Ethanol
	Glucocorticoids
	Griseofulvin
	Perhexiline maleate
	Vitamin A

References

Kanel GC. Conditions resembling alcoholic liver disease. In: Peters RL, Craig JR, eds. Liver Pathology. New York: Churchill Livingstone, 1986:286.

Zimmerman HJ, Ishak KG. Hepatic injury due to drugs and toxins. In: MacSween RNM, Anthony PP, Scheuer PJ, eds. Pathology of the Liver, 2nd ed. Edinburgh: Churchill Livingstone, 1987:528–531.

General References

Ishak KG, Mullick FG. Drug-induced and toxic liver injury. In: Peters RL, Craig JR, eds. Liver Pathology. New York: Churchill Livingstone, 1986:221–254.

Kaplowitz N. Drug-induced hepatotoxicity. Ann Intern Med 1986;104:826–839.

Mitchell JR, Jollows DJ. Metabolic activation of drugs to toxic substances. Gastroenterology 1975;68:392–410.

Zimmerman HJ. Chemical hepatic injury and its detection. In: Plaa GL, Hewitt WR, eds. Toxicology of the Liver. New York: Raven Press, 1982:1–45.

Zimmerman HJ. Hepatotoxicity. New York: Appleton-Century-Crofts, 1978.

Zimmerman HJ, Ishak KG. Hepatic injury due to drugs and toxins. In: MacSween RNM, Anthony PP, Scheuer PJ, eds. Pathology of the Liver. 2nd ed. Edinburgh: Churchill Livingstone, 1987:503–573.

CHAPTER 6

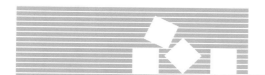

Vascular Disorders

■ Hepatic Venous Outflow Obstruction

Venous Congestion Secondary to Heart Failure

Major Morphologic Features

Acute:
1. Sinusoidal dilatation and congestion are prominent in perivenular region (zone 3).

Chronic:
1. Perivenular sinusoidal dilatation and adjacent liver cell atrophy occur.
2. Sinusoidal collagen is present in perivenular zones, often with bridging fibrosis of adjacent lobules in long-standing lesions.

Other Features

1. Parenchymal and portal inflammatory changes are minimal to absent.
2. Severe acute changes may be associated with marked perivenular hemorrhage, often extending into midzonal regions, with associated coagulative (hypoxic) liver cell necrosis.
3. Lipochrome is present in macrophages and Kupffer cells secondary to phagocytosis of anoxic hepatocytes.
4. Cholestasis is usually absent.
5. Bridging perivenular fibrosis from adjacent lobules may form ''nodules'' containing uninvolved normal portal tracts in their center (reversed lobulation); as the lesion progresses, there may be eventual fibrous linking of portal tracts to perivenular zones, forming a micronodular (cardiac-type) cirrhosis.
6. Both eosinophilic sinusoidal and intracytoplasmic hyaline globules and inclusions have been identified in perivenular zones.

Differential Diagnosis

1. *Budd-Chiari syndrome:* Budd-Chiari lesions are more marked, with significant perivenular cell dropout and hemorrhage. Red blood cells may be seen within the space of Disse, but this change is not noted in passive congestion from heart failure.
2. *Cirrhosis, alcoholic or viral etiology:* End-stage cardiac cirrhosis is micronodular, but regenerative activity is not as prominent as in viral-induced or alcoholic cirrhosis. In addition, cardiac cirrhosis has minimal septal and parenchymal inflammatory changes, without ground-glass cells or alcoholic hyalin.

Special Stain

1. *Masson trichrome:* Sinusoidal dilatation is accentuated, with collagen evident adjacent to atrophic liver cells.

Clinical and Biologic Behavior

1. Most patients with heart failure demonstrate clinical signs of congestive heart failure. Patients with constrictive pericarditis, however, may present with ascites that may be mistaken for cirrhotic ascites.
2. Elevation of serum bilirubin level is not common and is seldom above 5 mg/dL, frequently in unconjugated form. Overt jaundice is quite uncommon.
3. Serum aminotransferase elevations are mild in one third of cases, and the alkaline phosphatase is usually normal. In severe heart failure, however, prominent anoxic change in perivenular regions caused by low output state results in moderate to marked (may be

89

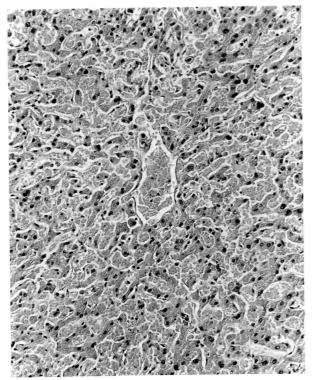

Figure 6–1. Venous congestion. The perivenular and midzonal hepatocytes are moderately atrophic. Dilated sinusoids are filled with red blood cells.

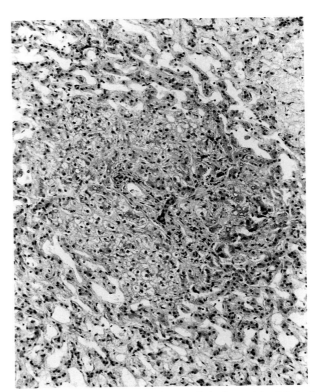

Figure 6–2. Venous congestion. A normal-sized portal tract is in the center of the field. The dilated sinusoids at the periphery have merged from adjacent lobules. The hepatocytes between these sinusoids are atrophic, with the individual cords now surrounded by pericellular collagen. As the disease progresses these hepatocytes are entirely replaced by collagen. The resultant nodules now contain portal tracts in their center (*reversed lobulation*).

greater than 1000 IU/L) elevations of serum aminotransferase activities, moderate hyperbilirubinemia, and significant decrease in prothrombin (20%–30% range) activity.

4. In chronic right-sided heart failure, persistent increased venous pressure may cause phlebosclerosis of medium and large hepatic venous structures.

5. Long-term congestion leading to the "cardiac" cirrhosis takes many years to develop and is not a true cirrhosis, since *regenerative* nodules do not form.

6. In cardiac failure, ascites can occur without portal hypertension and is caused by elevation in both free and wedged hepatic venous pressures. Once cardiac cirrhosis develops, portal hypertension may ensue, with the formation of esophageal varices in some patients.

7. Acute congestive cardiac failure usually results from congenital, ischemic, valvular heart disease or cardiomyopathy. In patients with presumed liver disease, alcoholic cardiomyopathy and iron overload need consideration.

Prognosis

1. Adequate treatment of heart failure will result in resolution of hepatic abnormalities.

2. Mortality is frequently related to severe heart failure rather than to hepatic failure.

References

Bras G. Aspects of hepatic vascular diseases. In: Gall EA, Mostofi FK, eds. The liver. Baltimore: Williams & Williams, 1973:408–412.

Dunn DG, Hayes P, Breen KJ, et al. The liver in congestive failure: A review. Am J Med Sci 1973;265:174–189.

Klatt EC, Koss MN, Young TS, et al. Hepatic hyaline globules associated with passive congestion. Arch Pathol Lab Med 1988;112:510–513.

Sherlock S. The liver in circulatory failure. In: Schiff L, Schiff ER, eds. Diseases of the Liver, 6th ed. Philadelphia: J.B. Lippincott, 1987:1051–1057.

Ware AJ. The liver when the heart fails. Gastroenterology 1978;74:627–628.

Budd-Chiari Syndrome

Major Morphologic Features

Acute

1. Severe sinusoidal dilatation, congestion, and hemorrhage occur in perivenular region (zone 3).

2. *Red blood cell–trabecular lesion:* Cord–sinusoid architecture is maintained, but red blood cells are present within the space of Disse, in many instances entirely filling the trabeculae by replacing necrotic liver cells (anoxic damage).

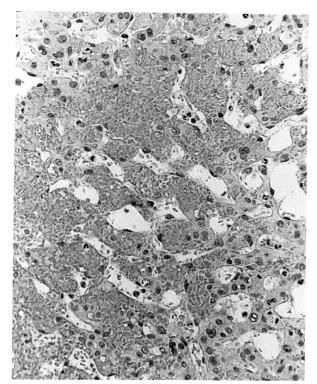

Figure 6–3. Budd-Chiari syndrome. The acute lesion often exhibits complete dropout of hepatocytes, with their replacement by red blood cells within the trabecular cords. The adjacent sinusoids remain open and may be somewhat dilated. This change is most prominent in the perivenular zone.

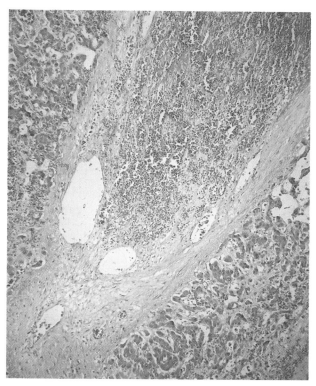

Figure 6–5. Budd-Chiari syndrome. The large sublobular vein exhibits thrombosis with recanalization. This feature is directly responsible for hepatic venous outflow obstruction.

Chronic
  1. Perivenular fibrosis and sinusoidal collagen deposition are prominent, with bridging fibrosis between perivenular regions.

Other Features

  1. Portal and parenchymal inflammatory changes are minimal to absent.
  2. The red blood cell–trabecular lesion, also seen in chronic outflow obstruction, may be difficult to identify when severe sinusoidal congestion and perivenular hemorrhage are also present.
  3. Variable degrees of acute changes, ranging from only mild sinusoidal dilatation to marked hemorrhagic necrosis, may occasionally be present within different lobules of the same liver biopsy specimen.
  4. Mild degrees of macrovesicular and microvesicular fat may be present in residual hepatocytes.
  5. Cholestasis is rare.
  6. Lipochrome is identified in macrophages and Kupffer cells secondary to phagocytosis of anoxic hepatocytes.
  7. In chronic obstruction, sinusoidal dilatation may not be present when collateral channels shunting blood proximal to the obstruction are established.
  8. The bridging fibrosis generally does not contain inflammatory cells.

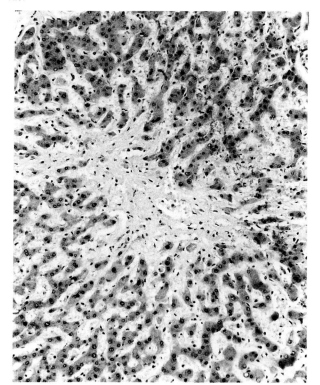

Figure 6–4. Budd-Chiari syndrome. In the more chronic form of this disorder there is fibrosis, which is initially concentrated in the perivenular region. Eventually there is a merging of the terminal hepatic veins by fibrosis.

9. Perivenular bridging fibrosis may lead to a "nodule" with a normal to only slightly fibrotic portal tract in the center *(reversed lobulation);* in long-term cases, portal-perivenular fibrosis may eventually occur, leading to a micronodular *(cardiac type)* cirrhosis.
10. Sublobular hepatic veins may exhibit thrombosis with fibrin deposition.

Differential Diagnosis

1. *Congestion secondary to heart failure:* Both acute and chronic Budd-Chiari syndrome may resemble right-sided congestive heart failure. The distinctive red blood cell–trabecular lesion may be seen in both Budd-Chiari syndrome as well as *left-sided heart failure* (see page 96) but is *not* seen in congestive right-sided heart failure. In addition, hemorrhagic lesions are less common in heart failure.
2. *Drug-induced and toxic necrosis* (e.g., pyrrolizidine alkaloids): Outflow obstruction of the terminal hepatic venules *(veno-occlusive disease)* caused by drugs and toxins may exhibit perivenular necrosis, fibrosis, and occasionally the red blood cell–trabecular lesion. Veno-occlusive disease is considered a variant of the Budd-Chiari syndrome.
3. *Cirrhosis of alcoholic or viral etiology:* Advanced cases of the Budd-Chiari syndrome may show a micronodular *cardiac-type* cirrhosis, sometimes difficult to differentiate from inactive advanced cirrhosis of other etiologies. Cardiac cirrhosis exhibits minimal regenerative activity, without significant septal or parenchymal inflammatory infiltration. Sinusoidal dilatation is often seen within the nodules.

Special Stains

1. *Masson trichrome:* This stain accenuates sinusoidal collagen in the space of Disse in both acute and chronic stages.
2. *Phosphotungstic acid hematoxylin:* Fibrin can be seen within sublobular veins.

Clinical and Biologic Behavior

1. *Budd-Chiari syndrome* is a clinicopathologic disorder caused by obstruction of the hepatic venous outflow at any site from the terminal hepatic venule to the entry of the major hepatic veins into the inferior vena cava. In membranous obstruction of the vena cava, the obstruction can occur at any site that extends from the confluence of the hepatic veins into the inferior vena cava to the entry of the inferior vena cava into the right atrium.
2. The incidence of hepatic outflow obstruction is variable. Membranous obstruction of the vena cava is more commonly seen in South Africa (6% of all liver biopsy specimens exhibit changes of the chronic lesion) and in Asia; in Western countries it is estimated that one case per year of the Budd-Chiari syndrome is seen in acute care facilities (500-bed hospitals).
3. The two most common causes are membranous obstruction of the large hepatic veins immediately superior to their entrance into the inferior vena cava (South Africa, Japan, India) and complete fibrous obliteration of major hepatic veins or ostia (44% in one series and the most common cause at the University of Southern California Liver Unit). Hepatocellular carcinoma was shown to be associated with almost 50% of cases of membranous obstruction in a South African series.
4. Clinical manifestations depend on the type and acuteness of the obstruction; these vary from a vague illness and mild abdominal distress of weeks to months in duration, to acute abdominal pain, hepatomegaly, ascites, and hepatic failure.
5. Laboratory data show variable degrees of serum aminotransferase elevations and hyperbilirubinemia, depending on the severity of the disease. In chronic disease, laboratory test results are similar to those seen in cirrhosis.
6. Other causes of hepatic vein thrombosis include hematologic abnormalities (myeloproliferative disorders, polycythemia vera, paroxysmal nocturnal hemoglobinuria), neoplasm (primary and metastatic), radiation, abscess formation, trauma, pregnancy, graft-versus-host reaction, chemotherapeutic agents and oral contraceptives.
7. Clinically apparent portal hypertension is present in all patients who survive long enough for collateral circulation between the portal and systemic circulations to develop; the most important collaterals that may lead to massive hemorrhage are through the coronary and left gastroepiploic veins, forming gastric and esophageal varices.
8. The drainage of the caudate lobe is often spared, resulting in marked enlargement secondary to a compensatory hyperplasia and can be identified on technetium-99m sulfur colloid and computed tomographic scans.

Prognosis

1. Extensive hepatic vein thrombus formation may lead to death within weeks to months after first symptoms.
2. In chronic disease, survival is similar to that in cirrhosis of uncertain etiology (e.g., "cryptogenic").

References

Parker RGF. Occlusion of the hepatic veins in man. Medicine 1959;38:369–402.
Rector WG, Xu Y, Goldstein L, et al. Membranous obstruction of the inferior vena cava in the United States. Medicine 1985;64:134–143.
Reynolds TB. Budd-Chiari syndrome. In: Schiff L, Schiff ER, eds. Dis-

eases of the liver, 6th ed. Philadelphia: J.B. Lippincott, 1987:1466–1473.

Simson IW. Membranous obstruction of the inferior vena cava and hepatocellular carcinoma in South Africa. Gastroenterology 1982;82:171–178.

Simson IW. Budd-Chiari syndrome and veno-occlusive disease. In: Peters RL, Craig JR, eds. Liver Pathology. New York: Churchill Livingstone, 1986:299–314.

Tavill AS, Wood EJ, Kreel L, et al. The Budd-Chiari syndrome: Correlation between hepatic scintigraphy and the clinical, radiological, and pathological findings in nineteen cases of hepatic venous outflow obstruction. Gastroenterology 1975;68:509–518.

Veno-occlusive Disease

Major Morphologic Features

Acute
1. Fibrous obliterative change involving terminal hepatic venules is present along with adjacent sinusoidal congestion and dilatation.

Chronic
1. Bridging fibrosis of adjacent perivenular regions (zone 3) occurs.

Other Features

1. Portal tracts are unremarkable; no significant inflammatory changes are present in the parenchyma or portal regions.

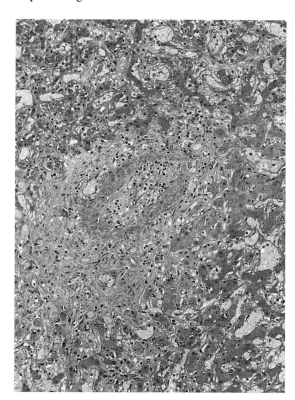

Figure 6–6. Veno-occlusive disease. The terminal hepatic vein is surrounded and the lumen totally replaced by loose collagen. The hepatocytes are slightly smaller than normal, with the sinusoids dilated.

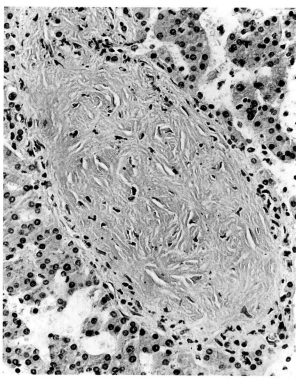

Figure 6–7. Veno-occlusive disease. The terminal hepatic vein is totally replaced by dense relatively acellular collagen in the latter form of the disease. Revascularization by small spindly vessels is present. The adjacent hepatocytes are small and the sinusoids markedly dilated.

2. *Red blood cell–trabecular lesion:* Red blood cells are present within the space of Disse in the perivenular zone, often entirely filling trabeculae by replacing anoxic hepatocytes.
3. Severe hemorrhage and necrosis with fibrin deposition may be present in perivenular regions.
4. Cholestasis may be present but is uncommon.
5. Atrophy of hepatocytes is seen adjacent to chronically dilated sinusoids.
6. Subintimal edema of sublobular veins occurs, with infiltration of the intima by red blood cells.
7. Although there may be some fibrosis involving sublobular veins, larger hepatic veins generally show no change.
8. The loose collagen in the perivenular region may exhibit hypertrophic fibroblasts; eventually, the collagen becomes more dense, with bridging fibrosis of portal–perivenular zones and formation of a micronodular *(cardiac-type)* cirrhosis.

Differential Diagnosis

1. *Lesions associated with the Budd-Chiari syndrome:* Outflow obstruction in the Budd-Chiari syndrome does not cause the obliterative fibrogenesis of terminal hepatic venules characteristic of veno-occlusive disease.

2. *Severe right-sided heart failure:* Acute perivenular sclerosis and fibrin deposition do not occur in heart failure.
3. *Acute sclerosing hyaline necrosis:* Extensive perivenular arachnoid fibrosis of the terminal hepatic venules is characteristically seen in acute sclerosing hyaline necrosis. Changes such as alcoholic hyalin surrounded by neutrophils are not seen in veno-occlusive disease.

Special Stains

1. *Masson trichrome:* Sclerosed terminal hepatic venules and subintimal lesions of the sublobular veins are accentuated.
2. *Phosphotungstic acid hematoxylin:* Fibrin is often present and stains blue in terminal hepatic venules and thrombosed veins.

Clinical and Biologic Behavior

1. Veno-occlusive disease may acutely present as a sudden onset of abdominal distention, ascites, and hepatomegaly, often leading to hepatic failure.
2. In chronic disease, presentation is insidious, occurring months to years after the inciting event; ascites, hepatosplenomegaly, and esophageal varices are usually present.
3. In acute disease, laboratory values depict features of acute liver cell injury, with moderately elevated serum aminotransferase levels, while hypoalbuminemia and decreased prothrombin activity are present with chronic disease.
4. Veno-occlusive disease is endemic in Jamaica, parts of Africa, the Middle East and India; in Jamaica, up to 30% of patients with chronic liver disease may have a cirrhosis secondary to chronic veno-occlusive disease.
5. In the West Indies the lesion is induced by ingestion of ''bush tea'' prepared from boiling leaves of *Crotalaria fulva* and *Senecio* containing toxic pyrrolizidine alkaloids.
6. Other causes include radiation therapy, chemotherapeutic agents (e.g., 6-thioguanine, 6-mercaptopurine), arsenicals, vinyl chloride monomer, and dimethyl busulfan. Veno-occlusive disease may occur in association with graft-versus-host disease following bone marrow transplantation, especially in those patients exposed to non-A, non-B hepatitis.
7. Veno-occlusive lesion has been reported in 74% and 52% of autopsy specimens of alcoholic cirrhosis and alcoholic hepatitis, respectively. Total occlusion of some hepatic venules was noted in 47%. Veno-occlusive disease complicating alcoholic liver disease may contribute to significant portal hypertension in patients with noncirrhotic disease.
8. Pathogenesis: Fibrin deposition causes obstruction

and liver cell damage; direct damage to endothelial lining cells occurs from toxic agents (alkaloids), with resultant fibrogenesis and eventual obliterative lesions.

Treatment and Prognosis

1. Treatment is symptomatic and directed to managing complications of chronic liver disease. In acute disease, withdrawal of the offending agent (e.g., chemotherapeutic agents) may result in amelioration.
2. In cases of hepatic failure from acute or chronic disease, hepatic transplantation should be offered.

References

Fajardo LF, Colby TV. Pathogenesis of veno-occlusive liver disease after radiation. Arch Pathol Lab Med 1980;104:584–588.
Goodman ZD, Ishak KG. Occlusive venous lesions in alcoholic liver disease: A study of 200 cases. Gastroenterology 1982;83:786–796.
Rider PM, Ohkuma S, McDermoktt WV, et al. Hepatic veno-occlusive disease associated with the consumption of pyrrolizidine-containing dietary supplements. Gastroenterology 1985;88:1050–1054.
Rollins BJ. Hepatic veno-occlusive disease. Am J Med 1986;81:297–306.
Simson IW. Budd-Chiari syndrome and veno-occlusive disease. In: Peters RL, Craig JR, eds. Liver Pathology. New York: Churchill Livingstone, 1986:299–314.

■ Decreased Arterial Blood Flow

Anoxia Secondary to Hypotension

Major Morphologic Features

1. Eosinophilic coagulative necrosis of hepatocytes is most prominent in the perivenular region (zone 3)
2. Eventual dropout of liver cells occurs after 4 to 6 days, with perivenular collapse.

Other Features

1. Macrophages and Kupffer cells, often containing lipochrome, are present in perivenular regions secondary to phagocytosis of necrotic liver cells.
2. Portal tracts show no significant abnormalities.
3. Neutrophils may be concentrated at borders of necrotic regions 1 to 2 days after ischemic event; the neutrophils are often fragmented (karyorrhectic).
4. Cholestasis is usually absent.
5. Kupffer cells are normal to minimally hyperplastic, depending on the degree of necrosis.
6. Cord–sinusoid pattern of uninvolved lobule is intact; regenerative activity is minimal to absent.
7. When right-sided heart failure is also present, perivenular sinusoidal dilatation and congestion are present; in chronic congestion, perivenular fibrosis may eventually occur.

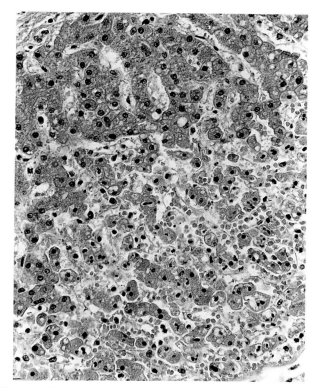

Figure 6–8. Anoxia secondary to hypotension. The liver cells in the perivenular and midzonal regions are slightly shrunken and eosinophilic, with small pyknotic nuclei, compared with the viable liver cells in the periportal zone *(above)*. The sinusoids are dilated and congested.

8. In a cirrhotic liver of any type, ischemic necrosis may involve part or an entire regenerative nodule, sparing adjacent nodules.
9. Large, well-defined areas of ischemic necrosis involving numerous lobules are generally known as *infarcts*.
10. Both sinusoidal and intracytoplasmic eosinophilic hyaline globules and inclusions have been identified in perivenular zones.

Differential Diagnosis

1. *Drug-induced liver injury* (e.g., acetaminophen): Early stage of acetaminophen toxicity exhibits coagulative-type necrosis, and in later stages there is perivenular collapse, both of which can occur in hypotension; however, neutrophils are not present in necrotic regions, regenerative activity is quite prominent, and sinusoidal dilatation and congestion are not present in drug-induced liver injury.
2. *Viral hepatitis* (e.g., yellow fever): Certain types of viral hepatitis exhibit a coagulative type of necrosis; however, the necrosis in yellow fever is midzonal, not perivenular. Herpesviruses and adenoviruses have no zonal preference of necrosis, and nuclear inclusions are usually present. These viruses may also have variable degrees of inflammatory activity in portal areas and parenchyma.

Special Stain

1. *Reticulin:* Intact cord-sinusoid pattern can be seen in perivenular regions with acute disease, and condensation occurs owing to collapse in later stages after necrotic cells have dropped out.

Clinical and Biologic Behavior

1. The majority of patients who are hypotensive do not develop significant hepatic dysfunction; in some cases, however, depending on the severity of the hypotension, mild jaundice may occur, and serum aminotransferase levels may be moderately to markedly elevated, sometimes exceeding 1000 IU/L with marked decrease in prothrombin activity.
2. Hepatomegaly and ascites are present when right-sided (congestive) heart failure is also present.
3. True infarction generally does not occur from hypotension alone; however, changes producing arterial occlusion, such as inadvertent or intended surgical ligation of hepatic artery (latter for severe hepatic bleeding from trauma), embolism, or polyarteritis nodosa, can cause infarction.
4. Ischemic necrosis may show variable degrees of change in the same biopsy specimen, with some lobules even being spared of liver cell damage; this change is most prominent in cirrhotic livers and is caused by variability in blood supply to different parts of the liver.
5. When ischemic necrosis of regenerative nodules is seen in a cirrhotic liver, the most common cause is severe gastrointestinal hemorrhage, frequently from esophageal or gastric varices.
6. Repeated episodes of hypotension will not lead to perivenular fibrosis in left-sided heart failure alone; if right-sided heart failure is also present, perivenular fibrosis will eventually occur.
7. Hepatic arterial blood flow is directly related to cardiac output, which is decreased significantly with low output states. Hepatocellular necrosis occurs in the perivenular zone, a zone with relatively low oxygen tension and, consequently, susceptibility to hypoxemic injury. If the blood flow is markedly reduced, only periportal hepatocytes are spared, leading to extensive necrosis involving the perivenular zone.

Treatment and Prognosis

1. In most instances, recovery from hepatocellular necrosis occurs when related to a single hypotensive episode.
2. Efforts to improve conditions of low cardiac output are important, with the outcome of possible liver dis-

ease depending on the severity of the cardiac disorder.

References

Bras G. Aspects of hepatic vascular diseases. In: Gall EA, Mostofi FK, eds. The liver. Baltimore: Williams & Williams 1973:408–412.

Dunn DG, Hayes P, Breen KJ, et al. The liver in congestive failure: A review. Am J Med Sci 1973;265:174–189.

Klatt EC, Koss MN, Young TS, et al. Hepatic hyaline globules associated with passive congestion. Arch Pathol Lab Med 1988;112:510–513.

Sherlock S. The liver in circulatory failure. In: Schiff L, Schiff ER, eds. Diseases of the Liver, 6th ed. Philadelphia: J.B. Lippincott, 1987:1051–1057.

Ware AJ. The liver when the heart fails. Gastroenterology 1978;74:627–628.

Red Blood Cell–Trabecular Lesion Secondary to Left-sided Heart Failure Without Hypotension

Major Morphologic Feature

1. Replacement of hepatocytes in perivenular regions by red blood cells occurs, with adjacent open sinusoids.

Other Features

1. Portal tracts are normal or exhibit minimal lymphocytic hyperplasia; fibrosis does not occur.
2. Cholestasis is minimal to absent.
3. Focal hepatocytolysis may be present in midzonal and periportal regions, but is scanty.
4. Cord–sinusoid pattern throughout the lobule is intact, with *no* perivenular collapse.
5. In the midzonal area at the border of the red blood cell–trabecular lesion, normal hepatic cords blend into the blood-filled trabeculae.
6. Lipochrome is often seen in atrophic perivenular liver cells and in Kupffer cells that have phagocytized the ischemic hepatocytes.
7. Red blood cells can often be seen at the border of the lesion within the space of Disse alone, without adjacent hepatocellular necrosis.
8. Perivenular sinusoids may be dilated and congested if right-sided heart failure is also present.

Differential Diagnosis

1. *Budd-Chiari syndrome:* In the acute Budd-Chiari syndrome, the red blood cell–trabecular lesion may be seen. Severe sinusoidal dilatation, congestion, and occasionally hemorrhage are present as well, which are features not typically found in left-sided heart failure without hypotension (unless concomitant right-sided heart failure is also present).
2. *Veno-occlusive disease:* The red blood cell–

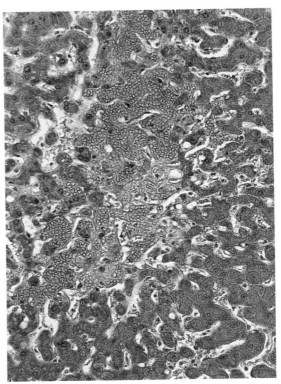

Figure 6–9. Red blood cell–trabecular lesion (trichrome). The hepatocytes in the perivenular zone have totally dropped out and are replaced by red blood cells. The adjacent sinusoids are dilated. This lesion has also been described in the acute Budd-Chiari syndrome (see Figure 6–3).

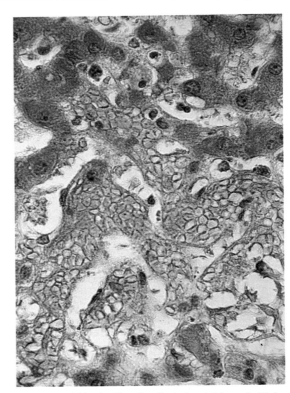

Figure 6–10. Red blood cell–trabecular lesion (trichrome). High power shows the red blood cells merging with intact hepatocytes *(above)*. The sinusoids are open and dilated. Thin strands of collagen are present at the sinusoidal margins.

trabecular lesion is seen in both disorders; however, the fibrotic obliterative perivenular changes of veno-occlusive disease are not present in left-sided heart failure without hypotension.

Special Stains

1. *Reticulin* and *Masson trichrome:* Both stains accentuate the intact and open cord–sinusoid pattern.

Clinical and Biologic Behavior

1. The patient's clinical presentation is that of left-sided heart failure (i.e., pulmonary congestion and dyspnea on exertion).
2. Laboratory data show a wide range of aminotransferase levels (100–2000 IU/L); jaundice is only rarely present, with hyperbilirubinemia generally below 5.0 mg/dL.
3. Pure left-sided heart failure rarely expresses overt hepatic disease unless there is concomitant hypotension; *without* hypotension, left-sided heart failure most likely produces the red blood cell–trabecular lesion by (a) maintaining blood pressure, with the sinusoids remaining open, and (b) causing ischemic damage in the perivenular zone owing to decrease in arterial blood flow. Red blood cells, under *normal* pressure, then replace necrotic hepatocytes within the empty cords.
4. In instances when the red blood cell–trabecular lesion is formed secondary to outflow obstruction (i.e., Budd-Chiari syndrome, veno-occlusive disease), the perivenular ischemia and increased sinusoidal pressure from the obstruction may ultimately lead to red blood cells within the trabeculae, establishing an extrasinusoidal circulatory plexus. It is presumed that sinusoidal blood flows coaxially with the terminal hepatic veins in an attempt to bypass the hepatic vein occlusion.
5. Patients recognized to be in heart failure are generally treated without the necessity of a liver biopsy; therefore this lesion may be more common than experienced.

Treatment and Prognosis

1. Treatment of heart failure (with digoxin, diuretics) results in resolution of liver test abnormalities without the development of chronic liver disease.

References

Cohen JA, Kaplan MM. Left-sided heart failure presenting as hepatitis. Gastroenterology 1978;74:583–587.
Kanel GC, Ucci AA, Kaplan MM, et al. A distinctive perivenular hepatic lesion associated with heart failure. Am J Clin Pathol 1980;73:235–239.
Killip T, Payne MA. High transaminase activity in heart disease. Circulation 1960;21:646–660.
Leopold JG, Parry TE, Storring FK. A change in the sinusoid-trabecular structure of the liver with hepatic venous outflow block. J Pathol 1970;100:87–97.

■ Inflammatory Vascular Lesions

Pylephlebitis

Major Morphologic Features

1. Inflammatory changes involve the portal *venous* system, with perivascular inflammatory infiltration (predominantly neutrophilic) and infiltration of vascular wall by inflammatory cells, with concomitant distortion and swelling of endothelial lining, often resulting in thrombosis.

Other Features

1. When abdominal infection is present, the parenchyma shows nonspecific changes such as Kupffer cell hyperplasia, mild focal necrosis, and increased circulating leukocytes within the sinusoids.
2. Portal tract may show variable degrees of inflamma-

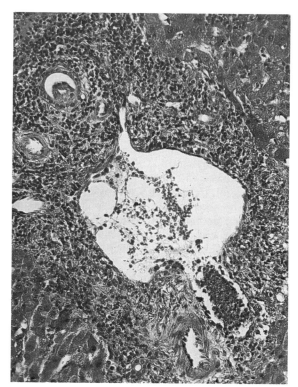

Figure 6–11. Pylephlebitis. The portal vein is surrounded by a mixture of mononuclear cells and neutrophils, with the latter infiltrating through the endothelium into the lumen and forming a small thrombus.

tory change away from an affected portal vein; the changes are usually mild.

3. In severe cases, microabscess formation may occur, with destruction of the vein.

Differential Diagnosis

1. *Acute cholangitis:* When neutrophils are oriented toward and invade duct structures, acute cholangitis is present. In severe cases of pylephlebitis, however, secondary duct inflammatory changes can also occur, morphologically resembling acute cholangitis.
2. *Thrombosis secondary to neoplasm:* Hepatocellular carcinoma as well as metastatic tumor may invade portal and hepatic venous structures. When tumor cells are necrotic, the changes may be difficult to differentiate from thrombosis secondary to infection; however, inflammatory cells do not characteristically invade the vascular wall with tumor thrombus formation.
3. *Endothelialitis* (associated with graft rejection following hepatic transplantation): Lymphocytes, not neutrophils, attach to and eventually invade the endothelial wall of portal and hepatic veins.

Clinical and Biologic Features

1. Pylephebitis, defined as inflammation of the portal vein, is usually caused by an infected thromboembolism of the intrahepatic or extrahepatic portal venous system secondary to an intra-abdominal suppurative infection.
2. The clinical onset may be identified by abdominal pain, distention, and vomiting, with chills and fever; hepatomegaly (60%), splenomegaly (10%–15%), and jaundice (50%) are often present.
3. In general, pylephlebitis will often begin in a thrombosed venous radicle of the splanchnic circulation draining an infected region; in the past, the most common cause was an appendicular abscess. Currently, causes such as diverticular and pelvic abscesses appear more likely.
4. Because of the dual (arterial and portal) blood supply to the liver, portal vein thrombosis alone generally will not lead to ischemic change; however, with severe hypotension or occlusion of both arterial and portal venous blood flow, *Zahn's infarct* may develop, caused by a backward flow from the hepatic venous system into portions of the liver not receiving enough blood, with resultant sinusoidal congestion. These areas are not true infarcts and are grossly well delineated triangular congested areas.

Treatment and Prognosis

1. Treatment of the primary focus of sepsis and possible hepatic abscesses is necessary. Mortality is high in untreated cases.
2. Visualization of gas in the portal vein on abdominal radiography is an ominous sign.

References

MacSween RNM. Vascular disorders. In: MacSween RNM, Anthony PP, Scheuer PJ, eds. Pathology of the Liver, 2nd ed. Edinburgh: Churchill Livingstone, 1987:480–481.

Scheuer PJ. Vascular disorders. In: Scheuer PJ, ed. Liver Biopsy Interpretation, 3rd ed. London: Baillière Tindall, 1980:156–157.

Polyarteritis

Major Morphologic Features

1. Segmented, destructive fibrinoid necrosis of the wall of medium-sized to large hepatic arteries occurs.
2. Mixed inflammatory infiltrate consists of neutrophils, eosinophils, and lymphocytes infiltrating the wall, often with secondary thrombosis of the lumen.

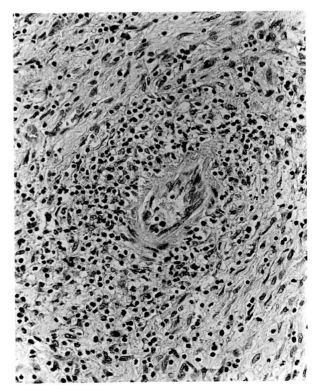

Figure 6–12. Polyarteritis. This large arteriole is completely surrounded and invaded by a mixture of lymphocytes, neutrophils, and occasional eosinophils.

Other Changes

1. Fibrosis and intimal proliferation with eventual scarring occur in more advanced (end-stage) lesions.
2. Periarterial granulomatous infiltration with occasional multinucleated giant cells may be seen.
3. Small arterioles are uninvolved, with small portal tracts usually showing no changes.
4. Parenchyma may exhibit coagulative necrosis and even well-defined areas of infarction when severe anoxic change is present.
5. Cholestasis and parenchymal inflammatory infiltration are not present.
6. Inflammatory involvement of adjacent portal venous branches may occur secondarily.

Differential Diagnosis

1. *Infarction from other causes:* Aneurysm, vascular thrombosis, embolism, and inadvertent surgical ligation of hepatic artery may result in infarction.
2. *Pylephlebitis:* Portal vein thrombosis with inflammation of portal venous radicles spares involvement of the arteries.

Special Stains

1. *Phosphotungstic acid hematoxylin:* Positive staining shows fibrin in walls of arteries and in lumina containing thrombi.
2. *Verhoeff's elastic stain:* Fragmentation of elastic tissue fibers in the vessel wall is evident, with gaps in the elastic lamina.

Immunohistochemistry

1. *HBsAg:* In rare instances there may be positive staining in the vessel wall when the polyarteritis is secondary to acute or chronic hepatitis B.

Clinical and Biologic Behavior

1. Polyarteritis (periarteritis, polyarteritis nodosa) is a necrotizing vasculitis involving small and medium-sized arteries throughout the body and involves hepatic arteries ranging from 50 μm to 5 mm in diameter.
2. The incidence is 1/100,000; it is twice as frequent in men and found at any age, including infancy.
3. Laboratory data may show elevated serum globulin levels, eosinophilia, and a decrease in serum complement factors.
4. The hepatic arteries are involved in two thirds of all cases; hepatic involvement is usually symptomatic, and dysfunction relates to the degree (if any) of anoxic necrosis.
5. Vascular thrombosis may lead to infarction in 15% of the cases.
6. Aneurysms may develop owing to segmental arterial involvement. Angiography is therefore the investigative method of choice in diagnosis.
7. Polyarteritis is immunologically related:
   a. It was described in soldiers following yellow fever vaccination in 1942.
   b. It is a manifestation of both acute and chronic hepatitis B in a small percentage of cases, with vasculitis secondary to deposition in arterial wall of antigen–antibody complexes of HBsAg.
   c. It is associated with other viral infections (herpesvirus, cytomegalovirus) and several bacterial antigens.

Treatment and Prognosis

1. Corticosteroids with or without chemotherapeutic agents (e.g., cyclophosphamide) are usually effective.
2. If chemotherapy is not effective, plasmapheresis is offered to remove circulating antigen–antibody complexes.
3. Polyarteritis can be serious and often fatal if not promptly treated; the 5-year survival is 50% or better, with death usually occurring within the first year and not related to hepatic involvement.

References

Gocke DJ, Morgan C, Lockshin M, et al. Association between polyarteritis and Australia antigen. Lancet 1970;2:1149–1153.

Mowrey FH, Lundbergh EA. The clinical manifestations of essential polyangitis (periarteritis nodosa) with emphasis on the hepatic manifestations. Ann Intern Med 1954;40:1145–1164.

Rose GA, Spencer H. Polyarteritis nodosa. Q J Med 1957;26:43–81.

■ Miscellaneous Disorders

Peliosis Hepatis

Major Morphologic Changes

1. Blood-filled parenchymal cysts without lining cells are seen, ranging from less than 1 mm to 1 cm in diameter.
2. Communication of cysts with adjacent dilated sinusoids occurs.

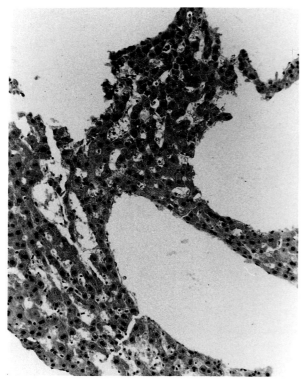

Figure 6–13. Peliosis hepatis. This needle biopsy specimen shows variably sized round to oval vascular structures that often merge with adjacent sinusoids. An endothelial lining is for the most part absent.

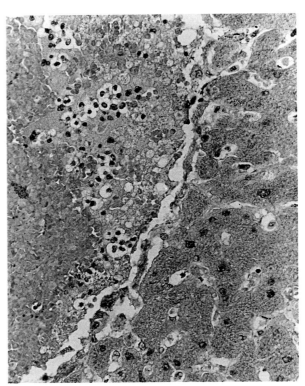

Figure 6–15. Peliosis hepatis. Higher power exhibits an absence of lining cells at the border of the hepatocytes and the large vascular space.

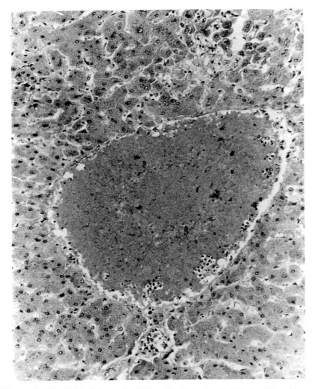

Figure 6–14. Peliosis hepatis. This peliotic lesion is filled with red blood cells. White blood cells are present in clusters toward the edge of the lesion.

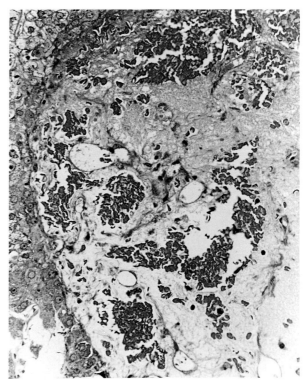

Figure 6–16. Peliosis hepatis. Red blood cells are seen within a loose fibrin network forming small vascular spaces.

Other Features

1. No distinct zonal distribution of cystic lesions is evident; however, perivenular accentuation may be slightly more common.
2. Cysts are occasionally lined by endothelial cells or thin collagen strands, with fibrin present along the cyst wall or throughout the cyst itself; formation of small new vascular spaces within the fibrin has been reported but is rare.
3. Sinusoidal dilatation occurs in areas away from cysts, often associated with liver cell atrophy.
4. Cholestasis may be present but is infrequent.
5. Portal areas show no significant changes.
6. Areas of parenchymal inflammation and hepatocytolysis are uncommon.

Differential Diagnosis

1. *Acute congestion with marked sinusoidal dilatation:* Peliosis may involve any zone of the lobule, while acute congestion always involves the perivenular region without formation of cystic structures.
2. *Simple hepatic cysts:* These cysts, when small, are lined by cuboidal epithelium and do not contain blood. The cystlike lesions of von Meyenberg complexes consist of multiple small but dilated duct structures within portal tracts.

Special Stains

1. *Phosphotungstic acid hematoxylin:* Fibrin is often deposited along the cyst wall.

Clinical and Biologic Behavior

1. Most patients are asymptomatic, with only hepatomegaly and normal to mildly elevated transaminase levels; cases may rarely occur, however, of severe hepatic dysfunction, jaundice, and hepatic failure.
2. Peliosis has been associated with the administration of drugs, most commonly androgenic/anabolic steroids (e.g., testosterone, oxymetholone, norethandrolone).
3. Peliosis has also been reported in patients who have undergone renal transplantation and in patients with tuberculosis or malignant neoplasms, after exposure to Thorotrast and vinyl chloride monomers, and in patients who are infected with human immunodeficiency virus.
4. Death occurs rarely secondary to rupture of subcapsular cysts with massive intraperitoneal bleeding.
5. Splenic cysts may also be present.

6. It is not known if liver biopsy is hazardous due to bleeding.
7. Possible pathophysiologic mechanisms include the following:
   a. Weakening of the sinusoidal reticulin network of the lobule due to drugs or toxins (the lesion has been experimentally induced in animals after the administration of phalloidin, a substance known to injure cell membranes)
   b. Focal liver cell necrosis with resultant sinusoidal outflow obstruction, endothelial damage, and eventual hemorrhagic cyst formation

Treatment and Prognosis

1. There is no specific treatment; when peliosis is associated with steroids, discontinuation of the drugs has been shown to result in complete regression of the lesions.

References

Anthony PP. Tumors and tumor-like lesions of the liver and biliary tract. In: MacSween RNM, Anthony PP, Scheuer PJ, eds. Pathology of the Liver, 2nd ed. Edinburgh: Churchill Livingstone, 1987:628–629.

Baghergi SA, Boyer JL. Peliosis hepatis associated with androgenic anabolic steroid therapy. Ann Intern Med 1974;81:610–618.

Czapar CA, Weldon-Linne M, Moore DM. Peliosis hepatis in the acquired immunodeficiency syndrome. Arch Pathol Lab Med 1986;110:611–613.

Yanoff M, Rawson AJ. Peliosis hepatis: An anatomic study with demonstration of two varieties. Arch Pathol 1964;77:159–165.

Zafrani ES, Pinaudeau Y, Dhumeaux D. Drug-induced vascular lesions of the liver. Arch Intern Med 1983;143:495–502.

Osler-Weber-Rendu Disease (Hereditary Hemorrhagic Telangiectasia)

Major Morphologic Features

1. Dilated and enlarged portal vascular channels are seen, often with increase in smaller portal and periportal venous structures.

Other Features

1. Variable degrees of portal fibrosis and even cirrhosis may be present.
2. Parenchyma exhibits focal sinusoidal dilatation.
3. Intimal proliferation and thrombus formation are occasionally present within arterioles.
4. Other portal changes are nonspecific, with no bile duct abnormalities or significant inflammatory infiltration.

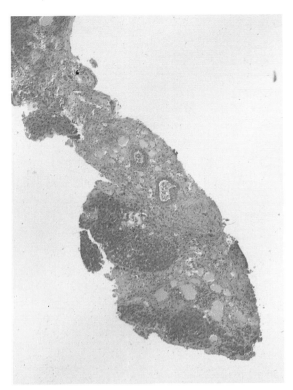

Figure 6–17. Osler-Weber-Rendu disease. A low power of this needle biopsy specimen demonstrates small hepatic nodules surrounded by fibrous septa containing numerous dilated vascular channels.

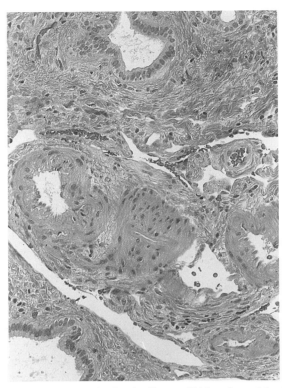

Figure 6–19. Osler-Weber-Rendu disease. Thickened arterioles have merged with a focally thin-walled vessel *(second from right)*, forming an arteriovenous malformation.

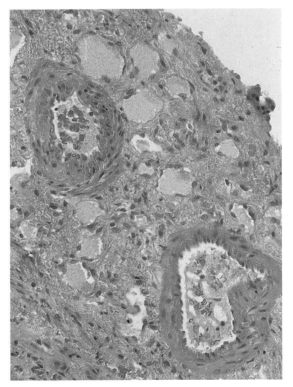

Figure 6–18. Osler-Weber-Rendu disease. High power of the septa reveals an arteriole *(upper left)* and thickened vein *(lower right)* surrounded by numerous small vascular structures.

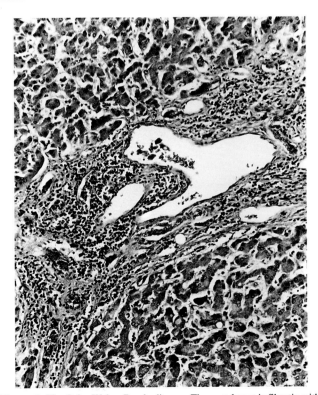

Figure 6–20. Osler-Weber-Rendu disease. The portal tract is fibrotic with a moderate lymphocytic infiltrate. Numerous variably sized vessels and dilated portal venous radicles are present. Although this feature can generally be seen in portal hypertension of numerous etiologies, dilatation of the veins to this degree is somewhat unusual.

Differential Diagnosis

1. *Idiopathic portal hypertension:* Dilated portal vascular channels, an indicator of portal hypertension, are a characteristic feature of idiopathic portal hypertension (noncirrhotic portal fibrosis); however, the clinical manifestations and systemic lesions seen in the two entities are quite different.
2. *Primary biliary cirrhosis:* The dilated vascular channels often seen in primary biliary cirrhosis with minimal fibrosis are caused by portal hypertension. Other morphologic changes, such as granuloma formation, primary nonsuppurative destructive cholangitis, decreased ducts, significant portal inflammatory change, and often periportal alcoholic hyalin, are not seen in Osler-Weber-Rendu disease.
3. *Fibrosis or cirrhosis of numerous etiologies:* With rare exceptions (e.g., congenital hepatic fibrosis), increased vascular channels are almost always seen in severe fibrosis or cirrhosis as a secondary manifestation of portal hypertension; however, other morphologic features relating to the cause of the cirrhosis (e.g., irregularly distributed parenchymal inflammatory changes and ground-glass cells in chronic hepatitis B infection; sinusoidal collagen and alcoholic hyalin in alcoholic liver disease) are absent in Osler-Weber-Rendu disease.

Clinical and Biologic Behavior

1. Osler-Weber-Rendu disease, also termed *hereditary hemorrhagic telangiectasia,* is an autosomal dominant disorder characterized by widespread capillary venous malformations with arteriovenous communications, most commonly seen as telangiectases in the skin (face, tongue, fingertips), nasopharynx, oral cavity, and gastrointestinal tract; pulmonary arteriovenous fistulas may also be present.
2. The disorder presents between the ages of 20 to 30 years, when epistaxis is noted owing to bleeding telangiectases; the number of vascular lesions increases with age, with gastrointestinal hemorrhage a later finding.
3. Osler-Weber-Rendu disease rarely produces clinically significant hepatic abnormalities; however, rapid blood flow from the hepatic artery to the hepatic vein through an arteriovenous fistula may yield a continuous bruit and palpable thrill over an enlarged liver.
4. Laboratory tests are not valuable; angiography, however, will demonstrate angiomas and arteriovenous fistulas in the gastrointestinal tract.
5. Small vascular structures are involved, including small arteries, arterioles, capillaries, and venules, with the vascular channels commonly dilated; the ultrastructure shows thrombosed endothelial gaps most commonly present in small venules.
6. Fibrosis and cirrhosis have been described as associated with the lesion, although there is controversy as to whether a true relationship exists. Cirrhotic livers may have prominent dilated vascular structures within the fibrous septa secondary to portal hypertension that may resemble telangiectases; it is possible that Osler-Weber-Rendu disease could be misdiagnosed or that incidental cirrhosis from other causes could be misinterpreted as secondary.
7. The cause is unknown; however, arterial intimal proliferation and contracture of well-developed muscular fibers surrounding some of the small vessels is speculated to lead to engorgment and formation of telangiectases.

Treatment

1. Surgical removal and selective embolization of clinically significant arteriovenous pulmonary fistulas have been described; however, there is no specific treatment for hepatic involvement

References

Daly JJ, Schiller AL. The liver in hereditary haemorrhagic telangiectasia (Osler-Weber-Rendu disease). Am J Med 1976;60:723–726.

Feizi O. Hereditary hemorrhagic telangiectasia with portal hypertension and cirrhosis of the liver. Gastroenterology 1972;63:660–664.

Martini GA. The liver in hereditary haemorrhagic telangiectasia: An inborn error of vascular structure with multiple manifestations: A reappraisal. Gut 1978;19:531–537.

Idiopathic Portal Hypertension (Noncirrhotic Portal Fibrosis)

Major Morphologic Features

1. Portal fibrosis with increased numbers of dilated vascular channels and minimal to absent portal or parenchymal inflammatory change occurs.
2. A consistent relationship between portal tracts and terminal hepatic venules is lacking.

Other Features

1. Stellate or arachnoid portal fibrosis is present.
2. Larger portal veins may show eccentric thickening.
3. Portal thrombi may be present.
4. There are no bile duct abnormalities.
5. Hepatocytes are often hydropic, with variable but minimal parenchymal regenerative activity.
6. Severe degrees of bridging portal fibrosis have been described.

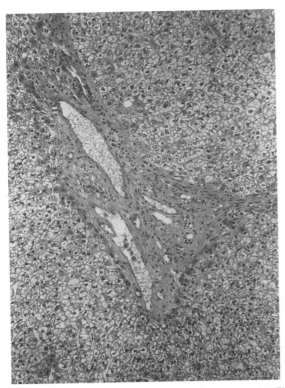

Figure 6–21. Idiopathic portal hypertension. The portal tract is fibrotic and contains numerous dilated vascular channels. Inflammatory infiltration is minimal.

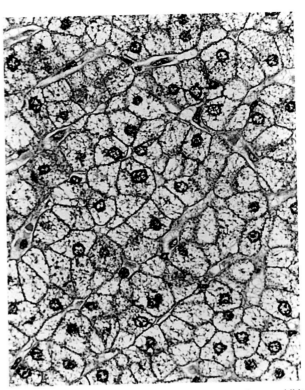

Figure 6–23. Idiopathic portal hypertension. The parenchyma exhibits a distorted cord–sinusoid pattern caused by marked hydropic change of the liver cells that represents regenerative activity. Inflammatory infiltration and Kupffer cell hyperplasia are not present.

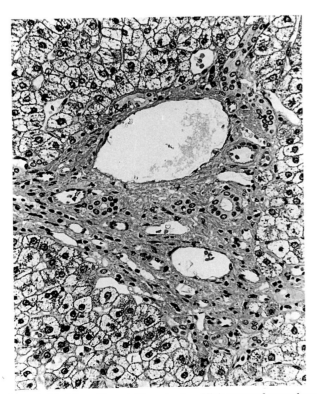

Figure 6–22. Idiopathic portal hypertension. High power of a portal tract exhibits numerous vascular channels even though portal fibrosis is minimal. Bile ducts are only slightly increased in number.

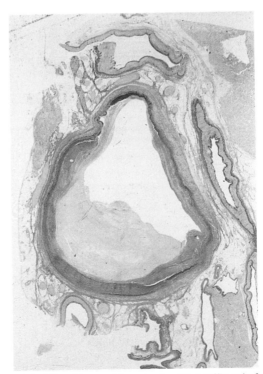

Figure 6–24. Idiopathic portal hypertension (Verhoeff's stain for elastic tissue). The low-power photomicrograph of this extrahepatic portal vein illustrates prominent eccentric proliferation of subintimal fibers, contributing to partial portal venous occlusion.

Differential Diagnosis

1. *Osler-Weber-Rendu disease:* Telangiectatic portal lesions may resemble portal lesions of idiopathic portal hypertension. Osler-Weber-Rendu disease may also exhibit periportal vascular dilatation.
2. *Primary biliary cirrhosis:* The early fibrotic stage of primary biliary cirrhosis can exhibit increased dilated vasculature related to portal hypertension but also may exhibit nonsuppurative destructive duct lesions, decreased ducts, granulomas, and chronic inflammatory infiltration, which are not seen in idiopathic portal hypertension.
3. *Toxins:* Chronic exposure to copper (vineyard sprays), arsenic (Fowler's solution, insecticides, water and indigenous medicinals in India), and vinyl chloride monomers (manufacture of polyvinyl chloride) may produce lesions morphologically identical to idiopathic portal hypertension.
4. *Schistosomiasis:* Degree of fibrosis in this parasitic infection is usually quite marked, with a "pipe-stem" fibrous lesion surrounding and eventually replacing the granulomatous inflammatory response to the ova. Organisms are also identified within portal tracts without an inflammatory response, as well as in portal venous radicles.
5. *Alcoholic liver disease:* Portal tracts also exhibit an arachnoid type of fibrosis with increased vasculature in alcoholic liver disease. Other lesions such as sinusoidal collagen, perivenular fibrosis, and superimposed changes of acute disease (alcoholic hyalin, neutrophilic infiltration in portal tracts and parenchyma) are not present in idiopathic portal hypertension.

Special Stain

1. *Verhoeff's elastic stain:* Elastic tissue delineates eccentric intimal thickening in some of the larger portal venous radicles.

Clinical and Biologic Behavior

1. Also more appropriately termed *noncirrhotic portal fibrosis,* idiopathic portal hypertension is rare in the United States but common in India (42% of all patients who underwent portacaval anastomosis between 1976 and 1982) and Japan (10.5% of all cases of portal hypertension between 1965 and 1980).
2. Idiopathic portal hypertension has an insidious onset more often in middle-aged women, with marked splenomegaly and recurrent bouts of hematemesis; ascites is uncommon and present only in advanced disease.

3. Laboratory tests are nonspecific; leukopenia (3,000/mm^3) and thrombocytopenia (92,000/mm^3) are usually due to hypersplenism. Serum albumin and aminotransferase levels are normal; however, for unclear reasons, prothrombin activity may be decreased to 60%.
4. Wedged hepatic venous pressure is normal or minimally increased, while portal venous pressure is significantly elevated, indicating presinusoidal portal hypertension.
5. Hepatic blood flow is normal to slightly increased, despite the marked splenomegaly (spleen weighs more than 500 g and often over 1000 g).
6. Angiography has demonstrated distortion and sudden diminution of the diameter of intrahepatic portal vein radicles with occasional complete cut-off of the channels, suggesting small venous occlusion; portal hypertension may be secondary to thrombosis of the portal veins with recanalization, resulting eventually in thickening of the intima and hypertensive changes.
7. Sclerosis of portal vein radicles may also occur in the absence of thrombosis, suggesting a primary disorder of the vascular system ("hepatoportal sclerosis").
8. Other disorders that may produce portal hypertension in a noncirrhotic liver include the following:
   a. *Infectious:* Schistosomiasis
   Leishmaniasis
   b. *Drugs/Toxins:* Alcohol
   Copper
   Arsenic
   Vinyl chloride
   Vitamin A
   c. *Vascular:* Budd-Chiari syndrome
   Arteriovenous fistulas
   Osler-Weber-Rendu disease
   d. *Congenital:* Congenital hepatic fibrosis
   e. *Miscellaneous:* Granulomatous (sarcoid)
   Primary biliary cirrhosis
   Myeloproliferative disorders
   Nodular regenerative hyperplasia
   Partial nodular transformation

Treatment and Prognosis

1. In the event of variceal hemorrhage, treatment includes endoscopic sclerotherapy or portosystemic shunt surgery. Since liver function is well preserved, devascularization is preferred to shunt surgery in some centers because of avoidance of post shunt encephalopathy.

2. Idiopathic portal hypertension has a better prognosis than cirrhosis:

	10-Year Survival	Mean Survival from Time of Diagnosis
Idiopathic portal hypertension	77%	25 years
Cirrhosis (predominantly viral, alcoholic etiologies)	29%	5.9 years

References

Mikkelsen, WP, Edmondson HA, Peters RL, et al. Extra- and intrahepatic portal hypertension without cirrhosis (hepatoportal sclerosis). Ann Surg 1965; 162:602–620.

Okuda K, Kono K, Ohnishi K, et al. Clinical study of eighty-six cases of idiopathic portal hypertension and comparison with cirrhosis with splenomegaly. Gastroenterology 1984;86:600–610.

Okuda K, Nakashima T, Okudaira M, et al. Liver pathology of idiopathic portal hypertension: Comparison with noncirrhotic portal fibrosis of India. Liver 1982;2:176–192.

Peters RL. Idiopathic portal hypertension, pathologic changes. In: Okuda K, Omata M, eds. Idiopathic portal hypertension: Proceedings of the International Symposium on Idiopathic Portal Hypertension. Tokyo: University of Tokyo Press, 1983:85–97.

Villeneuve JP, Huet P–M, Joly J–G, et al. Idiopathic portal hypertension. Am J Med 1976;61:459–464.

General References

Bras G, Brandt K-H. Vascular disorders. In: MacSween RNM, Anthony PP, Scheuer PJ, eds. Pathology of the Liver, 2nd ed. Edinburgh: Churchill Livingstone, 1987;478–502.

Edmondson HA, Peters RL. Liver. In: Kissane JM, Anderson WAD, eds. Pathology, 8th ed. St. Louis: C.V. Mosby, 1985:1172–1178.

Scheuer PJ. Vascular disorders. In: Scheuer PJ, ed. Liver Biopsy Interpretation, 3rd ed. London: Baillière Tindall, 1980:154–166.

CHAPTER 7

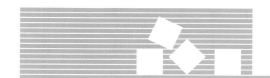

Nonviral Infectious Disorders

■ Bacterial Infection

Reactive and Pyogenic Bacterial Infection

Major Morphologic Features

1. Portal tracts show variable degrees of both acute and chronic inflammatory infiltration.
2. Variable degrees of focal hepatocytolysis, Kupffer cell hyperplasia, and scattered inflammatory infiltration are seen within the parenchyma.
3. An association with clinically severe cases of septicemia may exhibit:
   a. Dilated interlobular ducts and cholangioles, often with neutrophilic infiltration and acute cholangitis.
   b. Cholestasis and *microabscess* formation within the parenchyma.

Other Features

1. Edema of the portal tracts may be present.
2. Bile duct proliferation is mild.
3. Portal fibrosis is not typically seen.
4. Hepatocytes with variable degrees of hydropic change and mild macrovesicular fatty change are seen.
5. General maintenance of the cord–sinusoid pattern is present.
6. Circulating sinusoidal leukocytes are increased in number and associated with an elevated peripheral white cell count.
7. There is no particular zonal distribution of parenchymal changes; microabscesses, however, may tend to have a perivenular accentuation.
8. Large pyogenic abscess forms from coalescence of smaller microabscesses in untreated cases.

Differential Diagnosis

1. *Acute viral hepatitis:* Portal inflammatory changes are predominantly lymphocytic; focal necrosis, hydropic change, and disruption of the cord–sinusoid pattern typical of acute viral hepatitis are not prominent in reactive changes due to bacterial infection.
2. *Extrahepatic obstruction:* Perivenular cholestasis, bile duct dilatation and proliferation, and acute cholangitis are features of extrahepatic obstruction; in cases of severe bacterial sepsis, morphologic changes may resemble obstruction.
3. *Amebic versus pyogenic abscess:* Abscesses formed by bacteria and *Entamoeba histolytica* may attain huge sizes, with the following differential characteristics:

Feature	Amebic	Pyogenic
Jaundice	Rare	Common
Number	Single (usually)	Single or multiple
Associated acute cholangitis	No (enter through portal venous system)	Yes (enter through biliary tract)
Inflammatory change	Scanty to absent	Prominent neutrophils
Contents	Thick, yellow-brown, pasty; organisms often identified (periodic acid–Schiff)	White-yellow pus, malodorous; organisms seldom identified (Gram stain)
Amebic serology	Positive	Negative (unless previous exposure)
Abscess cultures for bacteria	Usually sterile; occasionally pus cultures are positive, suggestive of superinfection	Positive in up to 80% of cases

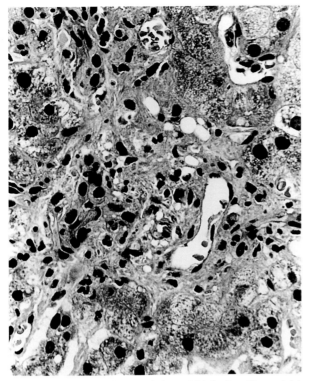

Figure 7–1. Reactive and pyogenic bacterial infection. The portal tract contains a mild to moderate inflammatory infiltrate consisting of both lymphocytes and neutrophils. Occasional fat globules are also seen within portal macrophages.

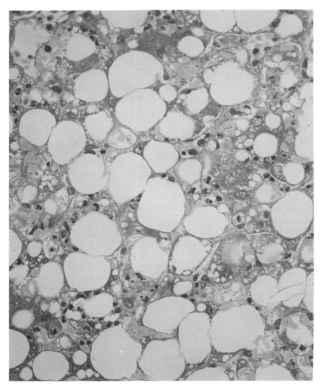

Figure 7–2. Reactive and pyogenic bacterial infection. The parenchyma shows macrovesicular fatty change and numerous single and small aggregates of neutrophils surrounding hepatocytes. Microabscesses may develop in untreated patients.

Special Stains

1. *Gram:* Results are always negative in reactive changes and usually negative in bacterial infection; they may be positive, however, on smears of aspirated material from large abscesses prior to antibiotic therapy.
2. *Periodic acid–Schiff:* This stain is useful in differentiating pyogenic versus amebic abscess, since the latter often exhibits positive cytoplasmic staining of *Entamoeba histolytica* located along the abscess wall.

Clinical and Biologic Behavior

1. The most frequent symptoms are malaise, anorexia, right upper quadrant abdominal pain, and fever. Diabetics are at greater risk.
2. Hepatomegaly is the most common physical finding; one third of patients with a liver abscess become jaundiced.
3. Serum aminotransferase levels are only minimally elevated in the majority of cases, although the alkaline phosphatase activity is often elevated. Serum albumin is decreased and levels below 2 g/dL carry a poor prognosis. Leukocytosis with left shift and anemia are frequent findings.
4. Neutrophilic reaction around ducts and cholangioles may itself cause an obstructive process at the lobular level and be in part responsible for cholestasis and jaundice.
5. Pyogenic abscesses are rare, the true incidence is unknown, and prevalence in autopsy series ranges from 0.3 to 1.5%. Causes include ascending cholangitis from biliary tract obstruction, blunt and penetrating trauma of the liver, and direct extension from adjacent organs (e.g., gallbladder). In a significant number of cases no obvious etiology is noted. Spread from an intestinal focus (e.g., appendix, diverticula) through the portal circulation may occur.

Aspiration Cytology

1. Aspiration of large pyogenic abscesses may be critically important for diagnosis (rule out neoplasm), with Gram stain, culture, and appropriate antibiotic therapy.
2. Abundant neutrophils and in some instances identification of gram-positive and gram-negative organisms are typical features of pyogenic abscesses.

Treatment and Prognosis

1. Abscess is treated with appropriate antibiotics.
2. Prognosis is related to the severity of infection, with mortality directly related to the infection itself and underlying or associated diseases in other organ systems.

References

Carcana JA, Montes M, Camara DS, et al. Functional and histopathological changes in the liver during sepsis. Surg Gynecol Obstet 1982;154:653–656.

Chopra S. Liver abscesses and cysts. In: Stein JH. Internal Medicine, 2nd ed. Boston: Little, Brown & Co, 1987:238–241.

DeCock KM, Reynolds TB. Amebic and pyogenic liver abscess. In: Schiff L, Schiff ER, eds. Diseases of the Liver, 6th ed. Philadelphia: J.B. Lippincott, 1987: 1235–1253.

Greenstein AJ, Lowenthal BA, Hammer GFS, et al. Continuing patterns of disease in pyogenic liver abscess: A study of 38 cases. Am J Gastroenterol 1984;79:217–226.

Perera MR, Kirk A, Noone P, et al. Presentation, diagnosis and management of liver abscess. Lancet 1980;2:629–632.

Brucellosis

Major Morphologic Features

1. Granulomas composed predominantly of lymphocytes, macrophages, Kupffer cells, and occasionally epithelioid cells are scattered throughout the parenchyma.
2. Kupffer cell hyperplasia is uniformly present.

Other Features

1. Portal tracts show mild lymphocytic hyperplasia and occasional infiltration by neutrophils.
2. Focal necrosis and hepatocytolysis without granuloma formation may be present.
3. Hepatocytes exhibit variable degrees of hydropic change.
4. Acidophil bodies may be present.
5. Larger granulomas rarely undergo central necrosis.
6. In later stages, granulomas may undergo healing with fibrosis and occasionally focal calcification.
7. Microabscess formation may occur in severe cases (*Brucella suis* infection).

Differential Diagnosis

1. *Granulomatous conditions of other etiologies:*
   a. *Salmonella typhi* (typhoid fever), *Francisella tularensis* (tularemia): A somewhat similar granulomatous type of necrosis may be seen; culture is necessary for diagnosis.

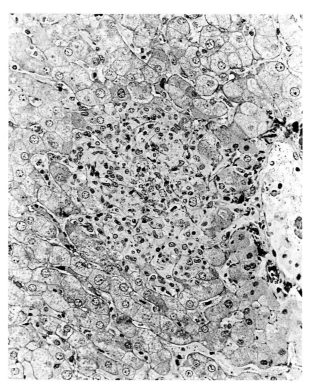

Figure 7–3. Brucellosis. A large aggregate of inflammatory cells consisting of lymphocytes, macrophages, and Kupffer cells is present adjacent to a terminal hepatic vein. The surrounding liver cells are slightly hydropic, with moderate Kupffer cell hyperplasia.

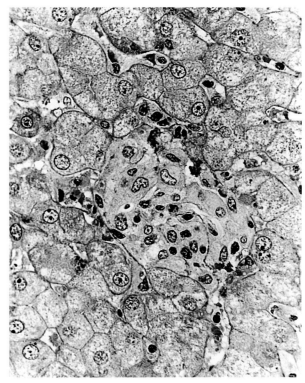

Figure 7–4. Brucellosis. High power shows a well-demarcated granuloma consisting of both mononuclear inflammatory cells and Kupffer cells. At the center of the granuloma are two large epithelioid cells having large pale nuclei and abundant cytoplasm.

b. *Acid-fast bacilli, fungi:* These organisms elicit well-defined and often large epithelioid granulomas. Multinucleated giant cells are often seen in these infections. In addition, central caseous necrosis may appear in larger granulomas of *Mycobacterium* infection.

c. *Drug-induced injury* (e.g., sulfasalazine): Certain drugs (see page 85) induce similar granulomatous reactions, although drug-related epithelioid cells and Kupffer cell hyperplasia are not as prominent as in brucellosis.

Special Stains

1. *Gram:* Gram-negative organisms (coccobacilli) of *Brucella* are rarely demonstrated within enlarged Kupffer cells and macrophages.
2. *Periodic acid–Schiff, methenamine silver, acid fast:* Positive staining rules out *Brucella* by confirming *Mycobacterium* or fungi as the cause of the granulomas.

Clinical and Biologic Behavior

1. *Brucella* is a gram-negative coccobacillus capable of invading all tissues and contracted by humans from close contact with infected cattle, goats, sheep, and swine; nonpasteurized dairy products are a minor source of contamination (e.g., cheese).
2. Four species are capable of infection in humans:
   a. *B. abortus:* Infection is mild and self-limited; severe complications are rare.
   b. *B. suis:* Suppurative destructive disease can occur and may become chronic.
   c. *B. melitensis:* This species is most virulent, with severe acute infection and highest mortality.
   d. *B. canis* (dogs, mainly beagles): This infection is rare in humans, but a mild disease may occur.
3. Infection occurs predominantly in men 20 to 50 years of age (e.g., workers in slaughter houses, farmers).
4. There are two types:
   a. *Acute:* Incubation period is 5 to 14 days with bacteremia and resultant chills, fever, and generalized lymphadenopathy; splenomegaly (10%–20%), hepatomegaly (5%–10%), and a tender liver are occasionally present; jaundice and hepatic abscess formation may occur but are rare.
   b. *Chronic:* In a small number of patients, chronic illness develops following acute infection, lasting months to years, with fatigue, vague pains, and intermittent fever; splenomegaly is the main physical finding. Although cirrhosis has been described, it is questionable as to its direct association with the infection.
5. Laboratory findings are of minimal value, with only slight elevation of aminotransferase activities; blood culture or culture from tissue (bone marrow, liver, lymph nodes) is necessary for a definitive diagnosis.
6. Pathophysiology: Experimental formation of granulomas in the liver has been shown in mice and guinea pigs. Intravenous injection of bacilli results in prominent Kupffer cell reaction within 3 hours; within 6 hours these cells contain abundant numbers of organisms, and by 24 hours neutrophils also contain bacilli. By 5 days, aggregates of epithelioid-type macrophages and large Kupffer cells collect in dilated sinusoids, forming granulomas; some fuse, the larger ones exhibiting central necrosis. After 1 year, the granulomas most often disappear.

Prognosis

1. In untreated patients, mortality is 3% to 5% and death is most often associated with endocarditis; treated patients have mortality less than 1%, with complications occurring in 1% to 2% of patients.
2. Liver failure is not a feature of *Brucella* infection.

References

Bruguera M, Cervantes F. Hepatic granulomas in brucellosis. Ann Intern Med 1980;92:571–572.

Cervantes F, Bruguera M, Carbonell J, et al. Liver disease in brucellosis: A clinical and pathological study of 40 cases. Postgrad Med J 1982;58:346–350.

Spink WW, Hoffbauer FW, Walker EE, et al. Histopathology of the liver in human brucellosis. J Lab Clin Med 1949;34:40–58.

Williams RK, Crossley K. Acute and chronic hepatic involvement of brucellosis. Gastroenterology 1982;83:455–458.

Wilson W, Geraci JE. Brucellosis. In: Stein JH, ed. Internal Medicine, 2nd ed. Boston: Little, Brown & Co, 1987:1696–1699.

Salmonellosis

Major Morphologic Features

1. Kupffer cell hyperplasia and hypertrophy are marked.
2. Focal necrosis and aggregates of Kupffer cells, lymphocytes and macrophages are present within the parenchyma, forming a "typhoid nodule."

Other Features

1. Portal tract shows moderate lymphohistiocytic infiltration and hyperplasia.
2. Inflammatory nodules are randomly distributed within the parenchyma, with a slight periportal accentuation.
3. Large inflammatory nodules may undergo a central necrosis.
4. Acidophil bodies may be present but are rare.
5. Kupffer cells may exhibit erythrophagocytosis.

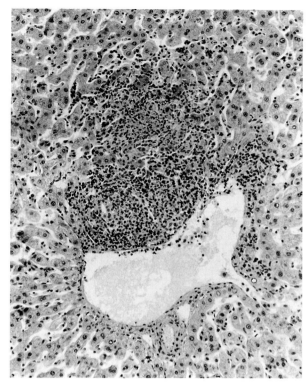

Figure 7–5. Typhoid fever. The portal tract exhibits prominent lymphocytic infiltration and hyperplasia. Spillover of the inflammatory cells into the adjacent parenchyma is evident.

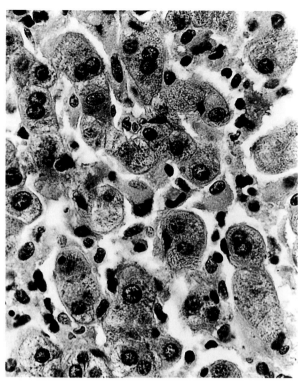

Figure 7–7. Typhoid fever. There is prominent Kupffer cell hyperplasia and hypertrophy uniformly distributed throughout the lobule.

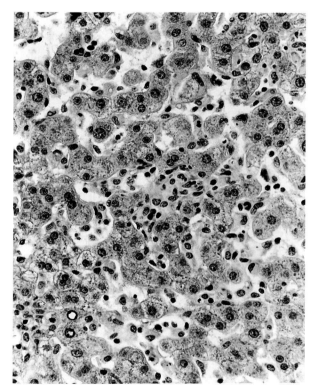

Figure 7–6. Typhoid fever. Focal necrosis is present within the lobule. The sinusoids are open, with an intact cord–sinusoid pattern.

6. Bile ducts rarely exhibit an acute cholangitis.
7. Cholestasis is uncommon.

Differential Diagnosis

1. *Reticuloendothelial neoplasm:* The marked hypertrophic and hyperplastic change of the Kupffer cells may suggest a malignant tumor of the reticuloendothelial system; however, there is minimal pleomorphism, with marked uniformity of changes throughout the liver in *Salmonella* infection.
2. *Infections secondary to other organisms:* Certain bacteria, such as *Brucella,* may evoke a granulomatous necrosis resembling the inflammatory nodule of salmonellosis; however, the prominence of the hypertrophic change of Kupffer cells is distinctive, although not diagnostic, of salmonellosis.

Special Stain

1. *Gram:* Gram-negative organisms may be identified within Kupffer cells.

Clinical and Biologic Behavior

1. *Salmonella* is a gram-negative anaerogenic bacterium with worldwide distribution: *S. typhi* is responsible for *typhoid fever* and *S. paratyphi* for *paratyphoid* infection.
2. The organisms are the most common etiologic agent responsible for food poisoning (*S. typhimurium* is most common organism); reservoirs have been isolated from virtually all domestic animals, with humans developing illness after ingestion of contaminated food products.
3. In *S. typhi* infection, humans are the only natural reservoir and spread occurs from one infected person to another through food, water, or contact.
4. In typhoid fever, the incubation period is 7 to 14 days; although asymptomatic infection is most common, a small proportion of patients will develop fever, headache, and abdominal pain, with one third having cough and one half nausea, vomiting, and diarrhea.
5. Hepatomegaly will develop in one third of the patients with typhoid fever, but jaundice is infrequent (0.4% to 7% in various series).
6. Laboratory tests are not useful for diagnosis of liver disease, with nonspecific elevations of serum aminotransferase levels and rarely of the bilirubin level.
7. Serologic testing (Widal test) is not helpful in early diagnosis; there are increased antibody titers to somatic (O) antigen (>1:80) in convalescent stage. In anamnestic reactions, increase in antibody titers to flagellar (H) antigen is seen.
8. Diagnosis is made by culture: blood is positive in 90% during first week, and stools (85%) and urine (25%) are positive during the third and fourth weeks.
9. Biliary tract disease may be involved, rarely with acute cholangitis; cholelithiasis and choledocholithiasis predispose to bacterial growth. A chronic carrier state may develop, leading to prolonged excretion of organisms in the stool (positive stool cultures for more than 1 year). Carriers have an increased incidence of gallbladder carcinoma.

Prognosis

1. At the present time untreated cases are exceedingly rare; in these cases, the mortality is 10% to 15%, with intestinal hemorrhage (5%–20%) or perforation (2%–5%) the most serious complications. Other complications include myocarditis, bone marrow suppression, localized infection (e.g., arthritis, meningitis), and liver cell injury.
2. Relapse may occur in 5% to 10% of untreated cases, with the symptoms usually mild.
3. Chronic carrier state occurs in 1% to 3%, with the gallbladder the focus of infection; therefore, cholecystectomy is indicated.
4. In treated patients, the mortality is less than 1%.

References

de Brito T, Vieira WT, Dias M. Jaundice in typhoid hepatitis: A light and electron microscopy study based on liver biopsies. Acta Hepatogastroenterol 1977;24:426–433.

Hornick RB, Greisman SE, Woodward TE, et al. Typhoid fever: Pathogenesis and immunological control. N Engl J Med 1970;283:686–691.

Johnson WD Jr, Pape JW. *Salmonella* and *Shigella* infections. In: Stein JH. Internal Medicine, 2nd ed. Boston: Little, Brown & Co, 1987:1691–1695.

McFadzean AJS, Ong GB. Intrahepatic typhoid carriers. Br Med J 1966;1:1567–1571.

Ramachandran S, Godfrey JJ, Perera MVF. Typhoid hepatitis. JAMA 1974;230:236–240.

■ Spirochetal Infection

Syphilis

Major Morphologic Features

Congenital
1. Severe portal and interstitial fibrosis surrounds individual and small groups of hepatocytes.

Secondary
1. Scattered epithelioid granulomas are present.
2. Vasculitis involves small arterioles and venules, with vaso-obliterative changes.

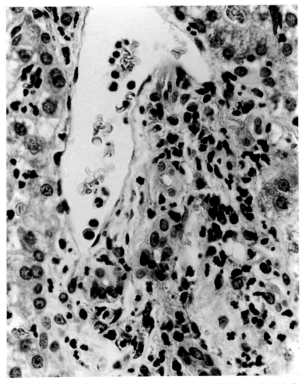

Figure 7–8. Secondary syphilis. A portal tract exhibits a mixed inflammatory infiltrate consisting of lymphocytes and neutrophils, the latter surrounding and in some areas infiltrating into the bile duct epithelium. Edema of the portal tract is also present.

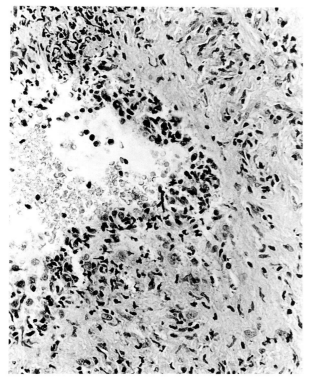

Figure 7–9. Secondary syphilis. A medium-sized vessel is surrounded and infiltrated by neutrophils, histiocytes, and lymphocytes, producing a vasculitis.

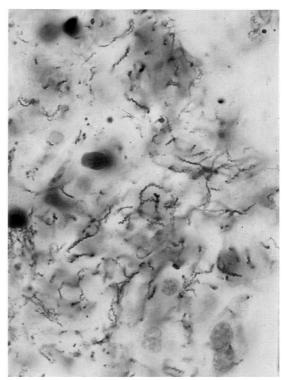

Figure 7–11. Congenital syphilis (Warthin-Starry). The silver stain demonstrates numerous elongated and helically coiled *Treponema* spirochetes. The organism is more difficult to identify in secondary and tertiary syphilis.

Tertiary

1. *Gumma formation:* Central necrosis is surrounded by a fibrous wall with adjacent chronic inflammatory infiltration, vascularization, and occasional giant cell formation.
2. Obliterative endarteritis occurs in small vessels adjacent to gumma.

Other Features

Congenital

1. Small epithelioid granulomas may be present in the parenchyma.
2. Regenerative changes are *not* present adjacent to interstitial fibrotic regions.
3. Focal necrosis and hepatocytolysis are present.

Secondary

1. Acute pericholangitic inflammatory reaction and portal edema are occasionally seen.
2. Epithelioid granulomas are present and usually perivenular.
3. Arterioles and venules may exhibit thickened walls.
4. Focal necrosis and hepatocytolysis occur, with infiltration by lymphocytes, eosinophils, and neutrophils.
5. Kupffer cell and endothelial cell hyperplasia is mild to moderate.
6. Cholestasis is rare.

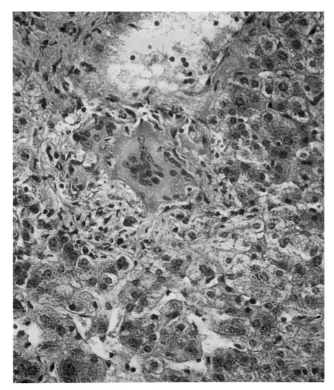

Figure 7–10. Secondary syphilis. A multinucleated giant cell surrounded by macrophages and lymphocytes is present immediately adjacent to a terminal hepatic vein.

Tertiary
1. Gummas may rarely undergo calcification.
2. Gummas may undergo severe fibrosis, with deep and relatively dense scar formation (*hepar lobatum*).
3. In some instances amyloid deposition may be seen.

Differential Diagnosis

1. *Neonatal giant cell hepatitis:* Congenital syphilis may exhibit prominent numbers of syncytial giant cells. Numerous organisms are typically demonstrated on silver stain.
2. *Granulomatous lesions of other etiologies* (e.g., *Brucella,* drug-induced): Vasculitis and demonstration of organisms in 50% of cases distinguish secondary syphilis from other etiologies.

Special Stain

1. *Warthin-Starry:* Silver stain demonstrates helically coiled *Treponema* with regular spirals around the axis. The degree of organism identification varies:
   a. *Congenital*—easily seen in vascular structures, fibrous tissue and focally within the parenchyma
   b. *Secondary*—difficult to identify but may be present in areas of necrosis in approximately 50% of cases
   c. *Tertiary*—scanty to absent

Immunohistochemistry

1. Antigenic determinants of *Treponema pallidum* may be demonstrated.

Clinical and Biologic Behavior

1. *Syphilis* is a highly infectious venereal disease caused by the obligate anaerobe spirochete *Treponema pallidum;* other *Treponema* species are normally present in the oral cavity (*T. macrodentium, T. ovale*) and genital region (*T. refringens*), while pathologic species include *T. pertenue* (yaws— a tropical disease), and *T. carateum* (pinta—a chronic skin disease).
2. Syphilis is most prevalent in the sexually active population in their early 20s.
3. Hepatic involvement can occur at any stage of the disease; 10% of patients in the secondary stage (hepatosplenomegaly, anemia, generalized lymphadenopathy, rash) have some degree of hepatic damage. Jaundice may be present, with moderate elevations of aminotransferase and alkaline phosphatase activities. This is the stage when most liver biopsies are performed.
4. Women acquiring syphilis in the third trimester of pregnancy may transmit the infection to the fetus; abortions and stillbirths are common, and although the infant may appear normal at birth, weeks to years later liver disease will become clinically manifest.
5. *Hepar lobatum* is a deeply scarred liver secondary to multiple fibrosed gumma and is often associated with ascites and varices; in the past this type of liver was erroneously confused with true cirrhosis.
6. The organism penetrates intact mucous membranes as well as defects in keratinized epithelium, forming a *chancre* (primary stage), which heals within 4 to 6 weeks. The secondary stage develops weeks to months later, followed by a latent period during which two thirds of the patients become spontaneously cured or remain asymptomatic; in the remaining one third, the tertiary stage will develop with gumma formation, aortic aneurysm, tabes dorsalis, and hepar lobatum.
7. Darkfield microscopy: Organisms can be identified on smears of moist lesions and chancre sores as thin 6 to 15 × 0.2-μm, tightly wound and corkscrew-shaped structures, with 4 to 14 uniform, rigid spirals exhibiting backward, forward, or corkscrew rotation about a long axis, sometimes with slight flexion.
8. Budd-Chiari syndrome has been described when a gumma forms immediately adjacent to the inferior vena cava and causes compression.

Prognosis

1. Consequences of tertiary disease, with cardiac insufficiency, neurologic abnormalities, and rarely portal hypertension, contribute to decreased survival.

References

Feher J, Somogyi T, Timmer M, et al. Early syphilitic hepatitis. Lancet 1975;2:896–899.

Lee RV, Thornton GF, Conn HO. Liver disease associated with secondary syphilis. N Engl J Med 1971;284:1423–1425.

Rein MF. Infections caused by *Treponema* (syphilis, yaws, pinta, bejel). In: Stein JH. Internal Medicine, 2nd ed. Boston: Little, Brown & Co, 1987:1719–1723.

Romen J, Rybak B, Dave P, et al. Spirochetal vasculitis and bile ductular damage in early hepatic syphilis. Am J Gastroenterol 1980;74:352–354.

■ Mycobacterium Infection

Tuberculosis

Major Morphologic Features

1. Portal and parenchymal epithelioid granulomas, often containing Langhans' multinucleated giant cells, are seen.
2. Central caseous necrosis of larger granulomas is indicative of active growth (acid-fast stain for *Mycobacterium tuberculosis* is often positive).

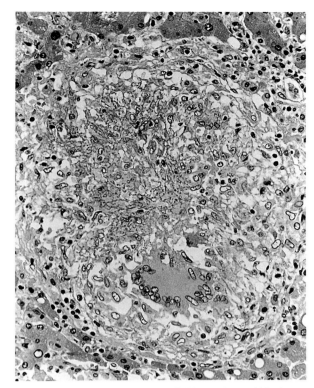

Figure 7–12. Tuberculosis. The epithelioid granuloma within the parenchyma consists of lymphocytes, enlarged macrophages, and Langhans' type multinucleated giant cell with peripherally located nuclei. Early necrosis is present above the giant cell and involves much of the granuloma.

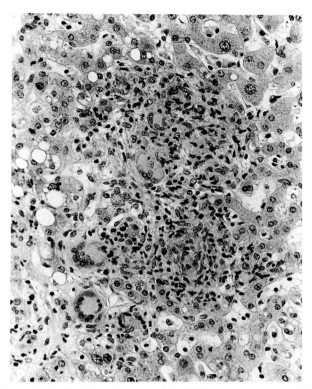

Figure 7–13. Bacillus Calmette-Guérin (BCG) immune response. The granulomas consist of numerous multinucleated giant cells, lymphocytes, and epithelioid cells. BCG, an immunostimulant derived from *Mycobacterium bovis,* elicits a granulomatous response in the liver morphologically identical to that caused by *M. tuberculosis.*

Other Features

1. Portal fibrosis is present in cases in which portal granulomas heal by fibrosis, occasionally with secondary calcification.
2. Granulomas are generally small without caseation; acid-fast stain is usually negative.
3. Focal hepatocytolysis and mild to moderate Kupffer cell hyperplasia are seen.
4. There are variable degrees of macrovesicular fatty change with no distinct zonal distribution; however, in cases of chronically ill patients, periportal fatty change is more common.
5. Cholestasis is uncommon.
6. In severe acute cases, a lymphocytic and neutrophilic destructive reaction can be seen in portal areas and parenchyma; acute cholangitis rarely may be demonstrated.

Differential Diagnosis

1. *Sarcoidosis:* Granulomas of sarcoid have a tendency to involve portal areas and often exhibit fibrous septate divisions. Sarcoidosis usually exhibits a greater inflammatory reaction in the parenchyma. Although a central type of necrosis may rarely be identified in sarcoid, acid-fast stains are always negative; in addition, asteroid and Schaumann bodies that are occasionally present in sarcoid granulomas are not seen in tuberculosis.
2. *Granulomatous reaction to other infectious agents:* Tuberculosis has well-defined epithelioid granulomas, while other organisms often have ill-defined granulomas (e.g., *Coxiella* in Q fever). Fungi within granulomas may be demonstrated by special stains (periodic acid–Schiff, methenamine silver). Caseous necrosis, when present, is typical, but not diagnostic, of tuberculosis.

Special Stain

1. *Acid-fast (Ziehl-Neelsen carbolfuchsin):* Bacilli stain deep red-purple and are most often seen in larger granulomas exhibiting caseous necrosis. When organisms are identified, usually only a small number are seen within a granuloma.

Clinical and Biologic Behavior

1. All *Mycobacterium* species have the following characteristics:

a. The organisms resist decolorization with acid-alcohol (''acid-fast'') after staining with carbolfuchsin.
b. The growth rates are relatively slow.
c. The organisms are obligate aerobes.
d. A granulomatous reaction is evoked.
2. Of all causes of granulomatous involvement of the liver, tuberculosis (*M. tuberculosis*) is the second most common (26.6%) at the University of Southern California Liver Unit, with the most common being sarcoidosis (28.3%).
3. Within 1 year of exposure, 3% to 5% of patients will develop clinical disease, while the remaining are asymptomatic with a positive skin test. Five percent of these will develop clinically active tuberculosis at a later time, and these cases are responsible for 95% of new cases per year.
4. Pulmonary disease is present in 84% of the cases; the incidence of hepatic involvement is as follows:

Percent	Type
71	Primary acute pulmonary
95	Miliary
25	Chronic pulmonary
Rare	Tuberculoma (aggregates of granulomas forming abscess)
Rare	Cholangitis (secondary to ruptured caseous granuloma into intrahepatic biliary system)

5. In only 1% of granulomas on liver biopsy can caseous necrosis be demonstrated; positive acid-fast staining is also relatively uncommon, and culture is positive in approximately 10% of cases.
6. Significant hepatic dysfunction is seldom present, with hepatomegaly (50%) and splenomegaly (25%–40%) usually the only physical signs of liver disease; biopsy is usually performed during workup of fever of unknown origin or for investigation of possible dissemination of pulmonary disease.
7. Laboratory values show elevation of alkaline phosphatase in 75% of cases with hepatic involvement; aminotransferase elevations are variable but low.
8. Infection of the fetus may occur by way of the umbilical cord from an infected mother, with the lesions often occurring in the porta hepatis as well as the parenchyma.
9. Bacillus Calmette-Guérin (BCG), an immunostimulant derived from a strain of *M. bovis* and used to vaccinate against tuberculosis in certain populations at high risk of infection, evokes an identical granulomatous response in the liver.
10. Mechanism of the granulomatous reaction: The organism (beaded rod 1–4 μm in length) is spread through the air, with the smaller droplets (<5 μm in diameter) entering and remaining in the pulmonary alveolar spaces; organisms are ingested by macrophages. Hematogenous spread and seeding of organs (brain, liver, joints) occur when organisms gain access to the bloodstream. Hypersensitivity develops 30 to 50 days after contact, at which time sensitized T lymphocytes evoke a granulomatous reaction, halting proliferation but not elimination of the organism.

Prognosis

1. Tuberculous involvement of the liver is rarely responsible for death.
2. Mortality in the United States is 1.4/100,000 but much higher in certain endemic areas (e.g., Philippines), where associated malnutrition may play a role.

References

Alexander JF, Galambos JT. Granulomatous hepatitis: The usefulness of liver biopsy in the diagnosis of tuberculosis and sarcoidosis. Am J Gastroenterol 1973;59:23–30.
Alvarez SZ, Carpio R. Hepatobiliary tuberculosis. Dig Dis Sci 1983;28:193–200.
Hopewell PC. Tuberculosis and nontuberculous mycobacterial infections. In: Stein JH, Internal Medicine, 2nd ed. Boston: Little, Brown & Co, 1987:1731–1746.
Hunt JS, Silverstein MJ, Sparks FC, et al. Granulomatous hepatitis: A complication of BCG immunotherapy. Lancet 1973;2:820–821.

Mycobacterium avium-intracellulare (MAI) Infection

Major Morphologic Features

1. Well to poorly defined small to medium-sized granulomatous lesions composed of histiocytes, lymphocytes, and occasional neutrophils are distributed in both portal tracts and parenchyma.
2. In immunocompromised patients, granulomas predominantly consist of foamy histiocytes.

Other Features

1. Portal mononuclear inflammatory infiltration is mild with no distinct bile duct changes; in immunocompromised patients, the portal reaction is minimal to absent.
2. Kupffer cell hyperplasia is mild.
3. Multinucleated giant cells may be present within the granulomas but are usually absent in immunocompromised patients.
4. No zonal orientation of the granulomatous lesions occurs.

Differential Diagnosis

1. *Granuloma formation secondary to M. tuberculosis:* Granulomas in tuberculosis are well defined, often with giant cell formation. Caseous necrosis may be

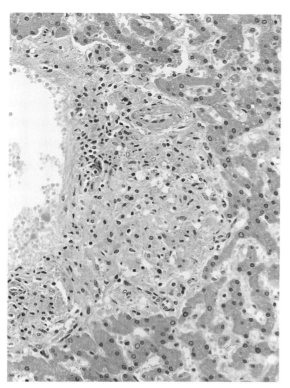

Figure 7-14. Mycobacterium avium-intracellulare infection (immunocompromised patient). A granuloma is present within a portal tract, and is composed of histiocytes having a foamy cytoplasm. The parenchyma exhibits an intact cord-sinusoid pattern, with no Kupffer cell hyperplasia or inflammatory infiltrate.

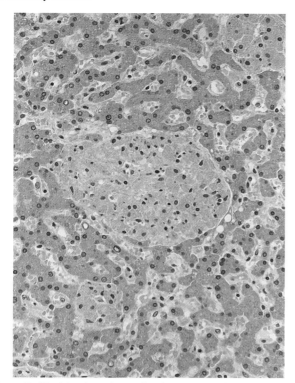

Figure 7-15. Mycobacterium avium-intracellulare infection (immunocompromised patient). A well-defined granuloma in the parenchyma is composed entirely of histiocytes having abundant foamy cytoplasm. Two smaller granulomas are also present.

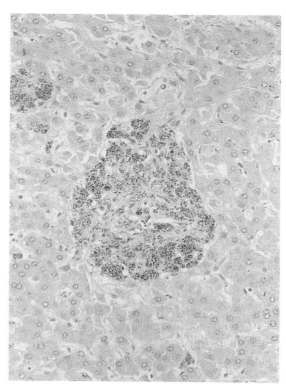

Figure 7-16. Mycobacterium avium-intracellulare infection (immunocompromised patient; acid-fast). All histiocytes comprising the granuloma are packed with acid-fast organisms, which also are positive with periodic acid–Schiff stain.

present in the larger granulomas. Although granulomas secondary to MAI may be indistinguishable from those seen in tuberculosis, in immunocompromised patients (e.g., those with the acquired immunodeficiency syndrome) giant cells are rare and caseous necrosis is not present. Tuberculosis seldom exhibits acid-fast bacilli on special stains in liver biopsy specimens, and when present the numbers of organisms are usually scanty. In contrast, granulomas in MAI infection, especially in immunocompromised patients, exhibit abundant numbers of acid-fast organisms that also stain positively with periodic acid–Schiff.

2. *Lesions with parenchymal histiocytic aggregates:* Lesions seen in Gaucher's disease, histiocytosis X, certain malignancies, and other nontuberculous granulomatous infections may resemble the lesions seen in MAI infection. Acid-fast and periodic acid–Schiff stains will rule out most of the above, and culture will differentiate between the different *Mycobacterium* species.

Special Stains

1. *Acid-fast (Ziehl-Neelsen carbolfuchsin):* Organisms are identified within both granulomas and individual Kupffer cells and are most abundant in immunocompromised patients.

2. *Periodic acid–Schiff:* Bacilli also are PAS positive (in contrast to *M. tuberculosis*).

Clinical and Biologic Behavior

1. *Mycobacterium-avium* complex (including *M. intracellulare*) is a slow-growing nontuberculous organism that may produce serious pulmonary dysfunction similar to tuberculosis but more often is clinically nonpathogenic; it commonly occurs, however, as a disseminated infection in patients with acquired immunodeficiency syndrome.
2. The infection in nonimmunocompromised patients is highly endemic in southeastern United States, western Australia, and Japan.
3. Hepatic involvement is present in over 50% of the cases when the organism is cultured in other organ systems; hepatomegaly, slight increases in aminotransferase and alkaline phosphatase activities, and normal bilirubin levels are generally the only hepatic manifestations of the disease.

Treatment and Prognosis

1. Response to multiple (usually four or five) drug combinations is often unsatisfactory in patients without the acquired immunodeficiency syndrome.
2. In acquired immunodeficiency syndrome, response to therapy is usually dismal; concomitant infection with cytomegalovirus, *Pneumocystis,* herpes, *Candida,* and numerous bacteria (*Staphylococcus aureus, Pseudomonas, Klebsiella, Salmonella*) makes assessment of treatment difficult.

References

Glasgow BJ, Anders K, Layfield LJ, et al. Clinical and pathologic findings of the liver in the acquired immune deficiency syndrome (AIDS). Am J Clin Pathol 1985;83:582–588.

Greene JB, Gurdip SS, Lewin S, et al. *Mycobacterium avium-intracellulare:* A cause of disseminated life-threatening infection in homosexuals and drug abusers. Ann Intern Med 1982;97:539–546.

Hopewell PC. Tuberculous and nontuberculous mycobacterial infections. In: Stein JH, ed. Internal Medicine, 2nd ed. Boston: Little, Brown & Co, 1987:1746–1748.

Reichert CM, O'Leary TJ, Levens DL, et al. Autopsy pathology in the acquired immune deficiency syndrome. Am J Pathol 1983;112:357–382.

Leprosy

Major Morphologic Features

1. *Tuberculoid type:* Well-formed epithelioid granulomas containing moderate numbers of lymphocytes, often with multinucleated giant cells, are present.
2. *Lepromatous type:* Collections of foamy, vacuolated histiocytes are seen in portal and parenchymal re-

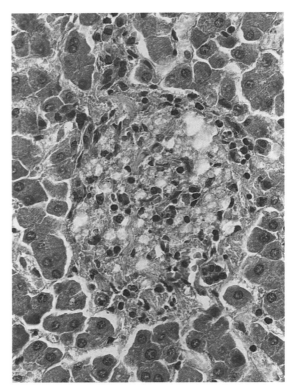

Figure 7–17. Leprosy, lepromatous type. The portal tract contains a large collection of both foamy and vacuolated histiocytes. Giant cells and lymphocytes are not present. These granulomas may also appear within the parenchyma.

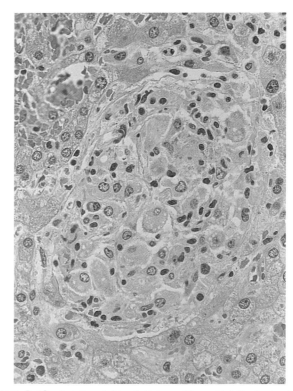

Figure 7–18. Leprosy, tuberculoid type. The well-defined granuloma within the parenchyma consists of numerous epithelioid histiocytes and scattered lymphocytes. Although not present in this photomicrograph, the granulomas may also contain multinucleated giant cells.

gions, with minimal to absent lymphocytic reaction and no giant cell formation.

3. *Intermediate type:* Granulomas exhibit epithelioid cells, but few lymphocytes; multinucleated giant cells are absent.

Other Features

1. Variable degrees of portal lymphocytic infiltration and hyperplasia are present.
2. Kupffer cell hyperplasia is mild.
3. Granulomas are more numerous in the lepromatous type.

Differential Diagnosis

1. *Noncaseating granulomas secondary to M. tuberculosis infection, sarcoidosis:* The tuberculoid type of granulomatous lesion seen in leprosy is similar to granulomas present in both of these entities; however, caseous necrosis of larger granulomas in tuberculosis, and septate and fibrotic granulomas of sarcoidosis, are not features of leprosy.

Special Stains

1. *Acid-fast (Ziehl-Neelsen carbolfuchsin, Fite):* Viable organisms (*M. leprae*) stain positively as parallel bacilli or globular masses; nonviable organisms are broken, beaded, or stain negatively.
   a. Tuberculoid type: Acid-fast stain is negative.
   b. Lepromatous type: Florid numbers of organisms occur in granulomas, portal macrophages, endothelial cells, Kupffer cells, and occasionally hepatocytes.
2. *Methenamine silver:* Positive staining occurs of nonviable organisms that are acid-fast negative.

Clinical and Biologic Behavior

1. *M. leprae* is an acid-fast obligate intracellular organism causing typical ulcerated skin lesions and associated neurotropic injury.
2. There are an estimated 15 to 20 million infected persons living predominantly in tropical and warm climate regions throughout the world. In the United States the disease may be found in residents of the southeastern states as well as in immigrants from the tropics, Philippines, Samoa, and Mexico.
3. Humans are the only reservoir of the bacillus, which is spread by release of organisms from skin lesions and from oronasal passageways through sneezing or coughing.
4. Hepatic granulomas are present from 10% to 90% of

the time, most frequently seen in the lepromatous type.
5. Although serum aminotransferase values may be slightly elevated, there are no clinical symptoms specific for hepatic dysfunction.
6. Type of reaction depends on the host response: tuberculoid type has heightened immune response and lepromatous type has increased immune tolerance.
7. Systemic amyloidosis is a frequent complication (46%) of chronic infection in the lepromatous type.

Treatment and Prognosis

1. Organisms may persist in histiocytes even after apparant cure.
2. Morbidity relates to nerve destruction, with localized damage in tuberculoid type and diffuse neuropathic injury leading to ulceration and loss of digits or extremities and disfigurement in lepromatous type. Blindness from exposure, keratitis, and amyloidosis can occur. Immune complex disease can be seen in lepromatous leprosy (no delayed hypersensitivity but abundant antibody response).

References

Chen TSN, Drutz DJ, Whelan GR. Hepatic granulomas in leprosy: Their relation to bacteremia. Arch Pathol Lab Med 1976;100:182–185.

Cooke M. Inections caused by *Mycobacterium leprae* (leprosy). In: Stein JH, ed. Internal Medicine, 2nd ed. Boston: Little, Brown & Co, 1987;1748–1752.

Desikan KV, Job CK. A review of postmortem findings in 37 cases of leprosy. Int J Leprosy 1968;36:32–44.

Karat ABA, Job CK, Rao PSS. Liver in leprosy: Histological and biochemical findings. Br Med J 1971;1:307–310.

Powell CS, Swan LL. Leprosy: Pathologic changes observed in fifty consecutive necropsies. Am J Pathol 1955;31:1131–1147.

■ Rickettsial Infection

Q Fever

Major Morphologic Features

1. Granulomatous necrosis within the parenchyma consists of lymphocytes, histiocytes, occasional eosinophils, and neutrophils, with a ring of fibrin surrounding a centrally located fat vacuole (lipogranuloma or ''*doughnut*'' lesion).

Other Features

1. Portal areas are widened but generally not fibrotic, with moderate numbers of lymphocytes and plasma cells.
2. Small foci of necrosis and hepatocytolysis are scattered throughout the parenchyma, often with plasma cell infiltration.

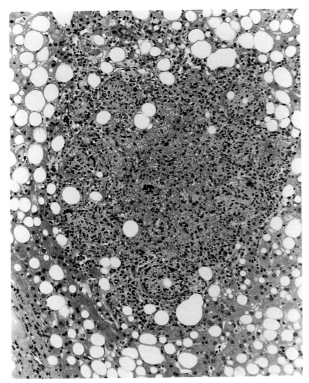

Figure 7–19. Q fever. The parenchyma exhibits a large aggregate of multinucleated giant cells, histiocytes, lymphocytes, plasma cells, and occasional neutrophils and eosinophils. Prominent macrovesicular fat is present in adjacent hepatocytes.

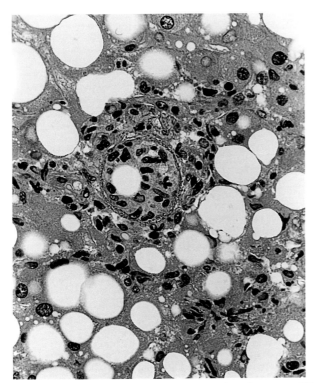

Figure 7–20. Q fever. A small inflammatory granuloma is present within the lobule and consists of histiocytes, lymphocytes, and occasional neutrophils. A uniformly circular ring of fibrin is present within the granuloma, as is a central fat vacuole (characteristic ''doughnut'' lesion).

3. Granulomatous necrosis may not exhibit fat and may be composed entirely of fibrin and inflammatory cells.
4. Inflammatory infiltrates may aggregate, forming large necroinflammatory lesions involving a large portion of the lobule.
5. Granulomas may exhibit a multinucleated giant cell reaction.
6. Granulomatous lesions may exhibit fibrous scarring after resolution.
7. Macrovesicular fat of variable degrees, with no zonal distribution, is present.
8. Kupffer cell hyperplasia is prominent.

Differential Diagnosis

1. *Bacterial infections:* Portal and nonspecific parenchymal inflammatory infiltration with plasma cells and occasional eosinophils and neutrophils can be seen in various bacterial infections. Presence of ''doughnut'' lesion is characteristic, although not diagnostic, for Q fever.
2. *Other conditions that may contain similar lipogranulomatous lesions:* Hodgkin's and non-Hodgkin's lymphomas, infectious mononucleosis, tuberculosis, cytomegalovirus, and *Salmonella* infections may rarely show somewhat similar types of lesions. A fibrin ring is usually not seen in these conditions.

Special Stain

1. *Phosphotungstic acid hematoxylin:* Stains fibrin ring of granulomatous lesion.

Clinical and Biologic Behavior

1. *Coxiella burnetti,* a pleomorphic intracellular organism, is the etiologic agent for Q fever, first described in Australia in slaughterhouse and dairy farm workers; *Coxiella* infection is classified as rickettsial, the more common of which in the United States is *R. rickettsii,* the etiologic agent for Rocky Mountain spotted fever (i.e., liver necrosis that is usually mild).
2. The organism may be transferred by an arthropod vector (tick) but is most often acquired by rural workers and meat handlers through inhalation and less commonly by ingestion of infected food products derived from cattle, goats, sheep, and birds.
3. Although Q fever is primarily a respiratory tract infection, patients present with fever, headache, and often abnormal liver tests. Hepatomegaly (65%), which may be tender (11%), is the only significant finding; jaundice is infrequent (6%).
4. Liver test results are abnormal in 85% of cases, with

elevation of serum aminotransferase levels (three to four times normal) and alkaline phosphatase activity (usually twice normal). Phase II *C. burnetti* antibody by complement fixation is usually markedly elevated and helpful in the diagnosis. Direct immunofluorescence of liver biopsy using anti–*C. burnetti* antibody is not conclusive.

5. In chronic forms of Q fever, portal fibrosis and cirrhosis have been reported but a causal relationship is not clear.

Treatment and Prognosis

1. Antibiotic therapy will usually eradicate the disease; in untreated cases, the overall mortality is 5%, with death not directly caused by hepatic involvement.

References

Bernstein M, Edmondson HA, Barbour BH. The liver lesion in Q fever: Clinical and pathologic features. Arch Intern Med 1965;116:491–498.

Clark WH, Lenette EH, Railsback OC, et al. Q fever in California: VII. Clinical features in 180 cases. Arch Intern Med 1951;88:155–167.

Hofmann CE, Heaton JW Jr. Q fever hepatitis: Clinical manifestations and pathological findings. Gastroenterology 1982;83:474–479.

Pellgrin M, Delsol G, Auvergnat JC, et al. Granulomatous hepatitis in Q fever. Hum Pathol 1980;11:52–57.

Travis LB, Travis WD, Li C-Y, et al. Q fever: A clinicopathologic study of five cases. Arch Pathol Lab Med 1986;110:1017–1020.

■ Fungal Infection

Histoplasmosis

Major Morphologic Features

1. Granuloma formation within the parenchyma consists of inflammatory and epithelioid histiocytes; multinucleated cells are uncommon.
2. Intracytoplasmic encapsulated organisms 2 to 5 μm in diameter, with retracted clear space (''halo''), are present within histocytes and Kupffer cells in active lesions.
3. Fibrotic and calcified granulomas occur with resolution.

Other Features

1. Granulomas may exhibit central necrosis, with the larger nodules 1 to 3 mm in diameter surrounded by granulation tissue.
2. In rare instances granulomas contain Schaumann bodies (laminated concretions of calcium and protein) and asteroid bodies (stellate-shaped inclusions within cytoplasm).
3. Ossification is rarely identified in calcified granulomas.

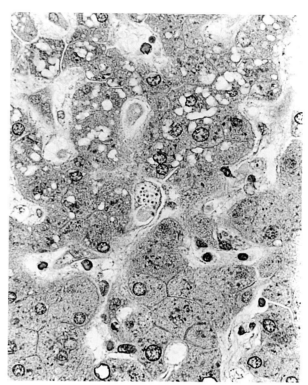

Figure 7–21. Histoplasmosis. Small intracytoplasmic organisms with a surrounding retracted clear space (halo appearance) is present in a Kupffer cell. Occasional hepatocytes contain numerous droplets of microvesicular fat.

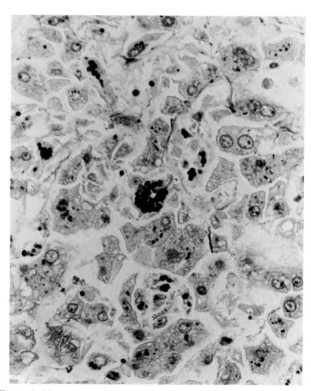

Figure 7–22. Histoplasmosis (methenamine silver). The positively staining fungi are round and uniform and seen in the majority of Kupffer cells. The irregular granular staining within hepatocytes does not represent organisms.

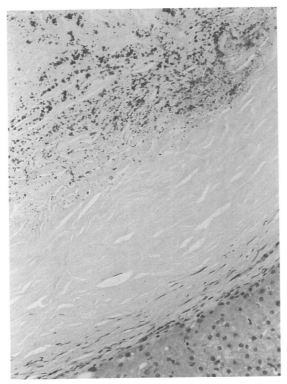

Figure 7–23. Histoplasmosis. A fibrotic granuloma, in this instance relatively acellular with calcification (*above*), is characteristic of resolution.

4. Portal tracts are normal or exhibit mild nonspecific inflammatory infiltration and bile duct proliferation.
5. Inflammatory reaction in immunocompromised patients may be minimal to absent, with abundant numbers of organisms present in hypertrophic Kupffer cells.

Differential Diagnosis

1. *Tuberculosis:* Central caseous necrosis may occur in both conditions. Identification of organisms by special stains and culture is necessary for diagnosis.
2. *Sarcoidosis:* Schaumann and asteroid bodies are characteristic, although not diagnostic, of sarcoid granulomas but can be seen in both conditions. Identification and culture of organisms are essential.
3. *Leishmaniasis: Leishmania donovani* are small intracytoplasmic parasites 2 to 3 μm in diameter present within Kupffer cells. Although resembling *Histoplasma capsulatum,* this organism does not stain with periodic acid–Schiff or methenamine silver.

Special Stains

1. *Periodic acid–Schiff, methenamine silver:* These stains are positive for the thin wall of the round to oval and occasionally budding yeast form. The

"halo" effect seen on hematoxylin and eosin stain is negative.

Clinical and Biologic Behavior

1. Histoplasmosis occurs worldwide and is caused by the dimorphic fungus *Histoplasma capsulatum.*
2. The disease is highly endemic in the Ohio and Mississippi River Valleys and in Guatemala, Mexico, Venezuela, and Peru.
3. The main carriers are birds, especially chickens, with spores present in bird droppings. Inhalation of the spores with development of yeast forms in the lung results in respiratory infection; spread of the organism through the blood and lymphatics may then lead to dissemination and hepatic involvement.
4. The organisms are 2 to 5 μm in diameter and reside in macrophages and Kupffer cells; on blood smear or aspirate, the organism has a basophilic cytoplasm that shows retraction from one side of a thin but rigid wall, giving a crescent or halo appearance.
5. Histoplasmosis is asymptomatic 90% of the time or presents as only a mild flulike illness, resolving without complication; depending on the host's immune status and the number of infecting organisms, this infection may present as an acute pulmonary illness and in less than 1% of cases may disseminate or become chronic.
6. Laboratory test results are nonspecific and show only mild elevations of serum aminotransferase levels and alkaline phosphatase activity.
7. In the *disseminated* form usually seen in immunocompromised or suppressed hosts, hepatosplenomegaly is almost always present; in chronic forms, hepatomegaly occurs in approximately one half of the cases and splenomegaly in one third.
8. *Hepatic candidiasis* may also occur as part of disseminated fungal infection in immunocompromised persons, forming granulomas or microabscesses; these fungi are identified in liver biopsy specimens by their characteristic hyphae (gram-positive pseudomycelial elements).

Prognosis

1. Mortality is high in clinically manifest acute, chronic, or disseminated infections (excludes mildly symptomatic patients) when not treated.

References

Graybill JR. Infections caused by fungi and the higher bacteria (actinomycosis and nocardiosis). In: Stein JH, ed. Internal Medicine, 2nd ed. Boston: Little, Brown & Co, 1987:1752–1756.

Mandell W, Goldberg DM, Neu HC. Histoplasmosis in patients with the acquired immune deficiency syndrome. Am J Med 1986;974–978.

Smith, JW, Utz JP. Progressive disseminated histoplasmosis. Ann Intern Med 1972;76:557–565.

Coccidioidomycoses

Major Morphologic Features

1. Epithelioid granuloma formation occurs with multinucleated giant cells containing characteristic spherules:
   a. 20 to 200 μm in diameter with wall 2 μm thick
   b. Filled with either endospores 2 to 5 μm in diameter or granular eosinophilic material

Other Features

1. Spherules may rupture, with endospores present immediately outside empty and often distorted spherules.
2. Smaller immature spherules 10 to 20 μm in diameter may also be present.
3. Although granulomas undergo some degree of fibrosis during resolution, calcification is not seen.
4. Portal tracts are normal or exhibit mild nonspecific inflammatory infiltration and bile duct proliferation.

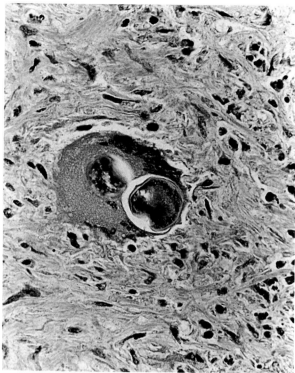

Figure 7–25. Coccidioidomycosis. High power shows the giant cell to contain a large spherule 80 to 100 μm in diameter that is filled with a granular eosinophilic material. The wall of the spherule is approximately 2 μm thick. Although not in this photomicrograph, the spherules may also contain endospores 2 to 5 μm in diameter.

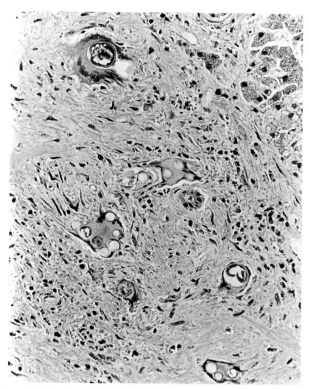

Figure 7–24. Coccidioidomycosis. Multinucleated giant cells are present within a fibrotic matrix containing a mild lymphocytic infiltrate.

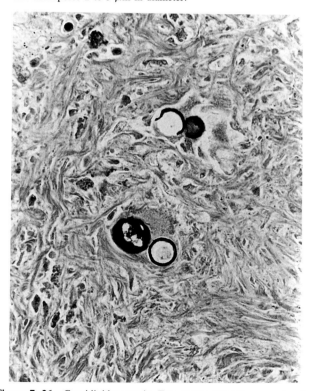

Figure 7–26. Coccidioidomycosis. Two empty spherules, one showing rupture of the cell wall, are present and represent release of the endospores. The two dark-staining immature spherules are relatively small and at times may be confused with nonbudding forms of *Blastomyces dermatitidis*.

Differential Diagnosis

1. *Tuberculosis, sarcoidosis:* Granulomas may morphologically be quite similar on hematoxylin and eosin stain. Special stains for identification of organisms may be necessary for diagnosis. In addition, division of granulomas by fibrous septa is often present in portal granulomas of sarcoidosis.
2. *Blastomycosis:* The small, immature spherules of *Coccidioides* may resemble the yeast form of *Blastomyces dermitiditis. Blastomyces* has a characteristic budding pattern and lacks the presence of large spherules seen in *Coccidioides* infection.

Special Stains

1. *Periodic acid–Schiff, methenamine silver:* The thick wall of the spherule stains positively, as well as the thin walls of the endospores.

Clinical and Biologic Behavior

1. *Coccidioides immitis* causes a benign, usually asymptomatic self-limited pulmonary infection, with no hepatic involvement.
2. The organism is endemic in southwestern United States, northern Mexico, and Central and South America.
3. Five per cent of the patients develop severe pulmonary injury, often with cavitation; less than 1% develop disseminated infection with multiple organ-system involvement.
4. Conditions related to severity include the following:
   a. Degree of intensity of exposure to organism
   b. Racial susceptibility (infection more frequent in blacks, Mexicans, and Filipinos)
   c. More frequent in immunocompromised patients (e.g., those with the acquired immunodeficiency syndrome)
   d. More severe in pregnant women
5. Hepatic involvement is usually present in disseminated infection; however, there are only mild serum aminotransferase elevations, consistent with minimal hepatic dysfunction.
6. Peritonitis presenting with ascites and fever has been reported, and at laparoscopy small white nodules similar to and confused with *Mycobacterium tuberculosis* can be seen on the parietal peritoneum.

Prognosis

1. In the disseminated form, fatality is greater than 50% if the infection is not treated.

References

Ampel NM, Ryan KJ, Carry PJ, et al. Fungemia due to *Coccidioides immitis:* An analysis of 16 episodes in 15 patients and a review of the literature. Medicine 1986;65:312–321.
Bronnimann DA, Adam RD, Galgiani JN, et al. Coccidioidomycosis in the acquired immunodeficiency syndrome. Ann Intern Med 1987;106:372–379.
Graybill JR. Infections caused by fungi and the higher bacteria (actinomycosis and nocardiosis). In: Stein JH, ed. Internal Medicine, 2nd ed. Boston: Little, Brown & Co, 1987:1756–1760.

■ Parasite Infection

Amebic Abscess

Major Morphologic Features

1. Cyst (abscess) formation is present with a fibrous wall and the following contents:
   a. Hepatocytes undergoing coagulative necrosis
   b. Amorphous eosinophilic debris (lysed liver cells)
   c. Trophozoites identifiable at edge of cyst wall:
      1) Round to oval, 10 to 60 μm in diameter
      2) Spherical nuclei approximately one fifth of the size of the organism
      3) Eosinophilic cytoplasm, often containing phagocytized debris and red blood cells
      4) If viable, surrounded by clear space (halo)
2. Minimal to absent inflammatory reaction occurs within abscess cavity and wall.

Other Features

1. Parasites may occasionally be identified in hepatic lobules immediately adjacent to the abscess, predominantly in sinusoids or in areas of focal necrosis.
2. Variable degrees of sinusoidal fibrosis occur in compressed lobules adjacent to the abscess wall.
3. Cholestasis is uncommon but occurs in instances of a large abscess compressing and obstructing large intrahepatic bile ducts.
4. Earliest change is focal necrosis with neutrophilic infiltration, eventually giving way to variable degrees of mononuclear inflammatory infiltration and formation of a rim of granulation tissue around necrotic debris.
5. Kupffer cell hyperplasia, focal hepatocytolysis, and macrovesicular fatty change are present in lobules distant to the abscess.
6. Prominent neutrophilic infiltration of the abscess occurs in the rare instances of bacterial superinfection.

Differential Diagnosis

1. *Amebic* and *pyogenic abscesses:* See page 107.
2. *Necrotic tumor mass:* Tumor cells that have under-

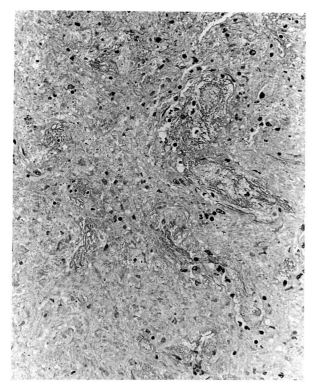

Figure 7–27. Amebiasis. The necrotic material present within an abscess is composed of a relatively amorphous eosinophilic debris owing to lysis of the hepatocytes. The inflammatory reaction is minimal.

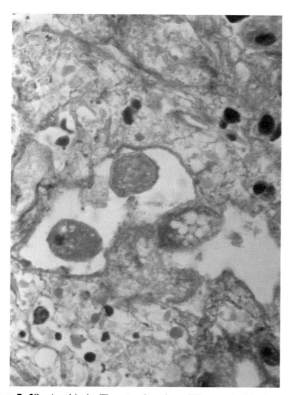

Figure 7–28. Amebiasis. Three trophozoites of *Entamoeba histolytica* are present at the edge of the cyst. The round to oval eosinophilic organisms measure approximately 50 μm in diameter, although the range for *E. histolytica* varies from 10 to 60 μm. A small spherical nucleus is present in one parasite (*left*), while another (*right*) contains a vacuolated cytoplasm.

gone ischemic necrosis, and necrotic hepatocytes in amebic abscesses, may appear morphologically similar. Trophozoites are usually not demonstrable in necrotic regions distant from the fibrous capsule, and in aspirated material, trophozoites are identified in only 20% to 50% of cases. Necrotic tumor may have a neutrophilic infiltration, a finding not typically seen in amebic abscesses. Examination of other tissue sections of the mass lesion for viable tumor, or tissue containing trophozoites, is often necessary.

Special Stains

1. *Periodic acid–Schiff:* Cytoplasmic staining of the trophozoite is positive.
2. *Gridley:* Organisms stain blue-green.

Immunohistochemistry

1. Immunoperoxidase and immunofluorescent staining may be helpful in identification of specific organisms.

Clinical and Biologic Behavior

1. *Entamoeba histolytica* is a microaerophilic protozoa present predominantly in the tropic and subtropical regions as an intestinal parasite, with a prevalence ranging from 5% to 50%, compared with 1% to 3% in industrialized countries.
2. In the United States, the disease is found more commonly in homosexuals, immigrants, refugees, and foreign travelers (Mexico).
3. The predominant clinical manifestation of amebic infection is colitis, often with typical flask-shaped ulcerations; the most common extraintestinal manifestation is hepatic abscess, occurring predominantly in men 40 to 60 years of age.
4. Access of the parasites into the portal venous system from the intestine leads to hepatic involvement; although most organisms initially do not lodge in the sinusoids, with time sinusoidal thrombosis traps the amebae which then invade the hepatic cords, release cytotoxins, and destroy liver cells.
5. Abscesses are usually single, range from 8 to 12 cm in diameter, and affect the right lobe approximately 70% of the time.
6. Clinical onset is gradual, with hepatomegaly and right upper quadrant tenderness; fever is usually present, and abdominal tenderness is sometimes referred to the shoulder when the abscess is adjacent to the diaphragm. About one half of patients presenting with hepatic abscess have no clinical symptoms of intestinal disease.

7. Laboratory tests reveal increased levels of serum aminotransferase (<100 IU/L) in 50% and of alkaline phosphatase in 80% of patients; hyperbilirubinemia is rare. Neutrophilic leukocytosis (>20,000/mm³) is present in about 50% but without eosinophilia. Amebic serology is positive in 95% of patients, with a 94% sensitivity of the indirect hemagglutination test.

8. With response to treatment, resolution occurs by shrinkage of the abscess and eventual complete obliteration or stellate scar formation.

9. Complications include systemic dissemination leading to pulmonary or cerebral abscesses; rupture into the pleural, pericardial, or peritoneal cavities; and fulminant infection. Hepatic failure is rare.

Aspiration Cytology

1. An "anchovy" chocolate-colored, non-foul-smelling pastelike material (bacterial culture negative) is present.
2. Contents may be cream colored owing to a combination of necrotic cells, bile, fat, red blood cells, and neutrophilic infiltration (secondary bacterial superinfection).
3. Trophozoite characteristics include the following:
   a. Usually 15 to 30 μm in diameter (range, 10–60 μm)
   b. Eosinophilic, refractile cytoplasm occasionally containing necrotic debris and red blood cells
   c. Single, eccentric nucleus with single karyosome and fine chromatin granules
4. Trophozoites are identified within aspirated contents in 20% to 50% of cases.

Prognosis

1. Mortality is increased in immunocompromised patients or if rupture into the pericardium or peritoneum occurs.

References

Brandt H, Perez Tamayo R. Pathology of human amebiasis. Hum Pathol 1970;1:351–385.

Datta DV, Saha S, Singh SA, et al. The clinical pattern and prognosis of patients with amebic liver abscess and jaundice. Am J Dig Dis 1973;18:887–898.

DeCock KM, Reynolds TB. Amebic and pyogenic liver abscess. In: Schiff L, Schiff ER, eds. Diseases of the Liver, 6th ed. Philadelphia: J.B. Lippincott 1987:1235–1253.

Leech JH. Infections caused by protozoa. In: Stein JH, ed. Internal Medicine, 2nd ed. Boston: Little, Brown & Co, 1987:1781–1785.

Malaria

Major Morphologic Features

1. Dark brown to gray-black pigment (*hemozoin*) is seen in Kupffer cells and, in later stages, in portal macrophages.
2. Sinusoidal congestion, with parasites (ring forms of *Plasmodium falciparum*) occurs in Kupffer cells and red blood cells.
3. Kupffer cell hyperplasia and hypertrophy may be marked.

Other Features

1. Portal infiltration by lymphocytes occurs accompanied by scanty numbers of histiocytes and plasma cells.
2. Focal hepatocytolysis is present.
3. In acute stages, sinusoidal congestion can be marked as parasitized red blood cells hug the sinusoidal border; focal areas of perivenular coagulative (anoxic) necrosis may be present.

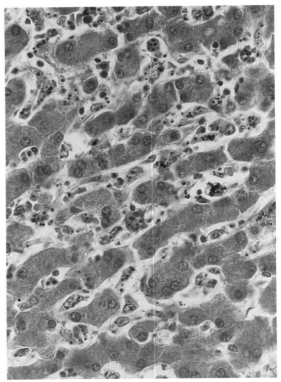

Figure 7–29. Malaria. The hyperplastic and hypertrophic Kupffer cells are filled with a granular dark brown to gray-black pigment (*hemozoin*, derived from breakdown of hemoglobin by *Plasmodium falciparum*), easily differentiated from hemosiderin by staining negatively with the Prussian blue iron reaction.

4. In resolving cases, hemozoin pigment is present only in portal macrophages, which eventually disappear.
5. Variable degrees of hemosiderin in Kupffer cells (secondary to hemolysis of red blood cells) are noted; hemosiderin may also be present in hepatocytes, predominantly periportal, in chronic infection (secondary to anemia).
6. Fatty change of macrovesicular type is mild.
7. Portal fibrosis is not typically seen; however, stellate fibrosis is described in long-term infection.
8. *Tropical splenomegaly syndrome* (hyperimmune reaction) includes the following:
   a. Marked portal lymphocytic infiltration and hyperplasia
   b. Mild portal fibrosis
   c. Lymphocytes in clusters or in single-file pattern within sinusoids
   d. Scanty to absent hemozoin pigment

Differential Diagnosis

1. *Disorders associated with marked hemosiderin deposition in Kupffer cells:* Patients with chronic hemolytic disorders (e.g., thalassemia major) or those having received multiple transfusions may accumulate considerable amounts of hemosiderin within Kupffer cells. Hemozoin is sharply defined, brown-black, birefringent, and negative on Prussian blue stain for iron, while hemosiderin is golden-brown and stains positively with Prussian blue. Both pigments may be present, however, within the same Kupffer cell.
2. *Schistosomiasis:* Schistosomal pigment resembles hemozoin on hematoxylin and eosin stain and is also negative with the Prussian blue stain. These pigments are different ultrastructurally and biochemically. Liver biopsy specimens will exhibit morphologic features of schistosomiasis, such as portal fibrosis, granuloma formation, and *Schistosoma* ova.
3. *Infectious mononucleosis (Epstein-Barr, cytomegalovirus infections), lymphocytic leukemia:* Chronic immune stimulation directed to the parasite (*tropical splenomegaly syndrome*) results in a prominent lymphocytic infiltration of portal and sinusoidal regions and often resembles infectious mononucleosis or even lymphocytic leukemia. Clinical and laboratory data, serology, and detection of antibodies to malarial antigens may be necessary for diagnosis.
4. *Anthracotic pigment:* Black anthracotic pigment may be seen in the liver in instances when thoracic lymph nodes containing this pigment rupture into adjacent pulmonary veins. The pigment then becomes phagocytized by Kupffer cells and morphologically resembles hemozoin. Unlike anthracotic pigment, hemozoin is birefringent.

Special Stain

1. *Prussian blue:* Hemozoin does *not* stain for iron in routine sections and is therefore useful to differentiate from hemosiderin.

Immunohistochemistry

1. Immunoperoxidase and immunofluorescent staining can identify antigens to specific *Plasmodium* species.

Clinical and Biologic Behavior

1. *Plasmodium* species are the most common parasitic infection worldwide, with over 100 million cases per year, and 1 million deaths per year in Africa alone.
2. Malaria is mainly found in tropical and subtropical regions and is most prevalent in sub-Saharan Africa and in South America, Haiti, and Southeast Asia; in the United States, it occurs predominantly in refugees and travelers to or military personnel who served in endemic areas.
3. Infection is spread through the insect vector *Anopheles* mosquito, leading to the following:
   a. Inoculation of sporozoite into blood
   b. Rapid invasion of the hepatocyte with proliferation (*exoerythrocytic stage*)
   c. Development asexually (schizogony) releasing merozoites that invade red blood cells (*erythrocytic stage*)
   d. Rupture of red blood cells, which releases merozoites (*febrile stage*) and is followed by invasion of other red cells cyclically
   e. Differentiation of some merozoites into gametocytes (*gametogony*), which are ingested by the mosquito, undergo sexual development into sporozoites, and infect human host at inoculation, thus completing the cycle
   f. Presence of small dormant forms (*hypnozoites:* e.g., *P. ovale, P. vivax*) within heptocytes capable of initiating nuclear division and perpetuating exoerythrocytic state
4. Four species infect humans: *P. falciparum* and *P. malariae* have no hepatic forms after initial exoerythrocytic stage; *P. ovale* and *P. vivax* maintain hepatic and red blood cell forms, which are responsible for relapses months to years after apparent resolution of infection.
5. *P. falciparum* is responsible for most fatalities, with adherence to postcapillary venules in liver, brain, and other organs, causing severe cerebral dysfunction (cerebral malaria), ischemic necrosis in liver (predominantly perivenular zone) and kidney (acute tubular necrosis), and massive hemolysis with

marked hemoglobinuria and renal failure (blackwater fever).

6. Patients present with cyclical symptoms of high fever (red blood cell hemolysis and release of parasites, toxins and pyrogens), nausea, vomiting, and headache, followed by sweats with defervescence every 72 hours for *P. vivax, P. ovale,* and *P. malariae* and 48 hours (less consistent) with *P. falciparum.*

7. Hepatomegaly and splenomegaly are almost always present, sometimes with abdominal pain; jaundice may be present.

8. Serum aminotransferase activities are three to four times normal and are higher when ischemic necrosis is prominent; serum bilirubin level is mildly elevated and is predominantly in the unconjugated form.

9. *Hemozoin* pigment, an iron porphyrin protein complex derived from anaerobic glucose metabolism and hemoglobin breakdown by the parasite, is commonly identified in Kupffer cells owing to hemolysis and erythrophagocytosis of parasitized red blood cells; because of hemolysis, *hemosiderin* to some degree is usually present in Kupffer cells and periportal hepatocytes (increased iron absorption in the chronically anemic state).

Prognosis

1. Increased mortality occurs in *P. falciparum* infections secondary to hemolysis and/or vascular occlusion by parasitized red blood cells; the cause of death is not due to hepatic disease.

References

Editorial. Tropical splenomegaly syndrome. Lancet 1976;1:1058–1059.
Hollingdale MR. Malaria and the liver. Hepatology 1985;5:327–335.
Joshi YK, Tandon BN, Acharya SK, et al. Acute hepatic failure due to *Plasmodium falciparum* liver injury. Liver 1986;6:357–360.
Leech JH. Infections caused by protozoa. In: Stein JH, ed. Internal Medicine, 2nd ed. Boston: Little, Brown & Co, 1987:1772–1777.

Hydatid Cyst

Major Morphologic Features

1. Unilocular or multilocular cyst formation occurs with the wall consisting of the following:
   a. Inner cellular germinal layer from which arise both smaller cyst replicas (endogenous *daughter cysts*) as well as multiple thin-walled bulblike processes (*brood capsules*) containing scolices (tapeworm heads of *Echinococcus*)
   b. Outer layer of laminated dense, hyalinized, and often calcified tissue, with adjacent granulation tissue, proliferation of fibroblasts, and chronic inflammatory infiltration merging into the bordering hepatic parenchyma

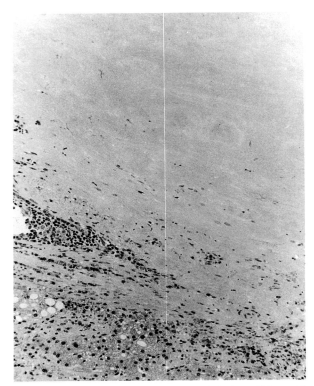

Figure 7–30. Hydatid cyst. The cyst wall is relatively acellular and hyalinized (*above*) with a chronic inflammatory infiltrate along its outer layer.

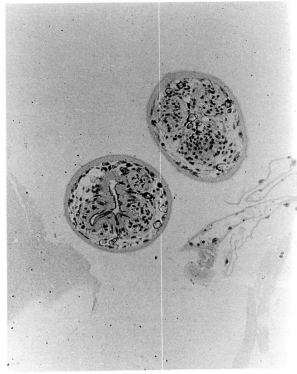

Figure 7–31. Hydatid cyst. The inner germinal layer of the cyst wall gives rise to *daughter cysts* and bulblike processes (*brood capsules*). This high-power photomicrograph of a capsule exhibits two scolices of *Echinococcus granulosus.*

Other Features

1. Amorphous eosinophilic and often calcified granular sediment occurs within the cyst (separation of brood capsules from the cyst wall).
2. Daughter cysts are present outside poorly formed cyst walls (typically seen with *E. multilocularis*).
3. Acute cholangitis is secondary to rupture of the cyst into the biliary tract.
4. Large cysts cause compression of adjacent hepatic parenchyma, with variable sinusoidal dilatation, congestion, and occasionally cholestasis.

Differential Diagnosis

1. *Amebic abscess:* The various layers of the capsule, with the inner brood capsules containing scolices, are diagnostic for *Echinococcus* infection. The fibrous wall, amorphous eosinophilic coagulative-type necrosis within the cyst, absence of inflammatory changes, and presence of amebic trophozoites at the edge of the cyst are diagnostic of an amebic abscess.

Special Stain

1. *Von Kossa:* Black calcium granules are often present in the outer cyst wall.

Clinical and Biologic Behavior

1. *Echinococcus* is a cestode (tapeworm) causing hepatic cyst formation in humans; the *E. granulosus* species is predominantly present in North Africa, Spain, Greece, the Middle East, Australia, New Zealand, and southern South American countries, while *E. multilocularis* species predominate in Alaska, Canada, the Soviet Union, and Central America.
2. The common host is the dog, in which the eggs are shed in the stools and ingested by humans (contaminated raw plants, soil). The larvae are freed in the duodenum and migrate through the mesenteric veins into the liver. Sixty per cent are retained in the sinusoids, while the rest continue into the inferior vena cava; 20% are then retained in the lungs and 20% in other organs through the systemic circulation.
3. The cyst presents as an enlarging, often palpable mass (may be larger than 20 cm in diameter), with 80% forming in the right lobe; the cyst is usually single.
4. Infection is often asymptomatic; when symptoms occur, the liver is most often involved (liver, 63%; lung, 23%; kidney, 3%; bone, 2%; brain, 1%).
5. Capsule and scolices of *E. granulosus* and *E. multilocularis* are quite similar; large cysts of *E.*

granulosus form *endogenous* daughter cysts; *E. multilocularis* species form *exogenous* cysts. Growth and clinical behavior pattern are much like that of invasive and metastatic carcinoma.
6. Encysted hepatic larvae form a characteristic lining of germinal and laminated zones. Proliferating *brood* capsules containing scolices form their own cyst lining (*daughter cysts*), eventually rupturing and forming ''hydatid sand'' (capsules, scolices). Degeneration of cysts and parasites leave a calcified amorphous debris.
7. Cysts forming just beneath Glisson's capsule may become pedunculated, with invasion of the diaphragm into the pleural cavity; peritoneal, pleural, or pericardial rupture may result in anaphylactic reaction, with delirium, syncope, and marked eosinophilia.
8. Complications include biliary obstruction from compression of large intrahepatic ducts, cholangitis due to rupture into the biliary tract, secondary infection, and anaphylaxis from ruptured cyst contents.
9. Appearance of cystic lesion with septations and calcifications on computed tomography is virtually diagnostic; on abdominal radiographs, sharply defined cysts and daughter cysts with calcification are seen 50% of the time. Serologic testing is positive in 90% of cases.

Aspiration Cytology

1. This procedure is contraindicated because of risk of intraperitoneal seeding of scolices. In a limited series, however, no sequelae were observed and quick diagnosis was established when aspirated fluid was stained with hematoxylin and eosin or Giemsa.
2. Presence of scolices in an unsuspected lesion is diagnostic.

Treatment and Prognosis

1. Ideal therapy is complete resection if the cyst is solitary and surgically accessible.
2. If the cyst is surgically unresectable, parasiticidal therapy prior to marsupialization is preferable.
3. In *E. multilocularis* infection, surgery is usually difficult because of multiloculations and exogenous daughter cyst formation; parasiticidal agents may be offered.
4. Prognosis is usually good; patients often live for years, with eventual death and calcification of the cyst; prognosis is also good when the cyst is surgically accessible and can be removed. Prognosis is worse with infected and ruptured cysts. With *E. multilocularis* infection, the majority of patients will die if the infection is not treated.

References

Leech JH. Infections caused by protozoa. In: Stein JH, ed. Internal Medicine, 2nd ed. Boston: Little, Brown & Co, 1987:1806–1807.

Marcial MA, Marcial-Rojas RA. Parasitic diseases of the liver. In: Schiff L, Schiff ER, eds. Diseases of the Liver, 6th ed. Philadelphia: J.B. Lippincott Co, 1987:1186–1188.

Van Steenbergen W, Fevery J, Broeckaert L, et al. Hepatic echinococcus ruptured into the biliary tract. J. Hepatol 1987;4:133–139.

Clonorchiasis

Major Morphologic Features

1. The liver fluke *Clonorchis (Opisthorchis) sinensis* is present within large dilated bile ducts.
2. Adenomatous proliferation of small glandular structures is marked, often with goblet cell metaplasia and increased mucin secretion immediately surrounding the large ducts.

Other Features

1. Variable degrees of acute and chronic inflammatory infiltration are seen within large duct walls, with prominent numbers of eosinophils.

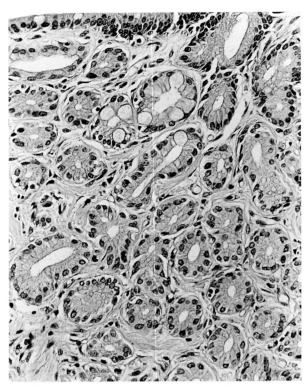

Figure 7–33. Clonorchiasis. High power of the bile duct wall exhibits numerous proliferating small glands, believed to be precursors in the development of cholangiocarcinoma.

2. Cysts may form in severe cases secondary to marked duct dilatation and contain clear bile and parasites.
3. Cholestasis is often present distal to duct involvement.
4. Ducts may become superinfected by colonic bacteria (*Escherichia coli*), with evidence of acute cholangitis, leading to abscess formation.
5. Portal tracts show variable degrees of duct proliferation and occasionally mild fibrosis but minimal inflammatory change (unless secondary cholangitis from obstruction occurs).

Differential Diagnosis

1. *Mechanical duct obstruction of other causes:* Cholestasis, bile duct proliferation and dilatation, and acute cholangitis are changes that can be seen in both *Clonorchis* infection and large duct obstruction as a result of more frequent conditions such as choledocholithiasis and strictures. The presence of a large duct in the biopsy specimen exhibiting adenomatous hyperplasia and prominent numbers of eosinophils suggests parasitic infection.
2. *Recurrent pyogenic cholangiohepatitis:* Cholangitis and abscess formation may occur in *Clonorchis* infection and are typical findings in recurrent pyogenic cholangiohepatitis (see page 47). Clonorchiasis is believed to be one of the etiologic factors in the de-

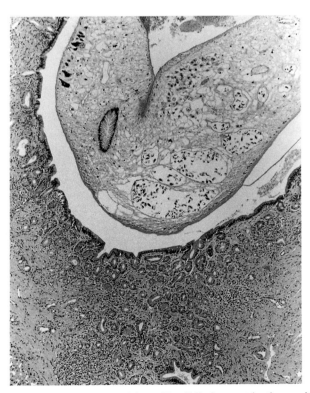

Figure 7–32. Clonorchiasis. A large dilated bile duct contains the parasite *Clonorchis (Opisthorchis) sinensis*. Numerous eggs are present within the organism. Small glandular structures are markedly increased within the wall of the large bile duct.

velopment of recurrent pyogenic cholangiohepatitis. However, about 50% of the cases do not have *Clonorchis* infection. Therefore, identification of the typical large duct lesions, and the parasite if possible, is essential for a definitive diagnosis of clonorchiasis.

Clinical and Biologic Behavior

1. *Clonorchis (Opisthorchis) sinensis* (Oriental liver fluke) is a common infection of man in the Far East, with humans as the definitive host; in some regions (Hong Kong) the parasite is present in up to 80% of persons in the 51- to 60-year age group.
2. The oblong (20 mm) parasite rests in major intrahepatic ducts. Although usually asymptomatic, severe infection may cause problems of mechanical duct obstruction and is associated 50% of the time with recurrent pyogenic cholangiohepatitis.
3. Patients present with recurrent attacks of fever, abdominal pain, and jaundice lasting 1 to 2 weeks; as the disease progresses, intervals between attacks shorten. Serum bilirubin, alkaline phosphatase activity, and the peripheral white cell count are significantly elevated with only mild to moderate elevations of serum aminotransferase levels.
4. The enlarged liver may reveal cysts beneath Glisson's capsule that are gray-white to pale blue (dilated ducts containing adult worms and clear bile).
5. The natural host is man, but other hosts include dogs, cats, and hogs; the eggs pass through feces into fresh water, are ingested by snails (intermediate host), and after development in the gut, larvae eventually leave the snails and penetrate the scales of fish, forming cysts. The worm develops from ingested cysts when raw or poorly cooked fish is eaten; the larvae travel to the biliary tree through the ampulla of Vater, where they mature.
6. Gallstones sometimes contain dead parasites, eggs, and inflammatory products, producing an amorphous green-brown material ("biliary mud").
7. Liver damage and bile duct injury are produced not only by obstructive change but also by direct mechanical injury to ducts from parasite suckers and chemical stimulants from metabolic byproducts of the parasite.
8. Complications include mechanical duct obstruction, often with intrahepatic gallstones, cholangitis, and abscess formation; cholangiocarcinoma may develop in a small percentage of patients (in large part due to chronic irritation of the bile ducts).

Aspiration Cytology

1. Clear mucoid fluid containing parasites may be present in aspirated cysts.

Prognosis

1. Complications such as cholangitis and abscess formation, and cholangiocarcinoma in long-term infections, increase mortality. Prognosis, however, is generally good since the majority of infections can be adequately managed.

References

Evans H, Bourgeois CH, Comer DS, et al. Biliary tract changes in opisthorchiasis. Am J Trop Med Hyg 1971;20:667–671.
Hou PC, Pang LSC. *Clonorchis sinensis* infestation in man in Hong Kong. J Pathol Bacteriol 1964;87:245–250.
Marcial MA, Marcial-Rojas RA. In: Schiff L, Schiff ER, eds. Diseases of the Liver, 6th ed. Philadelphia: J.B. Lippincott, 1987:1181–1182.
Sun T. Pathology and immunology of *Clonorchis sinensis* infection of the liver. Ann Clin Lab Sci 1984;14:208–215.

Schistosomiasis

Major Morphologic Features

1. Granulomatous reaction occurs in portal tracts to ova of *Schistosoma* parasite, with multinucleated giant cells, mononuclear inflammatory cells, and surrounding lamellar fibrosis ("*pipe-stem*" lesion).

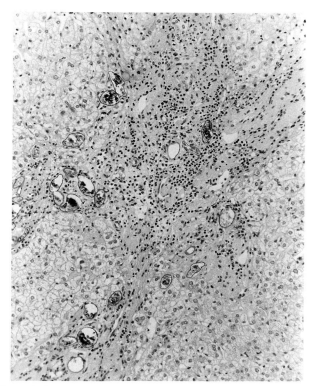

Figure 7–34. Schistosomiasis. Numerous eggs are scattered throughout the fibrotic portal tract. Mild lymphocytic infiltration is present, but there is no granulomatous reaction to the organisms.

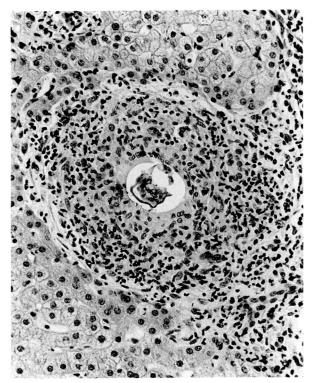

Figure 7–35. Schistosomiasis. The abundant inflammatory reaction, consisting predominantly of lymphocytes, epithelioid cells, and occasional neutrophils, uniformly surrounds the egg. Eventually a lamellar fibrosis appears, forming a typical *pipe-stem* lesion.

2. Variable degrees of portal fibrosis are noted in chronic disease, with a decrease in portal venous radicles.

Other Features

1. In early *acute* infection the following are noted:
   a. Portal tract often contains numerous inflammatory cells, predominantly eosinophils.
   b. Eosinophilic abscess may occur, with presence of Charcot-Leyden crystals.
   c. Kupffer cell hyperplasia and focal necrosis are present, with ova rarely identified within the parenchyma.
2. Ova may be seen in portal tracts and fibrous septa without inflammatory reaction.
3. Periportal sinusoidal collagen deposition is occasionally identified.
4. As the ova eventually disappear, the portal areas exhibit dense collagen formation, often with focal areas of calcification.
5. Fibrous septa with increased lymphatic channels form in the more chronic stages; well-developed cirrhosis is not seen.
6. Gray-black pigment resembling hemozoin is sometimes identified within portal macrophages, Kupffer cells, and granulomas.

7. Ova and granulomas may be immediately adjacent to, and sometimes within, the portal veins, producing endophlebitis, often with thrombosis, occlusion, and fibrous obliteration.
8. Irregular intimal fibrosis within medium-sized portal veins may occur.
9. Proliferation of intrahepatic arterioles may be present.
10. Nerve trunks may appear hypertrophic in large fibrotic portal regions near the hilum.

Differential Diagnosis

1. *Granulomatous lesions of other etiologies:* Most granulomatous disorders do not exhibit the characteristic fibrous "pipe-stem" lesion seen with schistosomiasis. Sarcoidosis, however, may exhibit a segmental fibrosis of larger granulomas, with the older lesions eventually becoming totally sclerosed. Granulomas within the parenchyma are unusual for schistosomiasis while quite common in sarcoidosis. Special stains may be necessary for determining the etiology of granulomas caused by other infectious agents (e.g., fungi, *Mycobacterium*).
2. *Noncirrhotic portal fibrosis:* There are multiple causes of portal hypertension arising in a noncirrhotic liver, with schistosomiasis being one example. If a liver biopsy specimen does not contain ova or typical granuloma, it may be difficult to differentiate fibrosis from other causes (e.g., idiopathic portal hypertension, see page 103).

Special Stains

1. *Acid-fast (Ziehl-Neelsen carbolfuchsin):* All *Schistosoma* species except *S. haematobium* stain positively.
2. *Prussian blue:* Schistosome pigment does *not* pick up this stain for iron.

Clinical and Biologic Behavior

1. Three species of the nematode *Schistosoma* infect humans:
   a. *S. mansoni:* Tropical and subtropical Africa, Middle East, Central and South America, Caribbean
   b. *S. japonicum:* Far East
   c. *S. haematobium:* Africa, Indian Ocean islands
2. *S. mansoni* and *S. japonicum* settle in the portal venous system and are responsible for the most common cause of portal hypertension throughout the world; *S. haematobium* settles in the vesicular venous plexus, causing urinary bladder disease and very seldom liver disease.
3. In *acute* schistosomiasis (Katayama disease), pa-

tients present with fever, chills, hepatomegaly, lymphadenopathy, and marked eosinophilia (serum sickness); the liver exhibits an acute inflammatory reaction; granulomas are not common on biopsy.

4. A small subset of patients may go on to develop *chronic* disease in which a marked portal granulomatous and fibrogenic reaction to the eggs leads to presinusoidal portal hypertension.

5. Patients may present with melena, hematemesis from esophageal variceal bleeding, hepatosplenomegaly (the spleen averaging 1000 g), ascites, and, rarely, jaundice; features of chronic liver disease such as vascular spiders, gynecomastia, and testicular atrophy are rare but may be present if liver disease from another cause is also present.

6. Alkaline phosphatase activity is mildly elevated, but serum aminotransferase activities and bilirubin level are usually normal.

7. Man contracts the parasite through bathing or wading in contaminated waters; the intermediate host is the snail, where the fork-tailed cercariae develop, leave the snail, and infect humans by direct skin contact or invasion of mucous membranes after ingestion.

8. The organisms migrate through lymphatics and venules into the venous circulation, through the heart and lungs, eventually terminating in the intrahepatic portal venous radicles; the larva mature into the adult male and female worms and migrate into the mesenteric veins; ovulation occurs (*S. mansoni* 300 eggs/d, *S. japonicum* 3500 eggs/d), and some of these eggs are retained in the portal veins, eliciting the *acute* response.

9. The number of eggs in the feces often directly correlates with the degree of hepatic fibrosis in long-term infection.

10. Diagnosis is made by serology and identification of ova in feces or in biopsy specimens.

Aspiration Cytology

1. Eggs are not generally present within the lobule, and aspiration is usually not contributory; however, when seen, specific identification can be diagnostic:
   a. *S. mansoni:* Elliptical, 148 μm in length, very prominent lateral spine
   b. *S. japonicum:* Spherical, 91 μm in length, small lateral spine often difficult to identify
   c. *S. haematobium:* Elliptical, 152 μm in length, terminal spine

Prognosis

1. Mortality is usually related to problems of portal hypertension (e.g., variceal bleeding); except in advanced cases, however, the overall mortality is relatively low since liver function is well preserved

References

Dunn MA, Kamel R. Hepatic schistosomiasis. Hepatology 1981;1:653–661.

Leech JH. Infections caused by protozoa. In: Stein JH, ed. Internal Medicine, 2nd ed. Boston: Little, Brown & Co, 1987:1802–1805.

Warren KS. The kinetics of hepatosplenic schistosomiasis. Semin Liver Dis 1984;4:293–300.

Warren KS, Domingo EO, Cowan RBT. Granuloma formation around schistosome eggs as a manifestation of delayed hypersensitivity. Am J Pathol 1967;51:735–756.

General References

Brown HW. Parasitology, 3rd ed. New York: Meredith, 1969.

Finegold SM, Martin WJ, Scott EG. Diagnostic Microbiology, 5th ed. St. Louis: C.V. Mosby, 1978.

Grases PJ. Bacterial, protozoal, helminthic, and spirochaetal inflammatory diseases. In: Peters RL, Craig JR, eds. Liver Pathology. New York: Churchill Livingstone, 1986:125–145.

Simson, IW, Gear JHS. Other viral and infectious diseases. In: MacSween RNM, Anthony PP, Scheuer PJ, eds. Pathology of the Liver, 2nd ed. Edinburgh: Churchill Livingstone, 1987:233–264.

CHAPTER 8

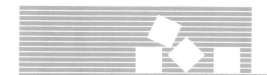

Developmental, Familial, and Metabolic Disorders

■ Biliary Tract Disorders

Biliary Atresia

EXTRAHEPATIC TYPE

Major Morphologic Features

1. Interlobular and cholangiolar bile duct proliferation and dilatation are marked.
2. Cholestasis is most prominent in the perivenular zone.
3. Portal fibrosis of the biliary type occurs, with eventual progression to secondary biliary cirrhosis.

Other Features

1. Portal tracts exhibit variable degrees of acute and chronic inflammatory infiltration.
2. Multinucleated giant cell transformation accentuated in the perivenular region is present in 15% to 25% of cases.
3. Kupffer cell hyperplasia is mild to moderate.
4. Bile plugs are often present in proliferating dilated interlobular duct structures.
5. The degree of portal fibrosis only slightly varies from one lobule to another.
6. Three types of duct structures at porta hepatis and extraheptic biliary tree are present:
   a. Type I—absence of lumen
   b. Type II—presence of lumen less than 50 μ in diameter, lined by cuboidal epithelium, with periductal neutrophilic infiltrate; cellular debris and cell necrosis in lumina of ducts more than 300 μ in diameter
   c. Type III—presence of altered duct incompletely lined by columnar epithelium
7. As the disease progresses the following are noted:
   a. Hepatocytes and Kupffer cells have a xanthomatous appearance.
   b. Bile lakes, bile infarcts, and alcoholic hyalin are seen in periportal or periseptal hepatocytes.
   c. Copper and copper-binding protein are increased in periportal and periseptal hepatocytes.
   d. Although ducts are generally present at the cirrhotic stage, cases occur in which ducts are decreased to absent.

Differential Diagnosis

1. *Neonatal giant cell hepatitis:* Fifteen to 25% of cases of extrahepatic biliary atresia exhibit some degree of syncytial giant cell transformation and may be difficult to differentiate from giant cell hepatitis. Interlobular and cholangiolar duct proliferation is marked in extrahepatic atresia, with the ducts often containing bile plugs, changes not see in giant cell hepatitis. In addition, giant cell hepatitis usually exhibits more prominent giant cell transformation without concomitant portal fibrosis.
2. *Choledochal cyst:* Cystic dilatation of the common bile duct may be associated with morphologic intrahepatic changes indistinguishable from those seen in extrahepatic biliary atresia. However, the hepatic lesions may not be manifest until childhood or even adulthood, while in biliary atresia jaundice is present in the neonate, with biliary cirrhosis present at ages 6 months to 2 years in untreated cases.

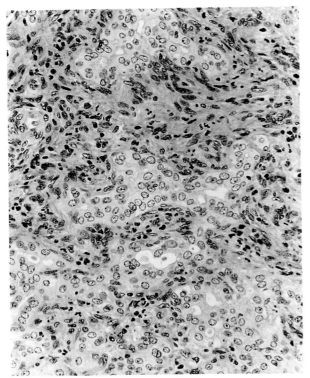

Figure 8-1. Extrahepatic biliary atresia. The portal tracts are fibrotic, with marked proliferation of duct structures. Some ducts are dilated, contain bile, and are surrounded by both lymphocytes and neutrophils.

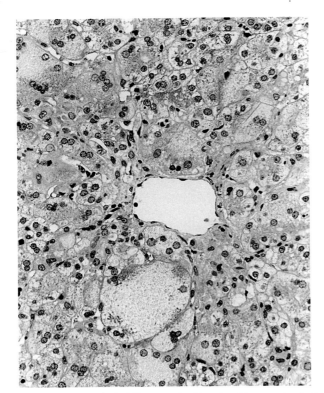

Figure 8-2. Extrahepatic biliary atresia. Occasional hepatocytes in the perivenular zone are swollen and contain multiple nuclei. Kupffer cell hyperplasia is present.

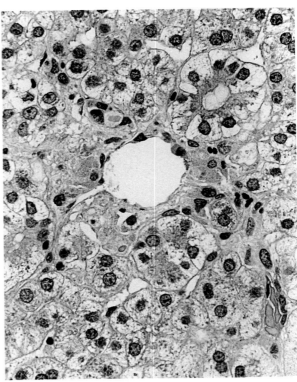

Figure 8-3. Extrahepatic biliary atresia. High power shows focal necrosis and aggregates of macrophages and Kupffer cells around the terminal hepatic venule. Dilated canaliculi containing bile are present.

Special Stains

1. *Orcein:* Brown-black granules in periportal or periseptal hepatocytes are secondary to an increase in copper-binding protein.
2. *Rhodamine:* Green-black granules represent copper in periportal or periseptal hepatocytes.
3. *Van Gieson:* Green-staining bile is identified in perivenular hepatocytes and occasionally as bile plugs in dilated cholangioles.

Clinical and Biologic Behavior (Table 8-1)

1. Extrahepatic biliary atresia accounts for almost one half of all cases of neonatal cholestasis, with an overall incidence of 1/8,000 to 1/20,000 live births.
2. It is four to five times more common in Southeast Asia and the Far East with a predominance in Asian females.
3. Jaundice is *not* present at birth but develops 1 to 3 weeks later, with dark urine and acholic stools; pruritus and xanthoma formation are rare.
4. Hepatomegaly is common; splenomegaly is initially mild but becomes progressively more prominent as hepatic fibrosis sets in.
5. There is elevation of conjugated serum bilirubin lev-

Table 8–1
CAUSES OF NEONATAL CHOLESTASIS
IN 288 PATIENTS

	No. Patients	% of Total
Extrahepatic	**142**	**49.3**
Biliary atresia	133	46.2
Biliary hypoplasia	4	1.4
Spontaneous perforation of bile ducts	3	1.0
Choledochal cyst	2	0.7
Intrahepatic	**146**	**50.7**
Structural type abnormalities	57	19.8
Paucity of ducts:		
Syndromatic (Alagille's)	39	13.5
Nonsyndromatic	18	6.3
Nonstructural type abnormalities	89	30.9
Inspissated bile syndrome	3	1.0
Viral infection	17	5.9
Cytomegalovirus		
Rubella		
Hepatitis B		
Miscellaneous	31	10.8
Alpha-1-antitrypsin deficiency		
Byler's disease		
Cystic fibrosis		
Hereditary fructose intolerance		
Niemann-Pick disease		
Neonatal "giant cell" hepatitis (unknown etiology)	38	13.2

Modified from Alagille D. Cholestasis in the first three months of life. In Popper H, Schaffner F, eds. Progress in Liver Diseases, vol VI. New York: Grune & Stratton, 1979:471–485.

els and marked increase in alkaline phosphatase and 5'-nucleotidase activities; serum aminotransferase values, however, are only slightly elevated.
6. Associated anomalies are present 15% to 30% of the time (e.g., vascular, polysplenia syndrome, trisomy-21); an increased incidence of viral infection (e.g., cytomegalovirus, rubella, varicella) is also present.
7. Atresia usually presents as complete involvement of the entire extrahepatic biliary system in 75% to 85% of the cases, with the rest exhibiting partial atresia or hypoplasia.
8. Although originally believed to be congenital, evidence indicates that it is probably an acquired disorder:
   a. It is exceptionally rare in premature infants and stillbirths.
   b. Reports of dizygotic and monozygotic twins have shown one to have atresia, the other a normal biliary tract.
   c. Association with a continuing inflammatory infiltrate occurs in portal regions, with gradually *diminishing* ducts (obstructive, obliterative cholangiopathy).
   d. Association with viral infection (reovirus 3) is possible.
9. Diagnosis using rose bengal iodine-131, or HIDA scan, is highly sensitive in over 97% of cases; liver biopsy is diagnostic 60% to 95% of the time (most difficult in very early stage).

Treatment and Prognosis

1. Partial intact common duct is corrected by a roux-en-Y anastomosis; however, this is seen in only a small number of cases.
2. Absent common duct (75% to 85%) is corrected with hepatoportoenterostomy (Kasai procedure), anastomosing the jejunal loop to the porta hepatis.
3. Some patients derive long-term benefit from the Kasai procedure, although the majority still have poor biliary drainage, leading to biliary fibrosis; this temporizing procedure allows survival for eventual hepatic transplantation.
4. Prognostic indicators are as follows:
   a. Bile flow is reestablished 60% to 90% of the time if surgery is performed within 2 to 3 months of birth, but less than 20% of the time when surgery is delayed longer than 3 months after birth.
   b. Prognosis is good when duct size at the hilum is more than 150 μm in diameter (correctable type); when ducts are less than 150 μm, the Kasai procedure is performed to attempt to identify larger duct structures during hilar dissection.
5. Death in untreated or late-treated patients is secondary to biliary cirrhosis, hepatic failure, and consequences of portal hypertension (e.g., bleeding esophageal varices); 50% of untreated patients die within the first year, with cirrhosis developing as early as 6 months after birth.

References

Alagille D. Cholestasis in the first three months of life. In: Popper H, Schaffner F, eds. Progress in Liver Diseases, vol VI. New York: Grune & Stratton, 1979:471–485.
Alagille D. Extrahepatic biliary atresia. Hepatology 1984;4:7S–10S.
Desmet VJ. Cholangiopathies: Past, present and future. Semin Liver Dis 1987;7:67–76.
Gautier M, Eliot N. Extrahepatic biliary atresia: Morphological study of 98 biliary remnants. Arch Pathol Lab Med 1981;105:397–402.
Landing BH, Wells TR, Reed GB, et al. Diseases of the bile ducts in children. In: Gall EA, Mostofi FK, eds. The Liver. Baltimore: Williams & Wilkins, 1973:480–509.

INTRAHEPATIC TYPE

Major Morphologic Changes

Paucity of Ducts Syndrome
1. Portal tracts show decreased (<0.5 ducts per portal region) to absent interlobular bile ducts.
2. Intralobular cholestasis is most prominent in the perivenular region.

Intrahepatic Familial Cholestasis (Byler's Syndrome)
1. Portal tracts are normal in size to small, with duct proliferation in early stages.
2. Ducts are decreased to absent in later stages, with biliary fibrosis and eventual cirrhosis.

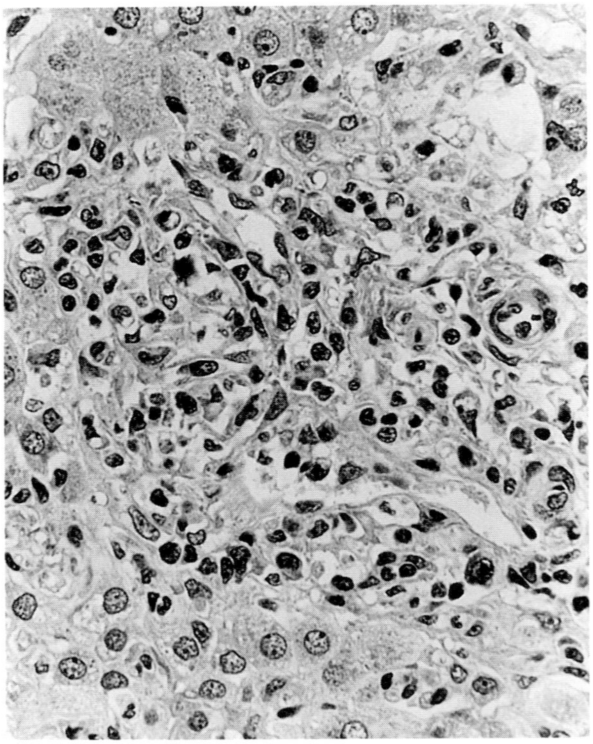

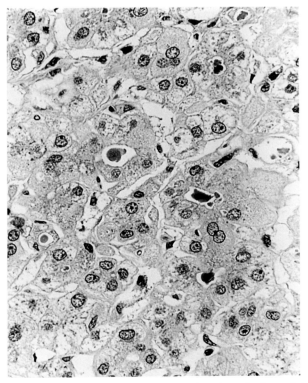

Figure 8–4. Paucity of ducts. The portal tract is normal in size, with a moderate lymphocytic infiltrate. Both interlobular bile ducts and cholangioles are absent.

Figure 8–5. Paucity of ducts. Marked dilatation of canaliculi containing bile is present in the perivenular zone.

3. Intralobular cholestasis is most prominent in the perivenular zone.

Other Features

Paucity of Ducts Syndrome
1. Portal areas may show variability in the number of ducts within the same biopsy specimen.
2. Mild chronic inflammatory infiltration occurs within portal tracts; the inflammatory cells are not oriented to duct structures.
3. Giant cell transformation, although not prominent, may be present in early stages.
4. Xanthomatous change occurs within hepatocytes and Kupffer cells.
5. Focal sinusoidal fibrosis is occasionally present.
6. Liver cell necrosis and lobular inflammation are uncommon.
7. Copper and copper-binding protein are slightly increased in periportal hepatocytes.
8. Mild portal fibrosis may occur, but without progression to cirrhosis in the majority of cases; however, biliary cirrhosis has been described and when present is usually seen at end stage of *nonsyndromatic* cases.

Intrahepatic Familial Cholestasis
1. Cholangiolar proliferation occurs in early stages; some cases, however, may present as decreased to absent ducts at this time.
2. Portal tracts show mild chronic inflammatory infiltration.
3. Copper and copper-binding protein are increased as the disease progresses.
4. Giant cell transformation is usually rare.

Differential Diagnosis

1. *Alpha-1-antitrypsin deficiency:* The chronic liver disease associated with alpha-1-antitrypsin deficiency may express itself in neonates with cholangiolar proliferation but a decrease in interlobular ducts, with eventual progression to biliary fibrosis and cirrhosis. Alpha-1-antitrypsin deficiency is distinguishable by the presence of eosinophilic cytoplasmic globules (abnormal alpha-1-antitrypsin protein) within periportal hepatocytes, confirmed with special staining (periodic acid–Schiff after diastase, immunoperoxidase) and serum quantitation and phenotyping of alpha-1-antitrypsin.
2. *Extrahepatic biliary atresia:* This disorder is not associated with concomitant intrahepatic atresia and presents with striking interlobular and cholangiolar duct proliferation and dilatation, the ducts often containing bile plugs.
3. *Neonatal giant cell hepatitis:* The degree of giant cell transformation and portal inflammatory change is much greater in giant cell hepatitis than in intrahepatic atresia. In addition, ducts are typically present

in giant cell hepatitis; however, there may be an overlap in morphologic changes between the two entities in the very early stages.

Special Stains

1. *Orcein:* Brown-black granules, representing copper-binding protein, may be present in periportal hepatocytes.
2. *Rhodamine:* Black-green granules represent copper in hepatocytes.
3. *Periodic acid–Schiff after diastase* (DiPAS): This stain is useful in differentiation from alpha-1-antitrypsin deficiency, with the latter exhibiting positive cytoplasmic inclusions in periportal hepatocytes.

Immunohistochemistry

1. *Alpha-1-antitrypsin:* This stain confirms the nature of DiPAS-positive inclusions in periportal hepatocytes for differential diagnosis.

Clinical and Biologic Behavior

Paucity of Ducts

1. Intrahepatic biliary atresia, also termed *arteriohepatic dysplasia,* is most likely an autosomal dominant disorder that can be divided into two subtypes: those *with* and *without* distinct facial, vertebral, and cardiovascular abnormalities (*syndromatic* and *nonsyndromatic*); this disorder is responsible for approximately one fifth of all cases of neonatal cholestasis (see Table 8–1).
2. The *syndromatic* subgroup (*Alagille's syndrome*) exhibits facial features (hypertelorism, deep-set eyes, wide cheek bones, broad forehead), pulmonary artery stenosis, growth and mental retardation, and vertebral defects (butterfly vertebrae, hemivertebrae); one third of patients may not have facial deformities, however.
3. Alagille's syndrome affects both sexes equally, with the earliest signs and symptoms being jaundice during the first 3 months, intense pruritus, hepatomegaly, and sometimes splenomegaly.
4. Conjugated serum bilirubin is elevated, and there is a slight increase in aminotransferase levels and markedly elevated alkaline phosphatase, serum cholesterol (500–1000 mg/dL), and bile acid (predominantly cholic acid) values.
5. Although variable degrees of fibrosis may be present, cirrhosis does *not* occur in patients with Alagille's syndrome.
6. Other associated genetic abnormalities with Alagille's syndrome include trisomy-17, trisomy-18, trisomy-21, and defect 45/XO.
7. Although the majority of cases do not develop severe

fibrosis or cirrhosis, in a small number rapid progression to cirrhosis is seen. A subgroup of patients have been documented to have marked elevations of trihydroxycoprostanic acid (TCA) as the main bile acid (rather than cholic acid). In these patients a defect in an enzyme normally converting TCA to cholic acid may produce liver damage from the direct toxic effects of TCA.

Intrahepatic Familial Cholestasis

1. This autosomal recessive disorder, first described in an Amish family (Byler), presents with diarrhea and foul-smelling stools during the first few weeks, progressing to jaundice in the latter part of the first year.
2. Ductules proliferate early in life, although portal tracts can be small with absent ducts; biliary cirrhosis and death from hepatic failure and consequences of portal hypertension occur usually by age 10.
3. Microfilamentous structures adjacent to the pericanalicular regions of the liver cell suggest a possible defect in bile acid transport.

Prognosis

1. In nonsyndromatic intrahepatic biliary atresia, the prognosis is poor, with cirrhosis developing in 40% to 73% of cases within 13 years.
2. Prognosis of Byler's syndrome likewise is poor, with death usually occurring within the first few years (although there are rare instances of survival into the second decade).
3. In cholestatic diseases of childhood progressing to hepatic failure, hepatic transplantation must be considered.

References

Alagille D. Intrahepatic biliary atresia (hepatic ductular hypoplasia). In: Berenberg SR, ed. Liver Diseases in Infancy and Childhood. Baltimore: Williams & Wilkins, 1976:129–142.

Alagille D, Odievre M, Gautier M, et al. Hepatic ductular hypoplasia associated with characteristic facies, vertebral malformation, retarded physical, mental and sexual development, and cardiac murmur. J Pediatr 1975;86:63–71

Clayton RJ, Iber FL, Reubner BH, et al. Byler's disease. Am J Dis Child 1969;117:112–124.

Hashida Y, Yunis EJ. Syndromatic paucity of interlobular bile ducts: Hepatic histopathology of the early and end-stage liver. Pediatr Pathol 1988;8:1–15.

Kahy EI, Daum F, Markovitz J, et al. Arteriohepatic dysplasia: II. Hepatobiliary morphology. Hepatology 1983;3:77–84.

Riely CA. Familial intrahepatic cholestatic syndromes. Semin Liver Dis 1987;119–133.

Bile Duct Dilatation

Major Morphologic Features

Choledochal Cyst (Extrahepatic)
1. Cyst formation in common bile ducts occurs with fibrotic wall and variable degrees of predominantly chronic inflammatory infiltration.

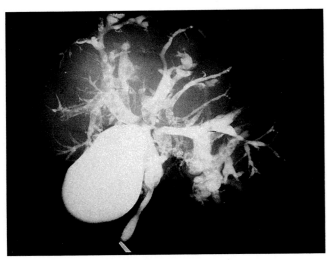

Figure 8–6. Caroli's syndrome (postmortem injection of extrahepatic and intrahepatic bile ducts). Marked segmental dilatation of intrahepatic ducts is present, with focal areas of cyst formation distally in both the right and left lobes. The gallbladder is dilated but does not contain stones.

2. Secondary hepatic changes include cholestasis, marked duct proliferation and dilatation, often acute cholangitis, and eventual fibrosis leading to biliary cirrhosis (changes similar to extrahepatic biliary atresia, see page 135).

Caroli's Syndrome (Intrahepatic)
1. Dilated ducts have cuboidal to columnar epithelium.
2. There are variable degrees of portal fibrosis.

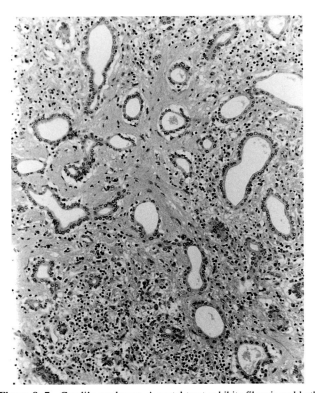

Figure 8–7. Caroli's syndrome. A portal tract exhibits fibrosis and both proliferation and dilatation of interlobular bile ducts.

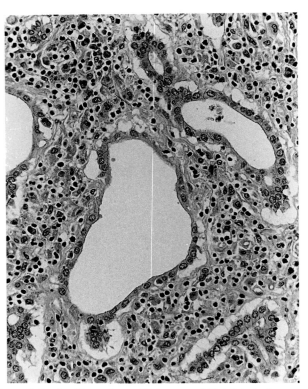

Figure 8–8. Caroli's syndrome. High power of dilated ducts shows variable degrees of thinning of the duct epithelium. Two smaller ducts (*upper and lower right*) exhibit periductal hydropic change, with occasional infiltration of the duct wall by lymphocytes.

Other Features

Choledochal Cyst
1. Cyst wall is composed predominantly of fibrous tissue; smooth muscle fibers can occasionally be identified.
2. Focal ulceration with neutrophilic infiltration of wall may occur.
3. Mucous glands are often present within the wall and at times are abundant.

Caroli's Syndrome
1. Ducts may form cystic lesions with focal ulceration.
2. Lumina of small cysts may contain inspissated bile.
3. Superimposed acute inflammation of duct and cystic structures occurs, with microabscess formation; lymphocytic infiltration of edematous duct epithelium may also be present.
4. Variable degrees of cholestasis occur within the parenchyma.

Differential Diagnosis

1. *Extrahepatic biliary atresia:* Both choledochal cyst and extrahepatic biliary atresia exhibit almost identical intrahepatic morphologic changes of prominent duct proliferation, cholestasis, and biliary fibrosis.

Further workup (e.g., ultrasound) may be necessary for diagnosis.

2. *Recurrent pyogenic cholangiohepatitis:* When super-infection and abscess develop in Caroli's syndrome the morphology resembles that seen in recurrent pyogenic cholangiohepatitis (see page 47). Recurrent pyogenic cholangiohepatitis is most often localized to the left lobe, and although Caroli's syndrome is usually diffuse, it may also be focal. Recurrent pyogenic cholangiohepatitis is most often found in the Asian population, a feature not seen with Caroli's syndrome. In addition, associated congenital malformations (e.g., microcystic renal disease) may also be seen in Caroli's syndrome.

Clinical and Biologic Behavior

Choledochal Cyst

1. The clinical presentation may occur at any age; 18% of cases occur during the first year of life.
2. Choledochal cysts are three times more frequent in females and are often associated with other duct anomalies (e.g., double common duct, double gallbladder, assessory hepatic duct); intrahepatic cystic dilatation (Caroli's syndrome) may also be present.
3. The neonate or young child usually presents with hepatic changes of progressive biliary disease that may be quite severe; older patients present more often with a mild form of obstructive jaundice.
4. Cysts vary in size; the larger ones contain 5 to 10 L of bile; they may be saccular or fusiform.
5. Cholangiocarcinoma may occur in 3% of the cysts, 2% in noninvolved major intrahepatic ducts, and in less than 1% as peripheral cholangiocarcinoma; when this tumor is present, Caroli's syndrome is usually present as well.
6. Pathogenesis: Reflux pancreatic enzymes cause injury and focal weakness to the duct wall, with resulting dilatation (developmental); it is part of a congenital spectrum including biliary atresia and neonatal hepatitis (obstructive cholangiopathy).

Caroli's Syndrome

1. Caroli's syndrome is diagnosed most often between 5 and 20 years of age during workup for jaundice and/or portal hypertension; however, it also may be seen in the older population or even be totally asymptomatic through life.
2. Hepatomegaly is present; serum aminotransferase levels are normal or only slightly elevated and alkaline phosphatase and gamma-glutamyl transpeptidase activities are moderately elevated; when associated with congenital hepatic fibrosis, portal hypertension may be present.
3. Diffuse, multifocal segmental dilatation of ducts is present interspersed with areas of normal ducts; associated abnormalities include congenital hepatic fibrosis, choledochal cyst, and polycystic or hypoplastic kidneys.

4. The incidence of cholangiocarcinoma is 3% of total cases.

Treatment and Prognosis

1. Since stones are usually of pigment type (bilirubinate), dissolution therapy is not effective. Dilatation of strictures to improve drainage may be attempted at endoscopy or surgery.
2. Surgical therapy:
   a. *Complete* resection of choledochal cyst and hepaticojejunostomy are preferable, since risk of cholangiocarcinoma increases if removal of cyst wall is partial.
   b. Partial lobectomy is considered when Caroli's syndrome affects only part of the liver.
   c. Abscesses should be drained percutaneously or at surgery.
   d. Hepatic transplantation is offered to patients with severe Caroli's syndrome.
3. Symptomatic choledochal cyst should be managed surgically; in Caroli's syndrome, surgery may be difficult in some, with death from sepsis occurring 5 to 10 years after initial biliary infection.

References

Barlow B, Tabor E, Blanc WA, et al. Choledochal cyst: A review of 19 cases. J Pediatr 1976;89:934–940.

Caroli J. Diseases of the intrahepatic biliary tree. Clin Gastroenterol 1973;2:147–161.

Landing BH, Wells TR, Reed GB, et al. Neonatal hepatitis, biliary atresia and choledochal cyst: The concept of infantile cholangiopathy. Prog Pediatr Surg 1974;6:113–119.

Summerfield JA, Nagafuchi Y, Sherlock S, et al. Hepatobiliary fibrocystic diseases: A clinical and histological review of 51 patients. J Hepatol 1986;2:141–156.

Cystic Disease

SOLITARY UNILOCULAR CYST

Major Morphologic Features

1. Benign cystic structure of variable size is lined by mature flattened to cuboidal epithelium and surrounded by multilayered mature collagen sharply demarcating the cyst from adjacent parenchyma.

Other Features

1. Inner lining may be absent secondary to sloughing.
2. The fibrous wall may be surrounded by nerves, ducts, and vascular elements.
3. Lumina contain the following:
   a. Variable types of fluid, most commonly serous or mucoid

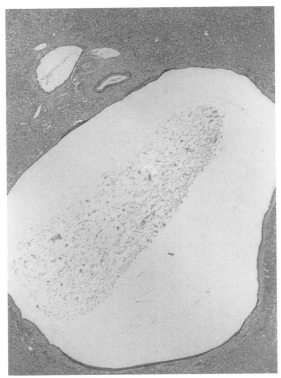

Figure 8–9. Unilocular cyst. The large round to oval cyst is lined by flattened epithelium. The lumen contains proteinaceous debris. A small portal tract containing a normal-appearing bile duct is also present (*upper left*).

    b. Blood products in instances of trauma
    c. Purulent debris in instances of superimposed infection
  4. Macrophages containing hemosiderin, cholesterol, or debris from within the cyst cavity may be present within the fibrous wall.
  5. Hepatic parenchyma may be atrophic immediately adjacent to larger cysts owing to compression.
  6. Von Meyenberg complexes (aggregates of dilated cystic structures predominantly in portal tracts) are occasionally present adjacent to the cyst wall.

Differential Diagnosis

1. *Cystadenoma:* This benign cystic neoplasm is distinguished from the simple cyst by commonly having a multiloculated pattern with papillary epithelial projections from the wall and is immediately surrounded by a mesenchymal stroma containing collagen, smooth muscle, fat, and benign glandular structures; however, it is possible that the simple cyst may be developmentally a type of cystadenoma.
2. *Cystic dilatation of intrahepatic ducts (Caroli's syndrome):* The cystlike structures in Caroli's syndrome represent dilated ducts that connect with the remainder of the biliary tree, unlike simple cysts that are structurally detached.

Clinical and Biologic Behavior

1. Solitary (nonparasitic) cysts are four times more common in women, occurring at all ages, but most often between the fourth and sixth decades; they are usually discovered incidentally during workup or laparotomy for other problems.
2. Most hepatic cysts are asymptomatic but may clinically present as a right upper quadrant mass, with pain, nausea, and vomiting due to compression of the adjacent stomach; rarely the cysts may spontaneously rupture.
3. Laboratory tests are usually normal, although alkaline phosphatase and bilirubin levels may be slightly elevated when the cysts are large and compress intrahepatic major bile ducts.
4. The cysts are round to elliptical and usually small, found twice as often in the right lobe, and are 95% unilocular and 5% multilocular; they are well circumscribed and may contain significant amounts of fluid (500 ml or more, one case reporting 17 L), which is usually clear (multiloculated cysts occasionally exhibit different physical properties in adjacent segments).
5. Cysts are both congenital and developmental and may arise from aberrant bile ducts.
6. Although calcification in the wall is rarely present, the hydatid (echinococcal) cyst needs exclusion when radiographs confirm calcification within a large cyst.
7. Papillomatosis may arise within the cyst wall, and in very rare instances, adenocarcinoma may develop.
8. Complications may present as abdominal emergencies (e.g., torsion, hemorrhage, rupture into the duct system or peritoneal cavity, infection).

Aspiration Cytology

1. Common findings include serous or mucous fluid sometimes containing blood, benign cuboidal to columnar epithelial cells, and cellular debris.

Treatment and Prognosis

1. When asymptomatic (incidental discovery), no treatment is necessary.
2. When large cysts produce significant symptoms, surgical resection is the best approach with excellent prognosis and very rare recurrence.
3. When surgical resection is not possible or desired, aspiration or drainage (surgical or percutaneous) may be tried.

References

Flagg RS, Robinson DW. Solitary nonparasitic hepatic cysts. Arch Surg 1967;95:964–973.
Ishak KG. Biliary cystadenoma. Cancer 1977;40:2400–2406.

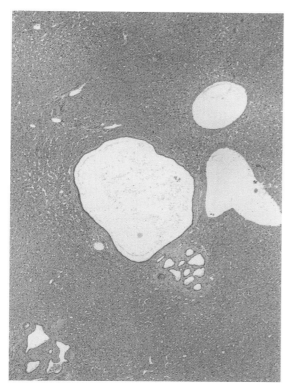

Figure 8–10. Polycystic disease. The multiple dilated ducts have a thin to cuboidal epithelium and form small cysts.

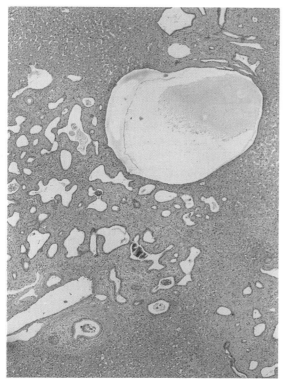

Figure 8–11. Polycystic disease. A single dilated duct and adjacent von Meyenberg complex containing bile are present.

POLYCYSTIC DISEASE

Major Morphologic Features

Infantile
1. Proliferation of dilated biliary channels that branch and anastomose, sometimes with polypoid projections, is present.

Adult
1. Multiple large cysts are lined by a single layer of flattened to cuboidal epithelium.

Other Features

Infantile
1. Biliary channels irregularly extend into the hepatic parenchyma.
2. Dilated ducts may contain a homogeneously eosinophilic material.
3. Prominent vascular and lymphatic channels are present within the fibroconnective network intertwining among the biliary channels.
4. Mild portal fibrosis may be present.
5. Normal interlobular bile ducts are usually absent.
6. Definite cyst formation is uncommon.

Adult
1. Atrophic hepatic parenchyma is immediately adjacent to large cysts secondary to compression.
2. Well-defined fibrous wall is not as apparent as in solitary cysts.
3. Von Meyenberg complexes (aggregate of markedly dilated irregularly shaped duct structures) are occasionally seen adjacent to larger cysts.
4. Minimal chronic inflammatory infiltate is present in surrounding fibroconnective tissue.

Differential Diagnosis

1. *Congenital hepatic fibrosis:* Congenital hepatic fibrosis exhibits proliferation of dilated duct structures within portal tracts; however, these portal regions also exhibit moderate to marked portal fibrosis with *decreased* venous and lymphatic channels; these changes are *not* features of polycystic disease.
2. *Von Meyenberg complexes:* The presence of these lesions can be suggestive of polycystic disease in instances in which the biopsy specimen is small and the degree of hepatic change cannot be assessed. Although von Meyenberg complexes are believed to be part of the spectrum of polycystic disease, these complexes may also be incidental findings in livers without clinical or other morphologic signs of polycystic disease.

Clinical and Biologic Behavior

Infantile

1. The disease presents clinically during the perinatal or infantile period; the degree of microcystic change increases when the disease presents after the first year of age.
2. Portal hypertension may be present, with the infant often dying of chronic renal failure and systemic hypertension.
3. The liver may grossly be normal or occasionally exhibit small cystic structures; however, the liver is usually firm due to the varying degrees of fibrosis.

Adult

1. Polycystic disease of the liver is rare, present in 0.07% to 0.15% of large autopsy series, and seen four to five times more frequently in women in their sixth decade.
2. Although the majority of patients are asymptomatic, hepatomegaly and right upper quadrant discomfort may be present with large lesions; serum aminotransferase levels are normal, and alkaline phosphatase and bilirubin values may rarely be elevated when large cysts cause obstruction to large intrahepatic ducts.
3. In 56% of cases, adult polycystic renal disease is also present; in addition, 37% of all patients with polycystic kidneys have concomitant polycystic liver involvement.
4. The liver is often diffusely involved by cysts ranging in size from less than 1 mm to greater than 12 cm; occasionally the left lobe alone may be involved.
5. The cyst fluid is clear to yellow and biochemically resembles the "bile salt–independent" fraction of human bile, supporting the hypothesis that the cyst wall is lined by functional biliary epithelium.
6. Embryologic maldevelopment and genetic predisposition (autosomal dominant) are probable etiologies; cysts are present not only in kidneys but rarely in other organ systems (e.g., pancreas, lung, spleen, brain, myocardium).
7. Complications are infrequent but include cyst rupture into the peritoneal cavity, hemorrhage, and infection; portal hypertension is rare.
8. Adult polycystic disease may develop from multiple von Meyenberg complexes present at birth, which gradually dilate over the years to form larger cystic structures.

Aspiration Cytology

1. In adult polycystic disease, cysts contain benign epithelium and amorphous material.

Treatment and Prognosis

1. Adult form of polycystic disease is usually asymptomatic and requires no treatment unless cysts enlarge, causing significant pain, hemorrhage or infection as the cysts develop. Aspiration and drainage (surgical or percutaneous) provides temporary relief and is of limited benefit.
2. Renal failure is a major cause of increasing morbidity and mortality with polycystic renal disease.

References

Blyth H, Ockenden BG. Polycystic disease of kidneys and liver presenting in childhood. J Med Genet 1971;81:257–284.

Comfort MW, Gray HK, Dahlin DC, et al. Polycystic disease of the liver: Study of 24 cases. Gastroenterology 1952;20:60–78.

Melnick PJ. Polycystic liver: Analysis of 70 cases. Arch Pathol 1955;59:162–172.

Summerfield JA, Nagafuchi Y, Sherlock S, et al. Hepatobiliary fibrocystic diseases: A clinical and histological review of 51 patients. J Hepatol 1986;2:141–156.

Van Erpecum KJ, Janssens AR, Terpstra JL, et al. Highly symptomatic adult polycystic disease of the liver: A report of fifteen cases. J Hepatol 1987;5:109–117.

CONGENITAL HEPATIC FIBROSIS

Major Morphologic Features

1. Extensive portal fibrosis and septa formation containing numerous markedly dilated anastomosing duct structures are present.
2. Regenerative parenchymal nodules are absent.
3. There is a marked decrease in portal vascular and lymphatic radicles.

Other Features

1. Minimal to absent inflammatory change occurs in areas of fibrosis.
2. Fibrotic regions are sharply demarcated from the parenchyma, with no arachnoid or sinusoidal fibrosis.
3. Duct structures are lined by cuboidal to columnar epithelium and often contain inspissated bile; however, cholestasis within the parenchyma is seldom present.
4. Duct lesions may appear singly or in small clusters within the parenchyma; fibrosis is minimal to absent adjacent to these ducts.
5. Parenchyma exhibits no significant inflammatory changes, with normal cord–sinusoid pattern; however, ducts may occasionally exhibit acute inflammatory changes secondary to superimposed infection.

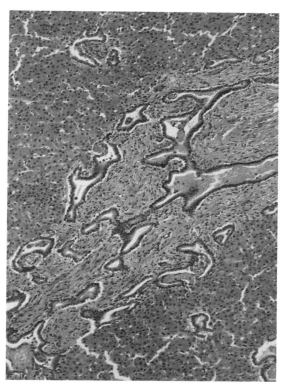

Figure 8–12. Congenital hepatic fibrosis. The liver is not cirrhotic but contains prominent portal fibrosis. Interlobular bile ducts are enlarged and dilated and contain an eosinophilic material.

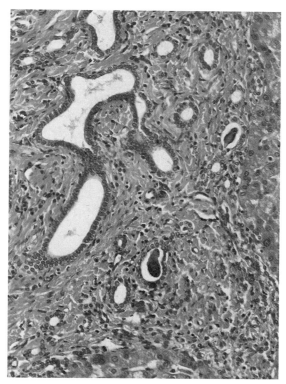

Figure 8–14. Congenital hepatic fibrosis. Occasional duct structures contain bile.

Differential Diagnosis

1. *Von Meyenberg complexes:* On needle biopsy congenital hepatic fibrosis may be misinterpreted as large or multiple von Meyenberg complexes; however, associated prominent portal fibrosis in a child or young adult with signs of portal hypertension strongly suggests congenital hepatic fibrosis as the leading diagnosis.
2. *Duct adenomas:* These consist of small mass lesions with proliferation of benign duct structures in a fibrous stroma. Congenital hepatic fibrosis has ectatic, branching ducts, often containing bile; duct adenomas are small with ducts that are not dilated and are devoid of bile.
3. *Cholangiocarcinoma or metastatic adenocarcinoma:* Congenital hepatic fibrosis may involve only one segment of a single lobe (*focal congenital hepatic fibrosis*) and may then present as a mass lesion. Morphologically, however, these focal lesions are identical to classic congenital hepatic fibrosis and therefore easy to differentiate from malignant lesions.

Clinical and Biologic Behavior

1. Congenital hepatic fibrosis is a rare congenital and autosomal recessive liver disease equally affecting

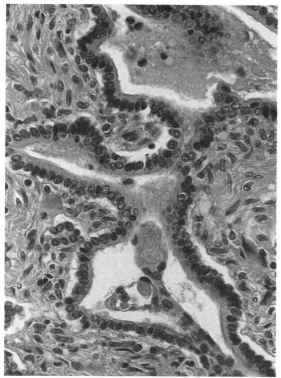

Figure 8–13. Congenital hepatic fibrosis. High power shows the duct to be dilated and surrounded by fibroblasts and occasional lymphocytes. The eosinophilic material within the duct consists of protein and mucin.

males and females; the disease is first discovered in patients between 5 and 20 years of age when bleeding from esophageal varices develops.

2. Patients usually have some degree of abdominal discomfort; hepatosplenomegaly and abdominal collateral veins are often identified secondary to portal hypertension, but ascites is unusual.

3. Laboratory findings are unremarkable except for a slight increase in alkaline phosphatase and gamma-glutamyl transpeptidase levels, especially with biliary tract infection; anemia may be present owing to hypersplenism.

4. One half of the patients may show variable renal changes ranging from polycystic kidneys to ectatic cortical and medullary tubules (in part resembling medullary sponge kidney).

5. In rare instances, only part of one lobe may be involved, clinically presenting as a mass lesion (*partial congenital hepatic fibrosis*).

6. The ductular lesions usually communicate with the biliary tree and resemble collapsed cysts, in contrast to adult polycystic disease in which ducts lose connection, have no drainage system, and therefore enlarge.

7. Congenital hepatic fibrosis represents one of the cystic diseases of the liver (i.e., von Meyenberg complexes, single and multiple cysts, duct ectasia) that develops from the same basic pathophysiologic process.

8. Associated duct disorders include *Caroli's syndrome,* in which collapsed microcysts do not form but instead ducts dilate *without* proliferation, and *choledochal cyst.*

9. Complications include infection of duct lesions (cholangitis) and, most importantly, consequences of portal hypertension (variceal hemorrhage); cholangiocarcinoma may occur but is rare.

Treatment and Prognosis

1. Although usually asymptomatic in early childhood, consequences of portal hypertension eventually occur; hemorrhage from esophagogastric varices is a major cause of death for which definitive therapy is offered (sclerotherapy or shunt surgery).

2. In patients who have associated renal cystic disease, renal failure is also a cause of death.

3. Caroli's syndrome and choledochal cyst may be responsible for cholangitis and sepsis.

References

DeVos M, Barbier F, Cuvelier C. Congenital hepatic fibrosis. J Hepatol 1988;6:222–228.

Ghishan FK, Younoszai MK. Congenital hepatic fibrosis: A disease with diverse manifestations. Am J Gastroenterol 1981;75:317–320.

McCarthy LJ, Baggenstoss AH, Logan GB. Congenital hepatic fibrosis. Gastroenterology 1965;49:27–36.

Sommerschild HC, Langmark F, Maurseth K. Congenital hepatic fibrosis: Report of two new cases and review of the literature. Surgery 1973;73:53–58.

Summerfield JA, Nagafuchi Y, Sherlock S, et al. Hepatobiliary fibrocystic diseases: A clinical and histological review of 51 patients. J Hepatol 1986;2:141–156.

Cystic Fibrosis (Mucoviscidosis)

Major Morphologic Features

1. Marked proliferation and dilatation of cholangioles containing amorphous eosinophilic concretions occur.

2. Multiple portal areas exhibit biliary type fibrosis (*focal biliary fibrosis*).

Other Features

1. Lining cells of cholangioles are generally atrophic secondary to compression by inspissated bile.

2. Rupture of cholangioles elicits a neutrophilic reaction.

3. Cholestasis within canaliculi and hepatocytes may be present in areas of biliary fibrosis.

4. Periportal fatty change, both macrovesicular and microvesicular, is present in 30% to 60% of cases.

5. Increased hemosiderin is occasionally seen in periportal hepatocytes.

6. Mucinous material is present in both extrahepatic

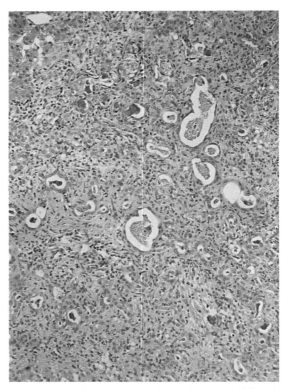

Figure 8–15. Cystic fibrosis. The portal tract shows marked fibrosis. Bile duct proliferation and dilatation are present, many containing pink to red inspissated material.

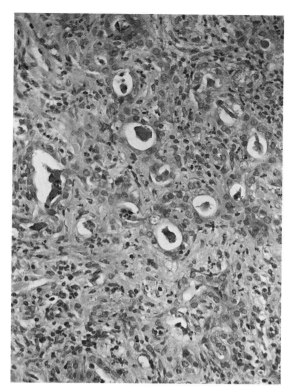

Figure 8–16. Cystic fibrosis. Many of the ducts are dilated with flattened to cuboidal epithelium and contain inspissated material. A moderate inflammatory infiltrate consisting predominantly of neutrophils is present.

and intrahepatic interlobular ducts in a minority of cases.

7. Multiple areas of biliary fibrosis eventually coalesce, forming *multilobular (multinodular) biliary fibrosis.*
8. Portal areas and parenchyma away from areas of fibrosis may be entirely normal.

Differential Diagnosis

1. *Extrahepatic large duct obstruction:* Portal fibrosis, bile duct proliferation and dilatation, cholangiolar proliferation, and cholestasis within the lobule are features seen in both cystic fibrosis and large duct obstruction. Initially the lesions in cystic fibrosis are focal, and a needle biopsy alone may miss characteristic morphologic changes. The presence of inspissated periodic acid–Schiff after diastase-positive material and mucin within ducts is characteristic of cystic fibrosis.

Special Stains

1. *Periodic acid–Schiff after diastase:* Biliary concretions in the cholangioles stain positively.
2. *Mucicarmine, Alcian blue:* Mucin, which is occasionally present within ducts, stains positively; however, the inspissated bile does not stain.

Clinical and Biologic Behavior

1. Cystic fibrosis is one of the most common lethal genetic disorders in the white population; it is inherited as an autosomal recessive disorder with an incidence of 1/2000 live births and a carrier gene frequency of 5%; the disorder is rare in the black population (1/17,000) and even rarer in Asians.
2. It presents clinically at any time from the neonatal period to adulthood; in the neonate, meconium ileus is present in approximately 50% of patients, with a small percentage of these cases developing an obstructive form of jaundice; neonatal hepatitis is present in approximately 5% of patients, usually caused by either cytomegalovirus infection or biliary tract obstruction.
3. Severe clinical problems related to pulmonary disease, including bronchiectasis and pneumonia (*Pseudomonas* and *S. aureus* most common), are usually evident in later childhood and adolescence.
4. Hepatomegaly is frequently due to fatty change.
5. In one third of cases slight to moderate elevations of serum aminotransferase levels and moderate elevations of alkaline phosphatase suggest biliary tract obstruction; serum bilirubin value is mildly increased.
6. Malabsorption is present owing to pancreatic insufficiency.
7. *Focal biliary fibrosis,* a classic and virtually diagnostic lesion of cystic fibrosis, is present overall in 22% to 33% of patients; when cystic fibrosis is clinically present before 3 months of age, the lesion is seen in 10.6%; at 3 to 12 months, 15.6%; when older than 1 year, 26.9% (suggesting that it is a progressive fibrogenic lesion).
8. *Multilobular fibrosis* is a developmental lesion, seen in adolescents in 6% to 10% of cases; portal hypertension may be present but is uncommon, with clinical evidence of cirrhosis seen in 2% cases (ascites 0.15%–0.30%).
9. Patients with multilobular biliary fibrosis may exhibit gross changes resembling hepar lobatum.
10. Microgallbladder is present in 15% to 20% of patients; chronic cholecystitis and/or cholelithiasis is seen in up to 60% of patients older than 15 years of age.
11. Sweat test is done for diagnosis: values greater than 60 mEq of chloride per liter (when supported by a positive family history), with repeated pulmonary infections and steatorrhea, are diagnostic. An abnormal test result is also seen in other conditions (e.g., Addison's disease), hence clinical history is important; test abnormality is caused by inhibition of electrolyte reabsorption.
12. Etiology of the liver disease is related to highly viscous mucus production, resulting in plugging of the interlobular bile ducts and inhibiting normal biliary excretion; gallstone production is secondary to malabsorption of bile acids and a decrease in the bile acid pool, with cholesterol stone formation.

Prognosis

1. Death is related to pulmonary problems, with the majority of patients not living past 30 years of age.

References

Huang NN, Schidlow DV, Szatrowski TH, et al. Clinical features, survival rates, and prognostic factors in young adults with cystic fibrosis. Am J Med 1987;82:871–879.

Hultcrantz R, Mengarelli S, Strandvik B. Morphological findings in the liver of children with cystic fibrosis: A light and electron microscopical study. Hepatology 1986;6:881–889.

Oppenheimer DH, Esterly JR. Hepatic changes in young infants with cystic fibrosis: Possible relation to focal biliary cirrhosis. J Pediatr 1975;86:683–689.

Psacharopoulos HT, Howard ER, Postman B, et al. Hepatic complications of cystic fibrosis. Lancet 1981;2:78–80.

■ Alpha-1-Antitrypsin Deficiency

Major Morphologic Features

1. Abundant numbers of distinct round eosinophilic intracytoplasmic inclusions are seen in periportal hepatocytes.
2. Cirrhosis occurs, micronodular or mixed macronodular and micronodular type in adults, and biliary type

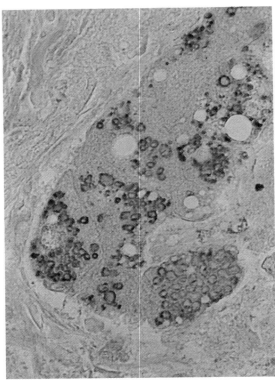

Figure 8–18. Alpha-1-antitrypsin deficiency (immunoperoxidase). The cytoplasmic inclusions are confirmed as alpha-1-antitrypsin. Note that the inclusions typically stain positive along their periphery but not in their center.

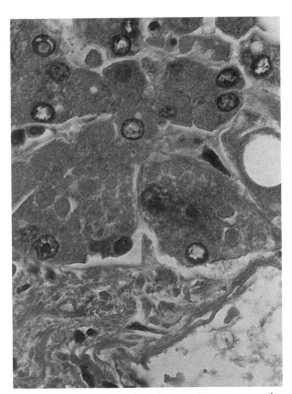

Figure 8–17. Alpha-1-antitrypsin deficiency. Numerous round eosinophilic cytoplasmic inclusions are present in these periportal hepatocytes, each inclusion smaller than the nucleus.

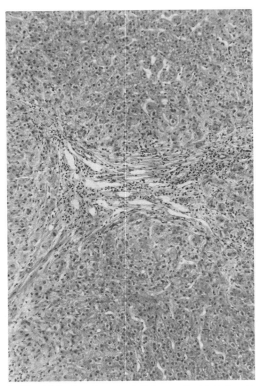

Figure 8–19. Alpha-1-antitrypsin deficiency. In this infant the biopsy specimen shows severe portal fibrosis with moderate lymphocytic infiltration, increase in vascular structures, but complete absence of bile ducts.

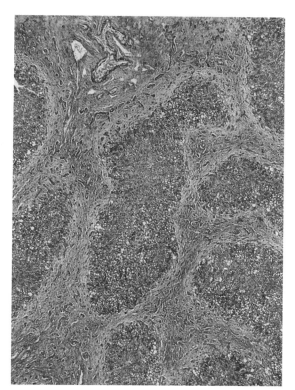

Figure 8–20. Alpha-1-antitrypsin deficiency (trichrome). The liver from this young child at the time of transplantation shows an advanced biliary cirrhosis. Slight edema surrounds all the regenerative nodules. A moderate degree of cholangiolar proliferation within the septa is present.

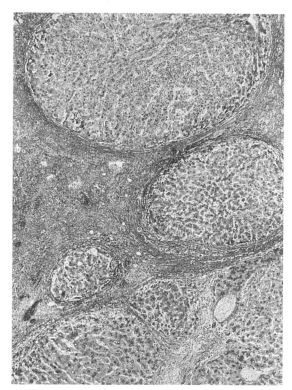

Figure 8–21. Alpha-1-antitrypsin deficiency (trichrome). The cirrhosis in this adult is a mixed macronodular and micronodular type. The nodules are well defined, with minimal inflammatory infiltration. Small duct structures are present within the septa.

in infants and young children, with inclusions present in periseptal liver cells and occasionally scattered within the regenerative nodules.

Other Features

1. In the neonate, giant cell hepatitis may be present, characterized by cholestasis, ballooning of hepatocytes, occasional acidophil bodies, and syncytial multinucleated hepatocytes.
2. Portal areas in the neonate exhibit mild mononuclear inflammatory infiltration.
3. Bile ducts initially proliferate; in latter stages there is atypical duct proliferation (serpentine growth pattern, flattened cells, absence of lumen) and eventual decrease to absence of interlobular ducts in severely fibrotic and cirrhotic stages. Cholangioles may be present in advanced stages.
4. Although inclusions in the neonate are not usually seen on routine staining before 12 weeks of age (may be weakly positive by immunoperoxidase), they gradually enlarge, ranging anywhere from less than 1 to 20 μm in diameter; inclusions are usually quite numerous in individual hepatocytes.
5. Inclusions may also be present in cytoplasm of bile duct epithelium.
6. Alcoholic hyalin may be identified, usually located in periportal or periseptal hepatocytes, when significant cholestasis is present.
7. Fatty change may be present.
8. Hyalinized collagen has been demonstrated in periseptal fibrous regions.
9. Inclusions may not be distributed evenly from one lobule to the next; in the cirrhotic stage, this finding is quite common, with some nodules totally lacking inclusions.
10. Cirrhosis in the adult exhibits little inflammatory change in the fibrous septa and parenchyma; however, in some instances features of chronic active hepatitis may be seen.
11. Inclusions are much more commonly seen *without* associated liver disease (heterozygous state); usually the number of hepatocytes exhibiting inclusions are less than in cases exhibiting liver disease.

Differential Diagnosis

1. In the neonate:
   a. *Giant cell hepatitis of viral etiology*
   b. *Extrahepatic biliary atresia*
   c. *Paucity of duct syndrome*

In each of the above disorders, cholestasis, giant cell transformation, and chronic inflammatory infiltrates can be seen, changes similar to alpha-1-antitrypsin deficiency. Giant cells are usually not as prominent in alpha-1-antitrypsin deficiency as in giant cell hepatitis secondary to virus or extrahepatic biliary atresia and not

present after the infant is 1 year of age. Since inclusions are often not identifiable before 12 weeks of age, distinction from the above disease entities on morphologic grounds alone may not be possible. Follow-up at a later date will, however, demonstrate inclusions. Serum alpha-1-antitrypsin levels and phenotyping is necessary to distinguish between the common benign heterozygous (e.g., PiMZ) and rare homozygous (PiZZ) states.
2. *Other disorders demonstrating cytoplasmic inclusions include the following:*
   a. *Anoxia:* Usually single, located predominantly within perivenular hepatocytes
   b. *Drug-induced liver disease* (e.g., procainamide): Accentuated in perivenular zone or has no distinct zonal distribution
   c. *Alcoholic liver disease:*
      1) *Lysosomes:* Hepatocytes and Kupffer cells contain numerous small cytoplasmic granular inclusions, the larger ones in Kupffer cells.
      2) *Megamitochondria:* This is usually single and of variable size (may become as large as nucleus), perivenular or scattered throughout all zones, and often present in acute alcoholic liver disease.
   d. *Familial hypofibrinogenemia:* Inclusions are present within cytoplasmic vacuoles.
   e. *Myoclonus epilepsy (Lafora's disease):* Single, relatively large inclusions are present in periportal hepatocytes and resemble ground-glass cells of chronic hepatitis B.
   NOTE: All of the above inclusions, except lysosomes, are periodic acid–Schiff after diastase–negative; in addition, all can be differentiated from alpha-1-antitrypsin inclusions by immunoperoxidase staining.

Special Stains

1. *Periodic acid-Schiff after diastase:* Inclusions are bright red to purple.
2. *Phosphotungstic acid hematoxylin:* Inclusions often stain blue.
3. *Orcein:* Brown-black granules in periportal and periseptal hepatocytes, representing copper-binding protein, are associated with chronic cholestasis and biliary-type fibrosis or cirrhosis.

Immunohistochemistry

1. *Alpha-1-antitrypsin:* Larger inclusions exhibit a pattern of positive staining along their outer margins but negative central staining.

Clinical and Biologic Behavior

1. Alpha-1-antitrypsin represents 90% of all alpha-1-globulins in human serum and is the major inhibitor of trypsin and other proteases; it is a glycoprotein (hence its positive staining with periodic acid–Schiff) with 33 codominant genetic alleles determining presence or absence of disease in humans.
2. Pi (protease inhibitor) MM phenotype is normal, with serum level of 220 to 450 mg/dL; PiZZ (incidence 0.03%–0.07%) is responsible for both hepatic and pulmonary disease, with serum levels less than 20%; heterozygous PiMZ (incidence 3%) with approximately 60% serum levels, is possibly related to liver disease as well, although this occurrence is very rare.
3. Approximately 20% PiZZ will present in neonate as cholestasis and/or acute liver cell injury, exhibiting giant cell hepatitis on biopsy; distinction between extrahepatic biliary atresia, viral hepatitis, or paucity of duct syndrome may not be possible on clinical grounds (hepatomegaly, jaundice) or routine laboratory testing (slight increase in aminotransferase levels, moderately elevated alkaline phosphatase activity) alone; quantitation of alpha-1-antitrypsin serum level and phenotyping (isoelectric focusing) are necessary.
4. Alpha-1-antitrypsin deficiency is responsible for between 5% and 10% of all cases of neonatal hepatitis.
5. Although only 20% are symptomatic, approximately one half of the remaining infants with PiZZ will have abnormal liver test results persisting for many years.
6. Although cholestasis and neonatal hepatitis usually resolve at about 6 months, 2.5% of patients will develop a rapidly progressive liver disease with cirrhosis and die within 2 to 4 years; 11% to 25% of symptomatic patients will develop cirrhosis and die of complications before age 10.
7. In adult with PiZZ, 10% to 12% will be cirrhotic (20% after age 50); 59% will have a chronic obstructive pulmonary disease (usually panlobular emphysema). Many patients with adult-onset liver disease are asymptomatic in childhood.
8. The adult may demonstrate features of portal hypertension (abdominal collaterals, esophageal varices, ascites); hepatocellular carcinoma has been associated with alpha-1-antitrypsin deficiency but is rare. It is important to note that alpha-1-antitrypsin globules may be present in both the tumor and nontumor portion of the liver in patients *without* alpha-1-antitrypsin deficiency (normal serum levels and PiMM).
9. In heterozygotes (PiMZ), inflammatory hepatic changes of any etiology usually cause a reactive increase in alpha-1-antitrypsin production, and patients then have a low normal to normal serum level.
10. Heterozygotes (PiMZ) have been shown to be twice as common as controls in patients with chronic active hepatitis (non-B); in addition, in a series of patients with hepatocellular carcinoma, 6% to 8% were PiMZ compared with 3.1% of controls.
11. Globules are shown under electron microscopy as

amorphous material within <u>dilated rough endoplasmic reticulum</u>, often with a peripheral halo.

12. Other phenotypes associated with liver disease are PiSZ and PiSS (very rare, with disagreement whether related or by chance).
13. Pathophysiology of liver injury is unknown. Substitution of glutamic acid for lysine in the peptide sequence and deficiency of normal sialic acid result in impaired secretion of alpha-1-antitrypsin from the hepatocyte; when proteolytic enzymes are released from white blood cells during inflammatory responses, the activity of their enzymes goes unchecked in liver (and lung) with continued damage.

Treatment and Prognosis

1. There is no specific therapy.
2. Infusion of pooled plasma will raise serum alpha-1-antitrypsin levels temporarily, but beneficial effects on liver disease are difficult to assess. Gene therapy is a possibility in the future.
3. At present, hepatic transplantation is the only definitive treatment of advanced liver disease and hepatic failure.
4. The prognosis in patients with PiZZ phenotype is uncertain, since not all affected patients develop liver or pulmonary disease.

References

Alagille D. Alpha-1-antitrypsin deficiency. Hepatology 1984;4:11S–14S.

Berg NO, Eriksson S. Liver disease in adults with alpha-1-antitrypsin deficiency. N Engl J Med 1972;287:1264–1267.

Hodges TR, Millward-Sadler GH, Barbatis C, et al. Heterozygous MZ alpha-1-antitrypsin deficiency in adults with chronic active hepatitis and cryptogenic cirrhosis. N Engl J Med 1981;304:557–560.

Larsson C. Natural history and life expectancy in severe alpha-1-antitrypsin deficiency, PiZ. Acta Med Scand 1978;204:345–351.

Qizilbash A, Young-Pong O. Alpha-1-antitrypsin liver disease differential diagnosis of PAS-positive, diastase-resistant globules in liver cells. Am J Clin Pathol 1983;79:697–702.

Sveger T. Liver disease in alpha-1-antitrypsin deficiency detected by screening of 200,000 infants. N Engl J Med 1976;294:1316–1321.

■ Hereditary Hyperbilirubinemias

With the exception of the Dubin-Johnson syndrome the hepatic morphology overall is not distinctive, with patients with Crigler-Najjar syndrome occasionally exhibiting bile plugs and patients with Gilbert's syndrome only rarely containing an increase in lipochrome-like pigment.

Dubin-Johnson Syndrome

Major Morphologic Features

1. Abundant granular, dark brown intracytoplasmic lipochrome-like pigment is seen within hepatocytes and concentrated around the canaliculi.
2. Pigment is most prominent in perivenular hepatocytes.
3. Portal tracts are unremarkable, and there is no significant necrosis or inflammatory change within the parenchyma.

Differential Diagnosis

1. *Conditions exhibiting increased lipochrome include the following:*
   a. *Older population:* Anisocytosis of hepatocytes is also present, and often prominent.
   b. *Drugs* (e.g., phenacetin)

Table 8–2
HEREDITARY HYPERBILIRUBINEMIAS

Syndrome	Age at Onset (yr)	Bilirubin			Deficiency	Clinical Presentation
		mg/dL	Conjugated	Unconjugated		
Inability to Conjugate Bilirubin						
Crigler-Najjar						
Type 1	Neonate	25–48	Absent	Increased	Glucuronyl transferase (total)	Kernicterus; death within 18 months
Type 2	Neonate	6–25	Trace	Increased	Glucuronyl transferase (partial)	May live past age 50
Gilbert's	Birth–18, but may be detected at any age	1–7	Normal	Increased	Transglucuronidation	Jaundice precipitated by fasting, infection, alcohol, stress
Inability to Secrete Conjugated Bilirubin						
Dubin-Johnson	15–25	2–10	Increased	Increased	Canalicular secretion	Hepatomegaly, fluctuation of jaundice
Rotor's	3–8	1–8	Increased	Increased	Canalicular secretion	Fluctuation of jaundice

Modified from Edmonson HA, Peters RL. Liver. In: Kissane JM, Anderson WAD, eds. Pathology, 8th ed. St. Louis: C.V. Mosby, 1985.

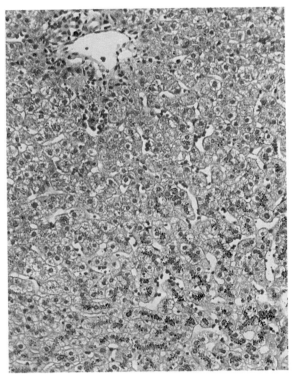

Figure 8–22. Dubin-Johnson syndrome. The architecture is intact. The portal tract is normal, with only a mild lymphocytic infiltration. The perivenular region shows a pigment within the liver cells.

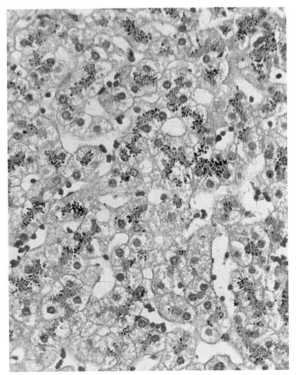

Figure 8–23. Dubin-Johnson syndrome. The hepatocytes are slightly hydropic. The granular brown intracytoplasmic pigment is concentrated around the canalicular border. Kupffer cell hyperplasia and inflammatory infiltration are not present.

NOTE: Pigment in the Dubin-Johnson syndrome is darker brown and usually more abundant and prominent than typical lipochrome.

Special Stains

1. *Periodic acid–Schiff after diastase, acid-fast (Ziehl-Neelsen carbolfuchsin):* The pigment exhibits variable degrees of positive staining; however, typical lipochrome exhibits similar staining characteristics.

Clinical and Biologic Behavior

1. Dubin-Johnson syndrome is an autosomal recessive disorder characterized by chronic and intermittent bouts of benign hyperbilirubinemia; 60% of the bilirubin is conjugated.
2. It is present worldwide, most prominent in the Middle East (approximately 1/1300), and twice as frequent in men, with characteristic onset of jaundice in the second to fourth decades.
3. Hepatomegaly and often abdominal discomfort are present in over one half of the symptomatic patients. Serum bilirubin is less than 10 mg/dL in 90% of the patients (has been reported as high as 27 mg/dL); serum aminotransferase levels are normal, and the alkaline phosphatase activity is only minimally elevated in up to 10% of patients. Prothrombin activity is usually normal but may be slightly decreased.
4. Jaundice may be precipitated by pregnancy, estrogen therapy (oral contraceptives), infection, trauma, and surgery.
5. The liver biopsy specimen grossly appears dark brown to black secondary to an increase in lipochrome-type pigment in perivenular hepatocytes; electron microscopy shows the granules to be present in lysosomes, to lack prominent lipid components, and to be slightly larger and not as dense or multilobulated as typical lipochrome.
6. Pigment is not always present or increased, however, in biopsy specimens obtained after many causes of rapid liver cell turnover (e.g., regeneration after viral hepatitis); the pigment will reappear in new hepatocytes after time.
7. The gallbladder does not opacify on oral cholecystography, and on technetium 99m HIDA scans only the extrahepatic biliary tract is visualized; urinary coproporphyrin I level is increased, coproporphyrin III is decreased, but total levels are normal. The diagnostic test is bromosulfopthalein (BSP) excretion; serum BSP values at 90 and 120 minutes greatly exceed values at 45 minutes, owing to reflux of BSP-glutathione conjugate from the liver cell to the plasma from failure of canalicular excretion.

Treatment and Prognosis

1. No therapy is usually needed except avoidance of precipitating factors; use of phenobarbital may improve bilirubin.

References

Billing BH. Bilirubin metabolism. In: Schiff L, Schiff ER, eds. Diseases of the Liver, 6th ed. Philadelphia: J.B. Lippincott, 1987:103–127.

Crigler JF, Najjar VA. Congenital familial nonhemolytic jaundice with kernicterus. Pediatrics 1952;10:169–179.

Dubin IN, Johnson FB. Chronic idiopathic jaundice with unidentified pigment in liver cells: New clinicopathologic entity with report of 12 cases. Medicine 1954;33:155–197.

Edmondson HA, Peters RL. Liver. In: Kissane JM, Anderson WAD, eds. Pathology, 8th ed. St. Louis: C.V. Mosby, 1985:1171.

Jansen PLM, Oude Elferink RPJ. Hereditary hyperbilirubinemias: A molecular and mechanistic approach. Semin Liver Dis 1988;8:168–178.

■ Storage Disorders

The disease entities listed in Table 8–3 are all attributable to enzyme deficiencies causing increased accumulation of metabolic byproducts in the liver. Morphologic changes on routine hematoxylin and eosin staining are not diagnostic of a disorder but may suggest an abnormal accumulation of substances within hepatocytes or Kupffer cells. Strong suggestion of a specific entity in some instances may occur (e.g., striated wrinkled cytoplasmic Kupffer cells in Gaucher's disease). The liver must be analyzed specifically for metabolic determinants and enzyme activities responsible for abnormal tissue deposition. Other organ systems are often involved as well, and hepatic failure is usually not the cause of death. Alpha-1-antitrypsin deficiency, porphyrias, and disorders in copper and iron metabolism are discussed in more detail elsewhere in this chapter.

References

Balistreri WF, Schubert WK. Liver disease in infancy and childhood. In: Schiff L, Schiff ER, eds. Diseases of the liver, 6th ed. Philadelphia: J.B. Lippincott, 1987:1337–1426.

Ishak KG, Sharp HL. Metabolic errors and liver disease. In: MacSween RNM, Anthony PP, Scheuer PJ, eds. Pathology of the liver, 2nd ed. Edinburgh: Churchill Livingstone, 1987:99–180.

Ruebner BH, Cox KL. Liver diseases in infancy. In: Peters RL, Craig JR, eds. Liver Pathology. New York: Churchill Livingstone, 1986:37–60.

■ Iron Storage Disorders

Basic Iron Metabolism

ABSORPTION

1. Approximately 1 mg/d is absorbed from a normal diet, most prominently at the level of the duodenum and proximal jejunum.
2. The iron is transferred to the bone marrow (hemoglobin), muscle (myoglobin), and other cells (enzymes)

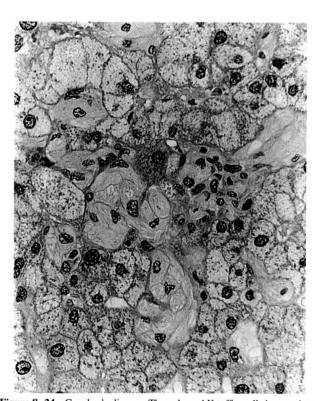

Figure 8–24. Gaucher's disease. The enlarged Kupffer cells have striated wrinkled cytoplasm containing abundant glucocerebroside.

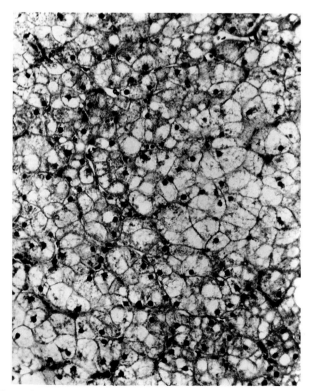

Figure 8–25. Glycogen storage disease type I. The hepatocytes are enlarged and hydropic. Variable degrees of fatty change are present. The cytoplasm of the liver cells, as well as cells of the proximal convoluted tubules of the kidney, are filled with glycogen owing to glucose-6-phosphatase deficiency. (Courtesy of Boris H. Reubner, MD)

Table 8–3
STORAGE DISORDERS

Disorder	Enzyme Deficiency	Hepatic Changes	Clinical Presentation
Glycogen Storage Disease			
I (von Gierke's)	Glucose-6-phosphatase	Glycogen within nuclei and cytoplasm; variable fatty change; liver cell adenomas reported	Stunted growth, recurrent infections, xanthomas, nephropathy
II (Pompe's)	Lysosomal alpha-1, 4-glucosidase (acid maltase)	Glycogen accumulation within lysosomes	Severe hypotonia of skeletal and cardiac musculature; renal failure; usually die in first year
III (Forbe's, Cori's)	Amylo-1, 6 glucosidase (debrancher)	Glycogen within nuclei and cytoplasm; portal fibrosis and cirrhosis may occur	Growth retardation, infections, metabolic abnormalities; consequences of portal hypertension in cirrhotics
IV (Andersen's)	Alpha-1, 4 glucon-6-glycosyl transferase (brancher)	Eosinophilic periportal inclusion-like material in liver cell cytoplasm; fibrosis and cirrhosis occur	Gastroenteritis, osteoporosis, failure to thrive; death from cirrhosis and cardiac failure
VI (Her's)	Hepatic phosphorylase	Glycogen within cytoplasm, nuclei	Growth retardation; no severe metabolic abnormalities
VIII	Phosphorylase activation	Glycogen within cytoplasm; fibrosis may occur	Mild symptomatology related to hepatomegaly
IX	Phosphorylase-6-kinase	Glycogen within cytoplasm	Mild symptomatology related to hepatomegaly
Mucopolysaccharidoses			
I (Hurler's)	Alpha-L-iduronidase (lysosomes)	Mucopolysaccharides as small lipid droplets in hepatocytes, Kupffer and Ito cells; fibrosis may be present	Mental retardation, cloudiness of cornea, skeletal deformities; death before age 10 from cardiorespiratory failure
III (Sanfilippo's)			
A	Heparin sulfatase	Similar to Hurler's	
B	N-Acety-1-alpha-D-glucosidase	Similar to Hurler's	
Neutral Lipid and Cholesterol Storage Disease			
Wolman's	Acid esterase and acid lipase (lysosomes)	Small droplet fat in hepatocytes and Kupffer cells; foamy macrophages with abundant cholesterol (demonstrable as crystals with polarized light, frozen sections) and triglycerides; cirrhosis has been described	Severe fat malabsorption, failure to thrive; hepatosplenomegaly, death by age 6 months
Cholesterol ester	Acid lipase (lysosomes)	Similar to Wolman's, with more abundant cholesterol	Much milder form than Wolman's, with hepatosplenomegaly; otherwise often asymptomatic
Familial High-density lipoprotein deficiency (Tangier's)	Lecithin cholesterol acyltransferase	Mild fatty change; cholesterol esters in Kupffer cells and macrophages (demonstrable as crystals with polarized light, frozen sections)	Hepatosplenomegaly, orange-yellow hyperplastic tonsils; peripheral neuropathy; absence of normal high-density lipoproteins
Gangliosidoses			
I (Tay-Sachs)	Hexosaminidase A	No change in light microscopy; electron microscopy shows laminated inclusions in hepatocytes (GM$_2$ gangliosides)	Psychomotor retardation, visual abnormalities, cherry-red spots in macula; decerebrate rigidity, death by age 3 years; adult form less severe
II (Sandoff's)	Hexosaminidase A and B	Kupffer cells with granules (periodic acid–Schiff and Luxol-fast blue positive); no other significant change; electron microscopy shows laminated inclusions in hepatocytes and Kupffer cells (GM$_2$ gangliosides and tetrahexosyl ceramide)	Similar to Tay-Sachs, with hepatomegaly
Glycosphingolipidoses			
Fabry's	Alpha-galactosidase	Hypertrophied portal macrophages, Kupffer and endothelial cells; electron microscopy shows whorled inclusions	Multiple cutaneous angiomas; renal, cardiac failure in third to fifth decade

Table 8–3 (*Continued*)

Disorder	Enzyme Deficiency	Hepatic Changes	Clinical Presentation
Glucocerebrosidoses			
Gaucher's	Glucocerebrosidase	Marked enlargement of Kupffer cells, with striated, wrinkled cytoplasm; fibrosis rare; autofluorescence, with intensive acid phosphatase activity	Hypertonia, failure to thrive; neurologic defects and death by age 2 years; adult form less severe, with hepatosplenomegaly and osteoporosis
Niemann-Pick	Sphingomyelinase	Foamy Kupffer cells, portal macrophages; hydropic hepatocytes; in adult, macrophages contain pigment with "sea-blue" appearance (sea blue histiocytosis); mild fibrosis can occur; autofluorescent foam cells	Neurologic abnormalities, failure to thrive; cherry-red spots in macula; adult forms may be asymptomatic

by way of the protein *transferrin;* any excess iron is incorporated into *ferritin,* which is synthesized on demand.

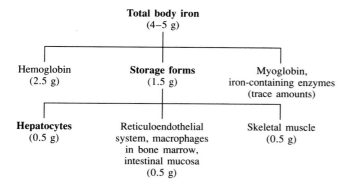

3. Abundant amounts of ferritin will eventually aggregate, denature from action of proteolytic enzymes, and form *hemosiderin.*

BODY LOSS

1. Approximately 1 mg/d is lost in sweat, urine, and feces.
2. Additional 10 to 30 mg is lost by menstruation.

TURNOVER

1. Main source is through senescent red blood cells (erythrophagocytosis by the reticuloendothelial system) and death of cells containing iron.
2. Approximately two thirds of this iron is immediately transferred to the bone marrow and other cells by transferrin.
3. Any excess iron will remain in the reticuloendothelial system as hemosiderin.

STORAGE FORMS
Ferritin
1. The primary storage form of iron, ferritin is present in the cytoplasm and lysosomes of all hepatocytes.

2. It is not visible by light microscopy with hematoxylin and eosin stain.
3. Prussian blue stain for iron is negative but may be diffusely although weakly positive when ferritin is present in significant amounts.

Hemosiderin
1. Hemosiderin is a heterogeneous water-insoluble granular material that has variable amounts of carbohydrates, protein, lipids, and iron.
2. It is golden-yellow on light microscopy, staining intensely with Prussian blue.
3. It is detectable predominantly surrounding canalicular poles in hepatocytes.

Conditions Associated With Increased Hepatic Iron (Table 8–4)

Table 8–4
CONDITIONS ASSOCIATED WITH INCREASED HEPATIC IRON GROUPED BY LOCATION OF IRON IN LIVER

Predominantly Hepatocellular	Predominantly Kupffer Cell	Mixed Hepatocellular and Kupffer Cell
Idiopathic hemochromatosis	Transfusions	Anemias secondary to ineffective erythropoiesis
Alcoholic liver disease	Bantu siderosis	Sideroblastic
Status post portacaval shunt	Hemolytic anemias: Hereditary spherocytosis	Megaloblastic
Porphyria cutanea tarda	Glucose-6-phosphate dehydrogenase deficiency	Anemias secondary to chronic infection
	Pyruvate kinase deficiency	Erythemic myelosis
	Anemias secondary to abnormal hemoglobins: Sickle cell (HbSS) Thalassemia (homozygous beta, intermedia)	Myelofibrosis

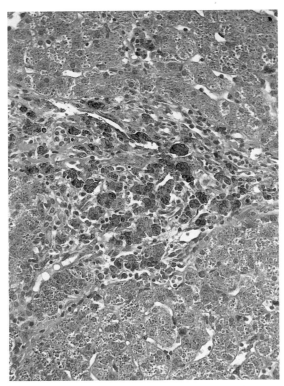

Figure 8-26. Hemosiderosis, thalassemia. Portal macrophages are distended and filled with a golden-brown pigment representing hemosiderin.

Idiopathic Hemochromatosis

Major Morphologic Features

1. Extensive hemosiderin deposition occurs in the cytoplasm of virtually all liver cells.
2. Portal fibrosis and eventual micronodular cirrhosis occur as the disease progresses.

Other Features

1. Hemosiderin is also present in bile duct epithelium and may be seen to variable degrees in endothelial cells as well as connective tissue in portal tracts.
2. Focal necrosis may be present within the lobule but is usually mild.
3. Kupffer cells and macrophages present in areas of parenchymal necrosis will contain hemosiderin; otherwise, Kupffer cells are devoid of the pigment.
4. Bile ducts show mild reduplication, with mild mononuclear portal inflammatory infiltration.
5. Hemosiderin is more concentrated in the pericanalicular regions of the hepatocytes.
6. Pigment resembling hemosiderin, but negative on iron stain, may be identified in hepatocytes and portal areas (hemofuscin).

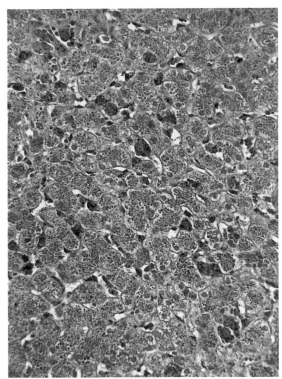

Figure 8-27. Hemosiderosis, thalassemia. The Kupffer cells are hyperplastic and hypertrophic and filled with golden-brown hemosiderin. Granular staining of the liver cell cytoplasm by hemosiderin is also present.

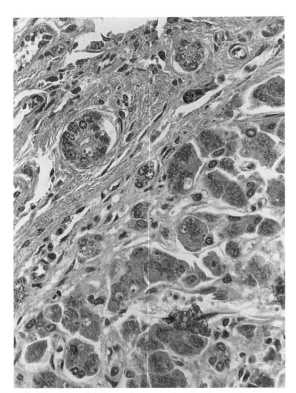

Figure 8-28. Idiopathic hemochromatosis. The liver cell cytoplasm and bile duct epithelium, but not Kupffer cells, contain abundant hemosiderin.

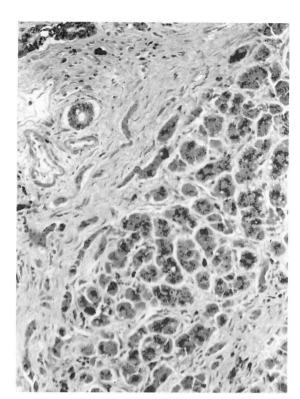

Figure 8–29. Idiopathic hemochromatosis (Prussian blue). This stain confirms that the abundant pigment is iron in both hepatocytes and interlobular bile ducts.

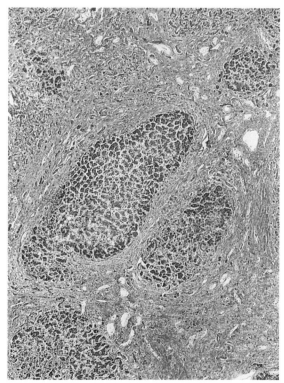

Figure 8–30. Idiopathic hemochromatosis (trichrome). The cirrhotic stage shows well-formed, small to medium-sized regenerative nodules. At this stage of the disease hepatocellular carcinoma may develop in up to one fourth of the patients.

7. Macrovesicular fatty change may be seen (more prevalent in diabetic patients).
8. Sinusoidal collagen deposition is minimal to absent.
9. In precirrhotic (early) stages, hemosiderin is concentrated in periportal hepatocytes; in cirrhosis, the regenerative nodules exhibit a periseptal accentuation of pigment deposition, depending on the degree of regenerative activity of the nodule (regenerative cells initially contain little pigment).
10. The cirrhotic nodules are usually small and fairly well defined.
11. Hepatocellular carcinoma may occur at the cirrhotic stage in up to one fourth of cases.

Differential Diagnosis

1. *Hemosiderosis from other etiologies:* Other causes of increased hepatic iron deposition have been listed in Table 8–4. The major differential features are the location (hepatocytes and not Kupffer cells) and quantity of iron.
   a. *Alcoholic liver disease:* A small percentage of patients with alcoholic liver disease exhibit moderate to marked amounts of hemosiderin in the cytoplasm of hepatocytes. In this patient with alcoholic cirrhosis who has been abstinent for at least 3 months, the morphologic changes (due to inflammatory inactivity) may resemble idiopathic hemochromatosis. Hemosiderin may also be seen in duct epithelium in the alcoholic; however, iron is not present in as great amounts in alcoholic liver disease, and thus iron stain is usually not as striking as in hemochromatosis. Any evidence of activity in the alcoholic, such as hyalin deposition in hepatocytes, neutrophilic infiltration of septa and parenchyma, and sinusoidal collagen, are features not seen in idiopathic hemochromatosis. Finally, the *hepatic iron index* (ratio of iron concentration to age) has been shown to clearly separate the precirrhotic patients with hemochromatosis from alcoholics with increased iron.

Special Stains

1. *Prussian blue:* Staining of hemosiderin granules in bile duct epithelium and virtually all liver cells is positive (4 +); the hemosiderin is often concentrated in pericanalicular regions of the hepatocyte.

Clinical and Biologic Behavior

1. Idiopathic hemochromatosis is an inherited autosomal recessive disorder characterized by massive deposits of iron stores within many organs, resulting in multiple organ dysfunction:

a. *Liver:* Cirrhosis is present in well-established cases, with complication of hepatocellular carcinoma 14% to 29% of the time.
b. *Pancreas:* Diabetes is found in approximately 63%.
c. *Heart:* Cardiomegaly and failure occur in 25%.
d. *Joints:* Chondrocalcinosis and degenerative arthritis are noted, commonly involving the second and third metacarpophalangeal joints of both hands in 25% to 75% of patients.
e. *Hypogonadism:* Loss of libido, impotence, amenorrhea, and testicular atrophy occur in approximately 50%; although cirrhosis may play a part, these features may be present before significant impairment of hepatic function.
f. *Skin:* Pigmentation present in almost all cases is slate-gray owing to iron deposition; increased melanin may also occur, giving the skin a bronze color.
g. Other sites of iron stores include thyroid, adrenal, anterior pituitary glands, lymph nodes, stomach, and kidneys.

2. The disorder presents clinically between ages 40 and 60 and is 10 times more frequent in men.

3. The disorder also presents earlier in men than women (35%–40% before age 46 in men, 20%–25% in women), most likely because of loss of iron in women from menstruation, pregnancy, and lactation. Patients present with hepatomegaly or bleeding esophageal varices; asymptomatic patients are identified incidentally by mild increase of serum aminotransferase levels.

4. Gene responsible for hemochromatosis is present on short arm of chromosome 6, tightly linked to HLA locus: HLA-A3, HLA-B7, and HLA-B14 are commonly present.

5. Relatives of affected patients have laboratory test results indicative of abnormal iron metabolism; increased iron is also present on liver biopsy, yet these patients are asymptyomatic.

6. The incidence of gene homozygosity is 0.25% to 0.31%, but clinical disease is seen in only 1/7000 deaths and 2 to 4/100,000 in autopsy series, which is evidence that full gene expression combined with multiple additional factors must play a role.

7. Liver test abnormalities are unimpressive, even in the presence of cirrhosis: serum albumin level is often normal, serum aminotransferase levels are normal or slightly elevated, and bilirubin is usually normal. Prothrombin activity is decreased in only one in four patients, and alkaline phosphatase activity is elevated only 20% of the time.

8. *Iron studies:* Plasma iron is greater than 200 μ/dL, transferrin saturation is greater than 85%, serum ferritin is greater than 2000 ng/dL, and hepatic iron is greater than 1% dry weight.

9. Ferritin concentration in plasma is usually a good indicator of iron stores, where 1 ng/mL equals approximately 8 mg iron stored (normal body storage is 1.5 g; in hemochromatosis it is 15 to 40 g); however, in many inflammatory conditions of the liver causing liver cell destruction and release of ferritin into plasma, ferritin concentrations may temporarily become elevated, even into the thousands (e.g., severe acute viral hepatitis).

10. Etiology of idiopathic hemochromatosis is unknown, but a number of factors contribute to the amount as well as rate of accumulation of iron:
a. *Genetic predisposition*
b. *Diet:* Substantial iron in diet (meat and byproducts), presence in cooking utensils, and vitamin supplements will contribute to earlier manifestations of the disease.
c. *Rate of iron loss:* Associated conditions resulting in considerable bleeding (e.g., variceal bleeding in cirrhosis, hematologic abnormality with hemorrhagic diathesis) may delay clinical onset.
d. *Other toxins:* Chronic alcoholics have more iron in the liver and a higher incidence of hemochromatosis than nonalcoholics; 10% to 40% of patients with hemochromatosis have some history of alcohol intake. Alcohol accelerates iron absorption as well as directly enhances liver cell injury.
e. *Iron toxicity:* Iron directly produces acute hepatotoxicity, causing necrosis of predominantly periportal hepatocytes; this is due to generation of free radicals by ferrous iron, which leads to lipid peroxidation and severe cell damage and is *not* due to iron stored as hemosiderin. Iron accumulates in lysosomes, possibly resulting in release of acid hydrolases into the cytoplasm with cell damage.

Aspiration Cytology

1. Because of the high incidence of hepatocellular carcinoma in hemochromatosis, workup of masses within the liver may reveal not only hepatocellular carcinoma but also massive hemosiderin deposits in hepatocytes from nontumor liver.

2. The tumor cells themselves lose the ability to incorporate hemosiderin into their cytoplasm.

Treatment and Prognosis

1. Therapy is supportive for patients with diabetes, cardiac failure, and arthritis.

2. Removal of iron is performed by phlebotomy or by chelating substances (e.g., desferrioxamine) when phlebotomy is contraindicated (e.g., cardiac failure).

3. Results show improvement in hepatic and cardiac function with treatment; however, cirrhosis will not resolve and the incidence of hepatocellular carcinoma in cirrhotics is the same in both treated and untreated patients.

4. When disease is treated, 5-year survival is 66%; 10-year survival, 32%. If disease is not treated, 5-year survival is 18%; 10-year survival, 6%.

References

Bassett ML, Halliday JW, Powell LW. Value of hepatic iron measurements in early hemochromatosis and determination of the critical iron level associated with fibrosis. Hepatology 1986;6:24–29.

Bothwell TH, Charlton RW. Hemochromatosis. In: Schiff L, Schiff ER, eds. Diseases of the Liver, 6th ed. Philadelphia: J.B. Lippincott, 1987:1001–1035.

Conte D, Piperno A, Mandelli C, et al. Clinical, biochemical and histological features of primary haemochromatosis: A report of 67 cases. Liver 1986;6:310–315.

Niederan C, Fischer R, Sonnenberg A, et al. Survival and causes of death in cirrhotic and in noncirrhotic patients with primary hemochromatosis. N Engl J Med 1985;313:1256–1262.

Searle JW, Kerr FR, Halliday JW, et al. Iron storage disease. In: MacSween RNM, Anthony PP, Scheuer PJ, eds. Pathology of the Liver, 2nd ed. Edinburgh: Churchill Livingstone, 1987:181–201.

■ Copper Storage Disorders

Basic Copper Metabolism

ABSORPTION

1. The daily requirement is approximately 2.5 mg.
2. Thirty to 60% is absorbed in the jejunum and then *loosely* bound to albumin.

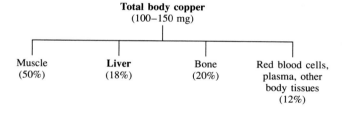

HEPATIC UPTAKE AND STORAGE

1. Copper is taken up by the liver and *firmly* bound to the alpha-2-globulin *ceruloplasmin* before being released into the plasma, with the end result being 6% loosely bound, 80% to 95% firmly bound, and trace amounts free and dialyzable.
2. Main excretory pathway is by way of the biliary system.
3. Copper is stored in the liver as hepatocuprein (*copper-binding protein*).

FUNCTIONS AS COMPONENT OF DIFFERENT ENZYME SYSTEMS

1. *Ceruloplasmin* aids in mobilization of iron from storage sites and functions as a ferroxidase enzyme in conversion of ferrous to ferric ions.
2. *Superoxide dismutase* protects red blood cells, liver, and brain by catalytically scavenging the toxic free radical superoxide (0_2^-) generated during aerobic metabolism.

3. Copper serves as a component of cytochrome c oxidase, tyrosinase, and dopamine beta-hydroxylase.

Conditions Associated With Elevated Copper Levels (Table 8–5)

Table 8–5
CONDITIONS WITH ELEVATED COPPER LEVELS

Hepatocytes	Plasma
Alpha-1-antitrypsin deficiency (neonatal)	Acute biliary tract obstruction
Chronic biliary tract obstruction	Acute and chronic infections
Drugs causing chronic cholestasis (e.g., chlorpromazine)	Leukemia, lymphoma (Hodgkin's)
Familial intrahepatic cholestasis	Oral contraceptives
Exposure to sprays containing copper sulfate (vineyard workers)	Pregnancy
	Rheumatoid arthritis
Indian childhood cirrhosis	Thyrotoxicosis
Primary biliary cirrhosis	Wilson's disease
Primary sclerosing cholangitis	
Wilson's disease	

Wilson's Disease

Major Morphologic Features

Precirrhotic
1. Variable degrees of nonspecific changes include the following:
   a. Macrovesicular and occasionally microvesicular fat, with no zonal distribution pattern
   b. Glycogen nuclei, predominantly periportal
   c. Increase in lipochrome pigment, predominantly periportal
2. Copper is demonstrable predominantly in periportal hepatocytes by special stains (40% cases).

Cirrhotic
1. Macronodular or mixed macronodular and micronodular types are noted.
2. Macrovesicular and occasional microvesicular fat (80%), cholestasis (65%), and alcoholic hyalin (40%) are present.
3. Copper is seen in hepatocytes (87%), with the distribution irregular from one nodule to another.

Other Features

1. In both precirrhotic and cirrhotic stages, focal necrosis and mononuclear inflammatory parenchymal changes are present and may be indistinguishable from those seen in chronic active hepatitis (6% to 38%).
2. Hepatocytes may exhibit hydropic change and occasional acidophil body formation.
3. Liver cell nuclei exhibit variable but sometimes marked anisocytosis.

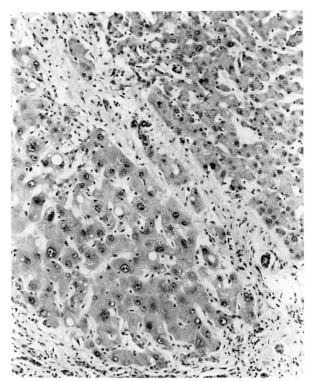

Figure 8–31. Wilson's disease. The cirrhotic liver shows prominent dysplastic change in one nodule (*lower left*) compared with the much smaller cells in the adjacent nodule. Scanty amounts of fat are present in the enlarged hepatocytes.

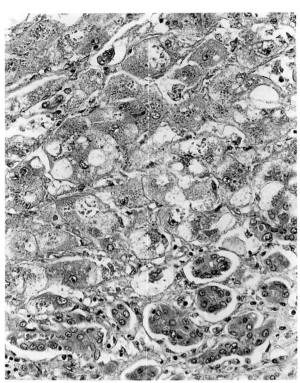

Figure 8–33. Wilson's disease. Many of the hepatocytes are hydropic, with some containing enlarged irregularly shaped cytoplasmic granular material representing increased lysosomes.

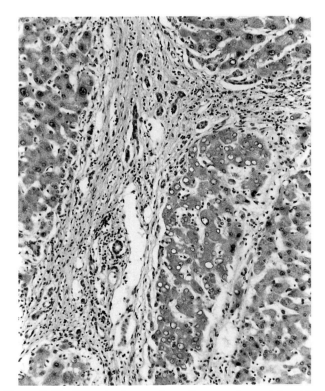

Figure 8–32. Wilson's disease. A small regenerative nodule exhibits numerous glycogen nuclei in virtually every hepatocyte.

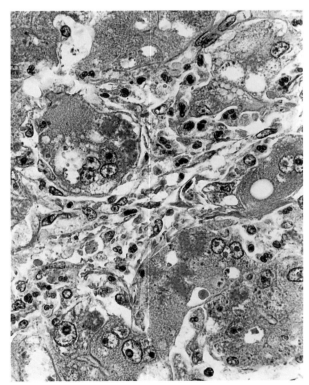

Figure 8–34. Wilson's disease. Alcoholic hyalin is identified in many of the hepatocytes. Scattered neutrophils are also present.

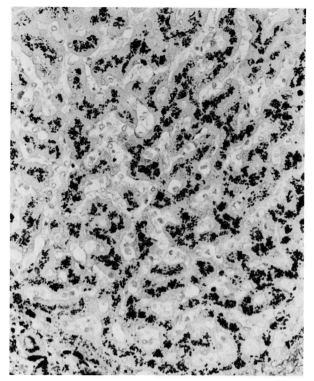

Figure 8–35. Wilson's disease (orcein). Copper-binding protein is abundantly present in all hepatocytes.

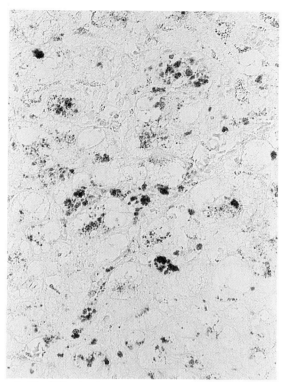

Figure 8–36. Wilson's disease (rubeanic acid). The copper is granular and stains dark blue-green in most of the hepatocytes.

4. The lipochrome pigment, present predominantly in periportal and periseptal hepatocytes, may be composed of larger granules than usually seen.
5. Kupffer cells may contain hemosiderin (hemolytic episodes) or small amounts of copper (secondary to hepatocytolysis).
6. Bile ducts show a mild to moderate degree of prolif-

eration in the early stages but less so in the cirrhotic stage.
7. In patients with fulminant hepatic failure and prominent liver cell necrosis, multiple small eosinophilic granular inclusion-like bodies may be seen in vacuolated, swollen hepatocytes.

Differential Diagnosis

	Alcoholic Hyalin	Fibrosis	Stainable Copper and Copper-Binding Protein	Fat	Glycogen Nuclei
Wilson's disease	+	+ +	+ +	+	+
Chronic cholestasis					
Mechanical duct obstruction	±	+	+	−	−
Primary biliary cirrhosis	+	+ +	+ +	−	−
Primary sclerosing cholangitis	−	+ +	+	−	−
Drugs (chlorpromazine)	−	−	+	−	−
Indian childhood cirrhosis	+ +	+ +	+ +	±	−
Alcoholic liver disease	+ +	+ +	±	+ +	±
Chronic active hepatitis, non-A, non-B	−	+	±	+	+
Diabetes mellitus	±	+	−	+ +	+ +

Special Stains

1. *Periodic acid–Schiff after diastase:* Lysosomes stain most prominently in perivenular hepatocytes in patients with acute hepatic failure.
2. *Rubeanic acid, rhodamine:* Copper stains granular black-green (rubeanic) or red (rhodamine), most prominently in periportal and periseptal hepatocytes.
3. *Orcein, Victoria blue:* Copper-binding protein, *not* copper, stains coarsely granular black-brown (orcein) or purple (Victoria blue), most prominently in periportal and periseptal hepatocytes.
4. *Prussian blue:* Hemosiderin may be present in Kupffer cells secondary to hemolytic episodes.

Clinical and Biologic Behavior

1. Wilson's disease (hepatolenticular degeneration) is an autosomal recessive metabolic disorder causing accumulation of copper principally within the liver and brain, most likely caused by failure of proper copper excretion by way of the biliary pathway rather than an abnormal increase in copper absorption.
2. The genetic defect is believed to be on chromosome no.13, with an incidence of 1 to 3/100,000 and a carrier rate of approximately 1/100.
3. There is a slight male predominance, with initial manifestation of liver disease between the ages of 3 and 33 (one case of cirrhosis was reported in a patient in the sixth decade).
4. Hepatic dysfunction presents as acute and/or chronic hepatitis or cirrhosis; it may even be relatively asymptomatic in 40% to 46% of patients, while psychiatric and/or neuromotor abnormalities (problems in gait, speech) are the first presenting signs in 41% to 45% of cases.
5. Patients presenting with liver disease may never develop clinical neurologic signs, perhaps because of diagnosis and therapy before significant copper accumulates in the brain; patients with neurologic signs *always* have liver disease (symptomatic or asymptomatic).
6. An acute episode may manifest as a Coombs-negative hemolytic crisis, with high mortality and death due to hepatic and renal failure; patients may also have recurrent episodes of hemolysis (accounting for hemosiderin in Kupffer cells).
7. Two ophthalmologic changes are characteristic for Wilson's disease:
   a. *Kayser-Fleischer ring:* Granular copper proteinate is deposited in Descemet's membrane of the cornea, appearing as a brown to gray and occasionally green crescent or ring at the periphery of the cornea (97% of patients).
   b. *Sunflower cataract:* Copper presents as petal-like fronds on the posterior capsule of the lens (7% of patients).

8. Liver tests show mild to moderate elevations of serum aminotransferase levels, even in instances of hepatic failure. Serum bilirubin may be mildly elevated except in severe or fulminant disease.
9. *Copper studies:*
   a. Serum ceruloplasmin level is less than 20 mg/dL (normal, 23–50 mg/dL) in 95% of patients (may also see low levels in fulminant viral hepatitis or advanced cirrhosis).
   b. Twenty-four-hour urinary copper value is greater than 100 μg/dL (normal, less than 30 μg/dL); with penicillamine therapy it is greater than 1200 μg/dL (normal, less than 500 μg/dL).
   c. Hepatic copper content is greater than 250 μg/g dry weight (normal 27 μg/g); however, elevated levels may also be seen in primary biliary cirrosis (441 μg/g), extrahepatic biliary obstruction (128 μg/g), and biliary atresia.
   d. Elevated levels of free serum copper are present.
10. Copper content of the liver is highest in the early stages of the disease; as hepatic storage becomes abundant, copper is released into the blood and picked up by other tissues (e.g., brain); release of copper may be sudden and responsible for acute massive hemolysis. The copper content of the liver afterwards may be slightly lower.
11. Basic defect is impaired excretion of copper from lysosomes into canaliculi; defect in synthesis of ceruloplasmin by injured hepatocytes is responsible for lower serum levels.
12. Hepatocellular carcinoma is not a complication of Wilson's disease.

Treatment and Prognosis

1. Therapy is low copper diet and administration of D-penicillamine (resulting in a negative copper balance).
2. In patients intolerant to penicillamine, zinc (inhibits copper absorption, promotes excretion) has been found by some investigators to be effective.
3. Hemofiltration for removal of copper has been used in patients with fulminant disease prior to transplantation.
4. Hepatic transplantation is offered for patients in hepatic failure or those with severe, apparently irreversible neurologic disease.
5. Prognosis is excellent in those patients responding to D-penicillamine; however, complications of portal hypertension result when cirrhosis is present.
6. Death from hemolytic crises and hepatic and renal failure invariably occurs in untreated cases.

References

Rector WJ Jr, Uchida T, Kanel GC, et al. Fulminant hepatic and renal failure complicating Wilson's disease. Liver 1984;4:341–347.

Sternlieb I, van den Hamer CJA, Morell AG, et al. Lysosomal defect of hepatic copper excretion in Wilson's disease (hepatolenticular degeneration). Gastroenterology 1973;64:99–105.

Stromeyer FW, Ishak KG. Histology of the liver in Wilson's disease: A study of 34 cases. Am J Clin Pathol 1980;73:12–24.

Sumithran E, Looi LM. Copper-binding protein in liver cells. Hum Pathol 1985;16:677–682.

Walshe JM. The liver in Wilson's disease (hepatolenticular degeneration). In: Schiff L, Schiff ER, eds. Diseases of the Liver, 6th ed. Philadelphia: J.B. Lippincott, 1987:1037–1050.

Indian Childhood Cirrhosis

Major Morphologic Features

1. Extensive portal, perivenular, and diffuse interstitial fibrosis is present.
2. Alcoholic hyalin is present in the majority of hepatocytes.

Other Features

1. Hepatocytes exhibit variable degrees of hydropic change, with focal hepatocytolysis and mild lymphocytic and occasional neutrophilic infiltration.
2. Portal tracts exhibit mild to moderate degrees of predominantly mononuclear inflammatory infiltration, with mild bile duct proliferation.
3. Cholestasis may be present but is rare.
4. Fat may be present in early stages but usually is absent in advanced disease.
5. Hyalin deposition is not present in early stages of the disease.

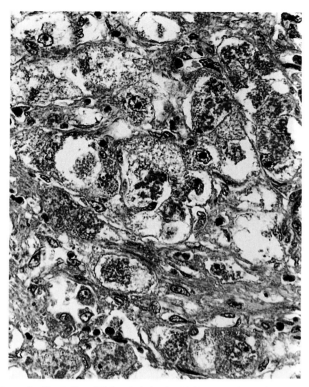

Figure 8–38. Indian childhood cirrhosis. High power shows the presence of alcoholic hyalin in many of the hydropic hepatocytes.

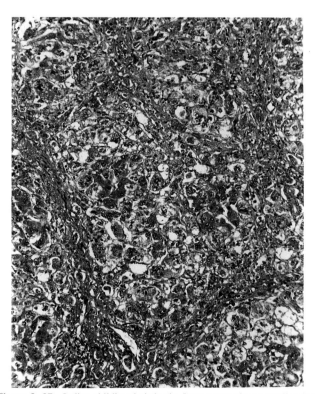

Figure 8–37. Indian childhood cirrhosis. Low power shows small rather ill-defined nodules. The fibrous septa are thin, with prominent periseptal and interstitial sinusoidal collagen deposition.

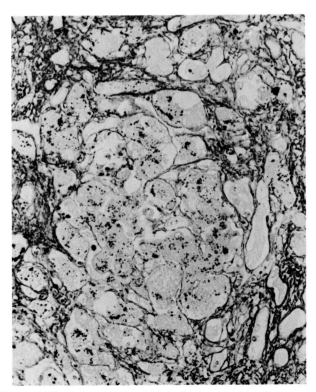

Figure 8–39. Indian childhood cirrhosis (orcein). Abundant copper-binding protein is present in all the hepatocytes.

6. Liver cells may contain two to three nuclei, but prominent giant cell transformation is not present.
7. Micronodular cirrhosis ultimately occurs, with the nodules poorly defined with scanty to absent regenerative change.
8. Increased copper and copper-binding protein is present and most prominent in periportal and periseptal hepatocytes.

Differential Diagnosis

1. *Alpha-1-antitrypsin deficiency:* Portal and to some degree sinusoidal fibrosis, occasional alcoholic hyalin deposition, and eventual biliary cirrhosis can be seen in infants with alpha-1-antitrypsin deficiency. Atypical duct formation, decreased ducts, and alpha-1-antitrypsin inclusions are characteristic of this disorder and are not seen in Indian childhood cirrhosis.
2. *Other causes of cirrhosis in infancy:* Rare metabolic defects (e.g., tyrosinemia, cystinosis, galactosemia, fructosemia, glycogen storage diseases III and IV, Wilson's disease) may be associated with cirrhosis in infancy and childhood. Indian childhood cirrhosis is distinctive, however, in being confined, with one exception, to the Indian subcontinent (similar type of cirrhosis reported in the United States). In addition, excluding Wilson's disease, abundant alcoholic hyalin is present only in Indian childhood cirrhosis.
3. *Acute sclerosing hyaline necrosis:* This form of acute alcoholic liver disease may morphologically resemble Indian childhood cirrhosis, although fat is much more abundant in the alcoholic; however, Indian childhood cirrhosis is not seen in the adult population.

Special Stains

1. *Rubeanic acid, rhodamine:* Copper stains granular green-black (rubeanic) or red (rhodamine), most prominently in periportal and periseptal hepatocytes.
2. *Orcein, Victoria blue:* Copper-binding protein, *not* copper, stains coarsely granular black-brown (orcein) or purple (Victoria blue), most prominently in periportal and periseptal hepatocytes.
3. *Masson:* Prominent diffuse interstitial fibrosis is emphasized.

Clinical and Biologic Behavior

1. Indian childhood cirrhosis is a generally fatal hepatic disorder found in children in India, usually of the Brahmin class, often having a familial predilection; there are case reports of similar disorders in the United States.
2. Clinical presentation is at 2 years of age (range, 6 months to 5 years) with a slight male predominance;

it has an insidious onset, with hepatosplenomegaly, rarely jaundice, and gradual progression to micronodular cirrhosis.
3. No distinct laboratory features are present, with only mild elevation of serum aminotransferase activities; bilirubin value is usually normal, with alpha-fetoprotein level elevated (from birth).
4. A defect in copper metabolism may play some part in the pathogenesis, since there are substantial amounts of copper in the liver; recent evidence suggests that copper toxicity develops in children ingesting milk with increased copper content (from boiling milk in copper vessels). There is no evidence to implicate malnutrition or viral infection as causal.

Prognosis

1. Death always occurs from cirrhosis with hepatic failure, usually within 1 to 2 years of diagnosis.

References

Lefkowitz JH, Honig CL, King ME, et al. Hepatic copper overload and features of Indian childhood cirrhosis. N Engl J Med 1982;307:271–277.
Mehrotra R, Pandey RK, Nath P. Hepatic copper in Indian childhood cirrhosis. Histopathology 1981;5:659–665.
Sumithran E, Looi LM. Copper-binding protein in liver cells. Hum Pathol 1985;16:677–682.
Tanner MS, Portmann B. Indian childhood cirrhosis. Arch Dis Child 1981;56:4–6.

■ Amyloidosis

Major Morphologic Features

1. Amorphous extracellular eosinophilic deposits are present:
   a. *Perireticular:* Deposits are sinusoidal within the space of Disse.
   b. *Pericollagenous:* Deposits are found among collagen fibers within portal tracts, in media of arterioles, and in sublobular and hepatic veins.

Other Features

1. In a small percentage of cases, amyloid may be seen as *globular type:*
   a. Round to oval structures 5 to 50 μm in diameter having a laminated pattern, often with intense central staining.
   b. Globules are present in portal tracts and sinusoids but not in arterioles.
   c. Amyloid often presents as a *mixed* form of perireticular, pericollagenous, and globular types.
2. Liver cells often exhibit atrophic changes adjacent to

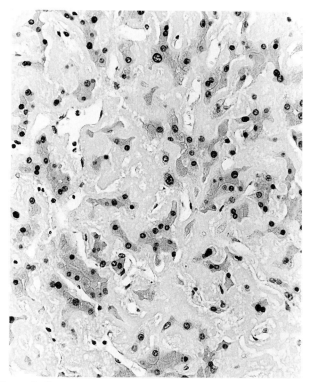

Figure 8–40. Amyloidosis. The extracellular amorphous eosinophilic deposits are present in all sinusoids and represent amyloid. Almost all of the hepatocytes are atrophic.

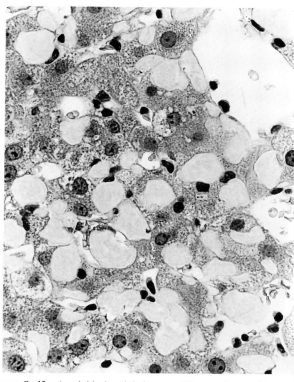

Figure 8–42. Amyloidosis, globular type. The round to oval irregularly shaped extracellular deposits represent globular amyloid. Typical forms of amyloid, as shown in Figure 8–40, are not present.

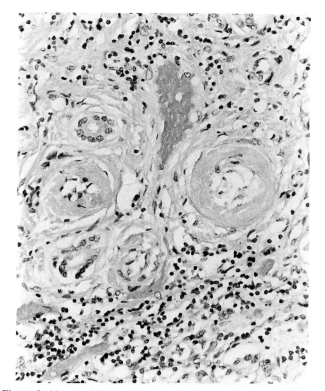

Figure 8–41. Amyloidosis. The arterioles in a portal tract are thickened by an amorphic eosinophilic material representing amyloid.

perireticular amyloid deposition; this change is quite striking in instances in which amyloid fills the entire sinusoid, pushing Kupffer and endothelial cells toward the center of the sinusoid.

3. Variability of degree of amyloid deposition may occur from one lobule to another, especially with the globular type.
4. Cholestasis is present in approximately 5% of cases.
5. Bile ducts show no features related to amyloidosis, although they may exhibit changes secondary to underlying disease entities.
6. Hepatic fibrosis is not a feature.

Differential Diagnosis

1. *Substances resembling perireticular and pericollagenous type of amyloid include the following:*
   a. *Collagen:* Collagen is fibrillar and often loose in appearance.
   b. *Fibrin:* Strands are deeply eosinophilic and fibrillar and stain positively with phosphotungstic acid hematoxylin.
   NOTE: Both substances are extracellular and do not stain with Congo red.
2. *Substances resembling globular type are listed below:*
   a. *Ground-glass cells:* In chronic hepatitis B

ground-glass cells stain positively with orcein and immunoperoxidase for HBsAg.

b. *Pale bodies:* Fibrolamellar hepatic carcinoma
c. *Periportal inclusions:* Myoclonus epilepsy (Lafora bodies)
d. *Drug-induced inclusions:* Phenytoin, phenobarbital, chlorpromazine, procainamide
e. *Perivenular inclusions:* Secondary to anoxia
NOTE: All of the above inclusions are *intracellular* and do *not* stain with Congo red.

Special Stains

1. *Congo red:* Positive pink-red staining of all types of amyloid is present, with apple-green birefringence on polarization microscopy (diagnostic).
2. *Congo red after trypsin digestion and potassium permanganate application:*
   a. *Resistant* to digestion: Positive staining with Congo red and green birefringence on polarization indicates amyloid is composed of immunoglobulin light-chain moieties.
   b. *Sensitive* to digestion: Negative staining with Congo red indicates amyloid of nonimmunoglobulin (AA) type.
3. *Periodic acid–Schiff:* Positive staining of various intensity is due to "P" (pentagonal) component in all forms of amyloid.
4. *Sirius red:* Positive red staining of various intensity is seen.

Fluorescence

1. *Thioflavin-T:* Amyloid stains intensely yellow-green.

Immunohistochemistry

1. *Anti-light chains:* Positive staining identifies amyloid composed of immunoglobulin *kappa* and *lambda* light chains (plasma cell dyscrasias, primary amyloidosis).
2. *Anti-AA:* Positive staining identifies amyloid composed of AA (amyloid-associated) protein (chronic inflammatory disorders, secondary amyloidosis).

Clinical and Biologic Behavior

1. *Amyloid* is best described in biophysical terms:
   a. Extracellular, homogeneously eosinophilic on hematoxylin and eosin stain, with apple-green birefringence on polarization after positive Congo red staining

   b. Characteristic fibrous, 7.5 to 10 nm in diameter, rigid, nonbranching linear aggregates of indefinite length on electron microscopy
   c. Cross beta-pleated sheet appearance on x-ray diffraction
2. Systemic amyloidosis has a worldwide distribution. It is present 0.1% to 0.7% of the time in autopsy studies; hepatic involvement is found in approximately 50% of these cases.
3. The clinical presentation is usually related to specific associated disorders (Glenner, 1980): *acquired systemic* (e.g., multiple myeloma, rheumatoid arthritis), *organ-limited* (e.g., cardiac), and *localized* (e.g., endocrine tumors such as medullary carcinoma of the thyroid).
4. Systemic amyloidosis is associated with chronic inflammatory disorders 5% to 11% of the time; 6% to 15% of patients with multiple myeloma develop amyloidosis.
5. In acquired systemic types, patients usually present in the fifth to seventh decade; the disorder is slightly more common in men.
6. Hepatic involvement results in hepatomegaly 47% to 57% of the time (weights ranging from 875 to 4880 g in one series, with reports up to 9000 g); splenomegaly is present in only 9% of total cases.
7. Stigmata of chronic liver disease are not present, and jaundice occurs in less than 5% of cases, with the serum bilirubin level usually below 5 mg/dL. Signs related to portal hypertension (ascites, esophageal varices) are rare, and splenomegaly is usually caused by direct amyloid involvement of the spleen.
8. Laboratory tests relative to liver involvement are nonspecific; the serum albumin level is occasionally slightly decreased, aminotranferase levels are normal or slightly elevated, and the bilirubin value is usually normal.
9. *Globular amyloidosis* is seldom associated with plasma cell dyscrasias, and most often involves the liver, spleen, kidneys, and adrenals; only the hepatic form of amyloid is globular, with the other organs demonstrating deposition patterns of typical amyloid; globular amyloid has been shown to be resistant to trypsin digestion and does not stain with antibodies to prealbumin, AA, or AL, possibly a pattern peculiar to the liver and local environmental conditions.
10. *Congo red* and *sirius red* are direct cotton dyes that do not stain all types of amyloid with the same intensity. In normal tissues, elastic fibers will bind the dyes, although birefringence does not occur. Certain organisms (*Mucor, Aspergillus, Candida, Blastomyces*) as well as materials such as cellulose and chitin can also bind the dyes and exhibit birefringence. It is necessary, therefore, to examine the pattern of morphologic change for diagnosis.
11. The fluorochrome *thioflavin-T* is useful in screening, since amyloid is easily identified on low power; false-positive results (*no* false-negative) occur (elastic lamina, fibrin, mucus, keratin, skele-

tal muscle), hence confirmation with Congo red is usually necessary.

12. Birefringence on polarized light after Congo red staining is caused by the fibrillar structure of amyloid and the orderly molecular arrangement of the dye after binding; nonspecific green birefringence is reported with Zenker's or Carnoy's fixation, *not* formalin.

13. Confirmation of amyloidosis by tissue biopsy: rectal biopsy 75% to 85% positive; biopsies of liver, kidney, gingiva, skin, bone marrow, and abdominal fat are also frequently positive. A rare complication of liver biopsy is rupture with bleeding (fracture of a somewhat "brittle" parenchyma).

14. Pathogenesis: Amyloid light chains are synthesized from plasma cells and lymphocytes (immunocytes), and AA protein is synthesized from chronic inflammatory cells; the latter are phagocytized (macrophages, Kupffer cells, synovial cells) and deposited as fibrils after proteolytic cleavage.

Aspiration Cytology

1. Presence of amorphous eosinophilic material and atrophic liver cells would be highly suggestive (confirmation by Congo red stain).

Prognosis

1. Treatment and eradication of underlying disease has been shown to stop amyloid production and possibly even cause slow resolution.

2. Most common causes of death from amyloid are renal failure and cardiac disease; hepatic failure can occur but is quite rare.

3. Length of survival is as follows:
   a. Primary amyloidosis: Mean survival is 14 months from time of diagnosis.
   b. Associated with myeloma: Mean survival is 4 months.
   c. Associated with chronic inflammation: Mean survival is 20 months and relates to underlying disorder.
   d. Associated with cardiac involvement and/or renal failure at time of diagnosis: Mean survival is less than 12 months.
   e. Hepatic, gastrointestinal, nerve involvement only: Survival is much longer; in instances when the specific disease is eradicated the survival is 5 to 10 years.

References

Glenner GG. Amyloid deposits and amyloidosis: The beta-fibrilloses. N Engl J Med 1980;302:1283–1292, 1333–1343.

Kanel GC, Peters RL. Globular hepatic amyloid: An unusual morphologic presentation. Hepatology 1981;1:647–652.

Kyle RA. Amyloidosis: Review of 236 cases. Medicine 1975;54:271–299.

Levine RA. Amyloid disease of the liver. Am J Med 1962;33:349–357.

Looi L-M. Sumithran E. Morphologic differences in the pattern of liver infiltration between systemic AL and AA amyloidosis. Hum Pathol 1988;19:732–735.

MacSween RNM. Liver pathology associated with diseases of other organs. In: MacSween RNM, Anthony PP, Scheuer PJ, eds. Pathology of the Liver, 2nd ed. Edinburgh: Churchill Livingstone, 1987:674–676.

■ Porphyrias

Porphyrins and Heme Synthesis

The porphyrias are inherited disorders of heme metabolism caused by enzyme defects at different stages of heme synthesis. They are usually classified as *hepatic* or *erythropoietic,* based on the predominant location of the biochemical defect. *Porphyria cutanea tarda (PCT)* and *erythropoietic protoporphyria (EPP)* are two porphyrias that may produce significant clinicopathologic liver disease.

Porphyria Cutanea Tarda (PCT)

Major Morphologic Features

1. Portal tracts are normal in size or exhibit variable degrees of fibrosis.
2. Intense red autofluorescence within hepatocytes is seen on frozen sections.

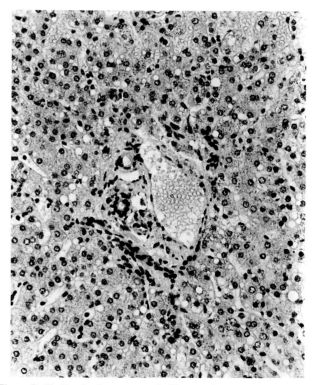

Figure 8–43. Porphyria cutanea tarda. The portal tracts are normal in size with a mild lymphocytic hyperplasia. Ducts are present and appear normal.

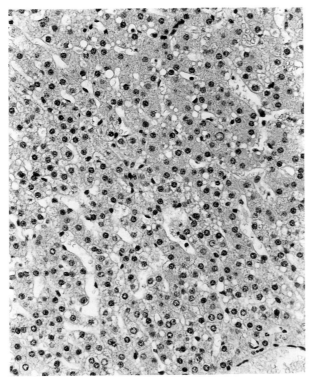

Figure 8-44. Porphyria cutanea tarda. The parenchyma exhibits a mild Kupffer cell hyperplasia. Scattered microvesicular fat is present.

Figure 8-46. Porphyria cutanea tarda (autofluorescence). Prominent red autofluorescence is present in every hepatocyte on frozen section and represents uroporphyrin.

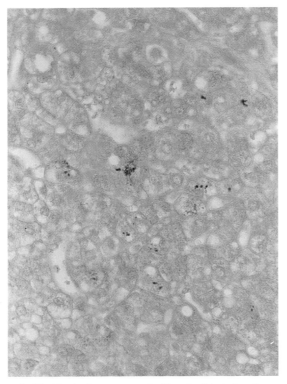

Figure 8-45. Porphyria cutanea tarda (Prussian blue). Iron is occasionally present within hepatocytes.

Other Features

1. Portal tracts show mild lymphocytic infiltration and hyperplasia; lymphocytes sometimes surround but do not invade interlobular ducts.
2. Increased macrovesicular fat, lipochrome, and hemosiderin may be present within hepatocytes.
3. Glycogen nuclei are seen in approximately 15% of cases.
4. Needle-shaped birefringent cytoplasmic inclusions (uroporphyrin crystals within lysosomes) can be identified, more often in unstained sections.
5. Focal necrosis and aggregates of Kupffer cells, fat, and iron may occasionally be identified in the lobule.
6. Cirrhosis has been identified in from less than 10% to 34% of cases.
7. In rare instances, hepatocellular carcinoma and inflammatory changes of chronic active hepatitis have been described.

Differential Diagnosis

1. *Chronic alcoholic liver disease, diabetes mellitus:* PCT may exhibit features seen in alcoholic liver disease (fibrosis and fat) and diabetes mellitus (fibrosis, fat, and glycogen nuclei). Because 70% to 90% of

patients with *clinically* manifest PCT are *also* alcoholics, and approximately 15% are diabetic, autofluorescence will help identify the presence of PCT but *not* rule out possible coexistence of other liver diseases.

2. *Disorders secondary to severe iron overload:* Iron may be quite abundant in PCT, both within hepatocytes and Kupffer cells. Autofluorescence is helpful in diagnosis.

3. *Other types of porphyrias:* With the exception of EPP, most of the other porphyrias exhibit mild nonspecific changes on liver biopsy. Autofluorescence is also present but usually weak. Clinical presentation, with a characteristic pattern of porphyrin excretion, is necessary for diagnosis.

Special Stains

1. *Prussian blue:* Iron is shown within cytoplasm of hepatocytes and occasionally of Kupffer cells.

Autofluorescence

1. Irradiation of nonfixed tissue (frozen sections) or dried smears of aspirates at wavelengths between 398 and 408 nm produces an intense red autofluorescence emitting between 620 and 630 nm (fluorescence of uroporphyrin) owing to intense absorption band near 400 nm (Soret band).

Clinical and Biologic Behavior

1. PCT occurs slightly more frequently in men, usually after age 35, with an incidence of approximately 5/100,000.
2. Clinical manifestations are predominantly cutaneous, commonly involving the face, feet, and backs of the hands.
3. The onset is usually insidious, with only a small number of patients having photosensitivity as the initiating factor; minor trauma can cause blistering, open vesicles with superinfection, poor healing, and scar formation.
4. Patients exhibit no signs of liver disease unless fibrosis or cirrhosis is present (minority of patients), either from PCT itself or coexisting alcoholic liver disease.
5. There is a slight increase in serum iron and iron saturation (60%), ferritin levels are at the upper limits of normal to slightly elevated, and total body iron stores are slightly increased (2–4 g).
6. Massive urinary uroporphyrin (largely subtype I) with moderate elevations of coproporphyrin (I and III) in red urine is virtually pathognomonic.
7. Exposure to certain toxins (hexachlorobenzene, seed

grain fungicide) may cause a clinical picture identical to PCT.

8. A deficiency in the enzyme *uroporphyrinogen decarboxylase* is present, with familial studies demonstrating an autosomal dominant inheritance pattern. However, a number of factors appear to play a role in the clinical expression of the disease:
   a. *Alcohol intake:* Seventy to 90% of patients are reported to have some form of chronic alcoholic liver disease; however, there is no direct correlation with the severity of alcoholic liver disease and PCT.
   b. *Estrogens:* PCT occurs more frequently in young women on oral contraceptives.
   c. *Iron deposits in the liver:* There are increased amounts of hemosiderin in hepatocytes in patients with PCT, although there is no correlation with the amount of iron and severity of the disease.
   d. *HLA:* Although a gene in HLA-linked primary hemochromatosis has previously been associated with the hemosiderosis found in PCT, recent studies are against a systemic association between the two entities.
9. Iron deposition, alcoholism, and estrogens may possibly induce expression of the disease in an otherwise asymptomatic patient.

Aspiration Cytology

1. Air-dried unfixed smears must be examined within a few hours, with individual cells exhibiting characteristic red autofluorescence (620–630 nm) of uroporphyrin moiety when irradiated at 398 to 408 nm.

Prognosis

1. Overall prognosis is good but dependent on whether fibrosis is present secondary to PCT and/or underlying chronic alcoholic liver disease.

References

Bloomer JR. The hepatic porphyrias: Pathogenesis, manifestations, and management. Gastroenterology 1976;71:689–701.

Beaumont C, Fauchet R, Phung LN, et al. Porphyria cutanea tarda and HLA-linked hemochromatosis: Evidence against a systemic association. Gastroenterology 1987;92:1833–1838.

Cortes JM, Oliva H, Paradinas FJ, et al. The pathology of the liver in porphyria cutanea tarda. Histopathology 1980;4:471–485.

Lefkowitch JH, Grossman ME. Hepatic pathology in porphyria cutanea tarda. Liver 1983;3:19–29.

Erythropoietic Protoporphyria (EPP)

Major Morphologic Features

1. Dark brown pigment (protoporphyrin crystals) is seen within hepatocytes, Kupffer cells, bile canalic-

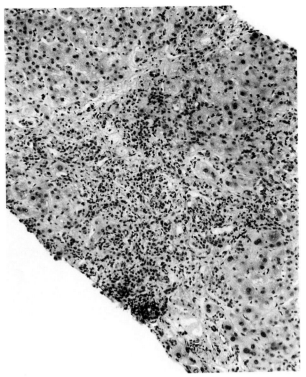

Figure 8–47. Erythropoietic protoporphyria. Portal fibrosis is present. A prominent portal lymphocytic infiltrate spills over into the parenchyma, surrounding hepatocytes and resembling a chronic active hepatitis-like picture. Cirrhosis may eventually develop.

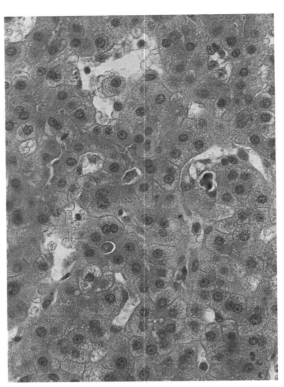

Figure 8–49. Erythropoietic protoporphyria. The liver, in addition to protoporphyrin, may also contain bile, present in this photomicrograph as green-yellow pigment within dilated canaliculi.

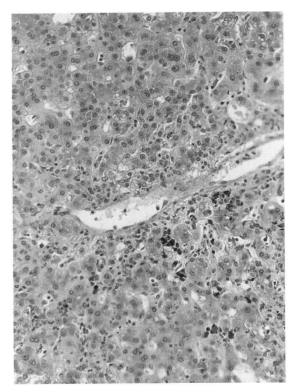

Figure 8–48. Erythropoietic protoporphyria. The Kupffer cells to the center and lower right of the field are enlarged and contain a dark brown pigment representing protoporphyrin crystals.

Figure 8–50. Erythropoietic protoporphyria (autofluorescence). The red to red-yellow autofluorescence in hepatocytes on frozen section represents protoporphyrin.

uli, portal macrophages, and rarely interlobular bile ducts.

2. Intense red to orange-red autofluorescence is present within hepatocytes on frozen sections.
3. Variable degrees of fibrosis, and occasionally cirrhosis, may be present.

Other Features

1. Pigment exhibits positive birefringence with polarization microscopy; the larger deposits are red to purple with central Maltese cross configurations (intralysosomal crystals).
2. Hemosiderin and lipochrome may be present in hepatocytes and Kupffer cells.
3. The parenchyma and portal areas may exhibit variable degrees of mononuclear inflammatory infiltration and focal necrosis.
4. Protoporphyrin pigment is not always present; however, it is quite abundant, as is cholestasis, in advanced cases.

Differential Diagnosis

1. *Disorders secondary to severe iron overload:* Iron may be quite abundant in EPP, both within hepatocytes and Kupffer cells. Close inspection, however, will reveal the predominant pigment to be dark brown, to be negative on iron stain, and to exhibit positive birefringence under polarized light. Autofluorescence is also helpful in differentiation.
2. *Other types of porphyrias:* EPP is the only porphyria with the characteristic dark brown birefringent pigment; in less severe cases, however, fibrosis and pigment deposition may not be present, necessitating the clinical setting with characteristic protoporphyrin for diagnosis.

Special Stains

1. *Prussian blue:* Iron (hemosiderin) is demonstrated within hepatocytes and Kupffer cells, and can be distinguished from the negative staining dark brown protoporphyrin pigment.

Autofluorescence

1. Irradiation of nonfixed tissue (frozen sections) or dried smears of aspirates at wavelengths between 398 and 408 nm produces an intense red to orange-red autofluorescence emitting between 620 and 630 nm (fluorescence of protoporphyrin) owing to intense absorption band near 400 nm (Soret band).

Clinical and Biologic Behavior

1. Although the overall incidence is not known, EPP can exist in a latent, asymptomatic form; it occurs slightly more commonly in males.
2. Predominant clinical features are cutaneous; manifestation is usually before 13 years of age (average onset at age 4 to 5 years) and is characterized by burning, swelling, and itching, predominantly of the nose, cheeks, fingers, and backs of hands. Clinical features can occur moments after sunlight exposure with formation of bullae, scabs, and scars.
3. Gallstones are present in 5% to 15% of patients; the stones contain considerable amounts of protoporphyrin.
4. Severe fibrosis and cirrhosis occur in a small percentage of patients and are clinically manifest as hepatomegaly, portal hypertension (esophageal varices), jaundice, and eventual hepatic failure.
5. Laboratory features consist of minimal elevations in liver test values unless hepatic failure sets in; increased proptoporphyrin IX is present in feces and red blood cells.
6. *Ferrochelatase,* involved in the final step of heme synthesis, is deficient in these patients; in addition, there is an overactivity of the enzyme *ALA synthetase* (converts succinyl CoA + glycine to ALA), since heme itself is involved in an inhibitory feedback mechanism of this enzyme.

Aspiration Cytology

1. Air-dried unfixed smears must be examined within a few hours, with individual cells exhibiting characteristic red to red-orange autofluorescence (620–630 nm) of the protoporphyrin moiety when irradiated at 398 to 408 nm.

Prognosis

1. Although the overall incidence of serious liver disease is relatively small, cirrhosis and death from hepatic failure are known to occur.

References

Bloomer JR. Protoporphyria. Semin Liver Dis 1982;2:143–153.
Bloomer JR. The liver in protoporphyria. Hepatology 1988;8:402–407.
Cripps DJ, Scheuer PJ. Hepatobiliary changes in erythropoietic protoporphyria. Arch Pathol 1965;80:500–508.
Klatskin G, Bloomer JR. Birefringence of hepatic pigment deposits in erythropoietic protoporphyria. Gastroenterology 1974;67:294–302.

■ Sickle Cell Anemia

Major Morphologic Features

1. Clumping of sickled red blood cells, occasionally admixed with fibrin, occurs in dilated sinusoids and is most prominent in the perivenular zone.

Other Features

1. Focal areas of necrosis, predominantly the coagulative type, may be present in the perivenular zone in instances of severe sludging and thrombi formation of sinusoidal red blood cells.
2. Kupffer cells are hyperplastic and often hypertrophic, containing hemosiderin and fragmented red blood cells.
3. Hemosiderin is present in hepatocytes (predominantly periportal) as well as Kupffer cells.
4. In cases in which there have been numerous episodes of severe sinusoidal outflow obstruction, thin strands of collagen may be deposited in the space of Disse in the perivenular zone.
5. Macrovesicular fat is occasionally present.
6. Cholestasis may occur in association with bile duct

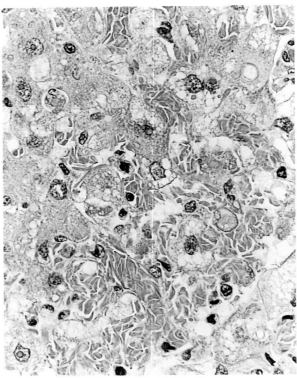

Figure 8–52. Sickle cell anemia. High power of the dilated sinusoids shows numerous enlarged and somewhat pointed sickled red blood cells.

obstruction caused by gallstones, the latter more common in patients with sickle cell disease.
7. Portal tracts exhibit only mild bile duct proliferation and mononuclear inflammatory infiltration.
8. Extramedullary hematopoiesis is present to some degree in 50% of cases (secondary to chronic hemolytic anemia).

Differential Diagnosis

1. *Acute viral hepatitis:* Sickle cell anemia may clinically resemble acute hepatitis. Prominent ischemic necrosis is responsible for enzyme elevations in these cases. The presence of perivenular coagulative necrosis, clumping of sickled red blood cells, and minimal portal tract changes easily distinguishes between the two entities.
2. *Passive congestion:* Perivenular congestion and sinusoidal dilatation are present in acute and chronic passive congestion as well as in sickle cell disease. Groups of sickled cells and fibrin are not found in passive congestion.
3. *Disseminated intravascular coagulation:* Fibrin may be present within sinusoids in disseminated intravascular coagulation, usually involving the periportal zone as well as small portal venous radicles. In sickle cell disease fibrin is usually perivenular.

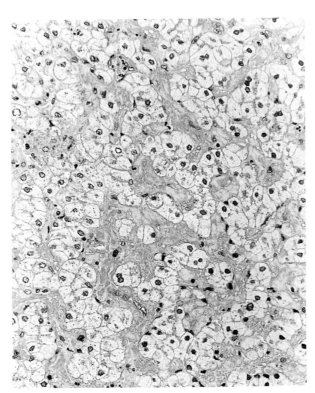

Figure 8–51. Sickle cell anemia. The sinusoids are dilated and filled with an eosinophilic material composed of sickled red blood cells. The individual sickled cells cannot be appreciated because of considerable clumping and mixture with fibrin.

Special Stains

1. *Prussian blue:* Hemosiderin is identified within Kupffer cells and to variable degrees within periportal hepatocytes.
2. *Phosphotungstic acid hematoxylin:* Fibrin deposition is accentuated in the sinusoids.

Clinical and Biologic Behavior

1. Sickle cell anemia (homozygous HbSS) is a severe inherited chronic hemolytic disorder that first manifests itself in early childhood: it is often fatal before age 30.
2. The sickle gene is present almost exclusively in the black population. The incidence of sickle cell anemia (homozygous) is 0.1% to 0.2% of all blacks in the United States, and the incidence of the carrier (heterozygous) state is approximately 8%.
3. Sickle cell hemoglobin (HbS) differs from normal (HbA) by substitution of the amino acid valine for glutamic acid in the sixth position of hemoglobin's beta-chain; HbS may polymerize and distort (sickle) the shape of the red cell in HbSS, HbSC, sickle-beta thalassemia, and other rarer forms.
4. *Acute sickle crises* occur in the homozygous patient and are characterized by abdominal pain in 50%, chest syndrome (clinically similar to pneumonia) in 10% to 20%, priapism in 10% to 40% of males, cerebrovascular accident in 5% to 10% children, and liver disease in less than 2%.
5. Chronic disease is characterized by aseptic necrosis (hips and shoulders) in 10% to 25% of adults, proliferative retinopathy in 50%, leg ulcers in 10% to 20%, functional asplenia in more than 90%, nephropathy with nephrotic syndrome, and renal failure in older patients.
6. The heterozygous person is asymptomatic, only occasionally demonstrating hematuria from sickling in the renal medulla.
7. Acute liver disease may clinically resemble acute viral hepatitis, with aminotransferase levels sometimes in the thousands and marked hyperbilirubinemia (predominantly indirect from hemolysis, but may see up to 50% direct fraction if concomitant liver disease is severe).
8. Gallstones are present in approximately 50% of patients; persistent hyperbilirubinemia may be due to a combination of chronic hemolysis, recurrent liver disease from biliary obstruction (gallstones), and anoxic liver cell necrosis.
9. The fibrosis and cirrhosis occasionally seen in patients with sickle cell anemia are most likely due to post-transfusion chronic hepatitis.
10. Liver injury is predominantly due to anoxic-type necrosis; the basic pathophysiology involves obstruction of sinusoidal blood flow due to aggregation of red blood cells and fibrin, with these cells having an elongated, curved sickled shape that is two to three times larger in greatest dimension than the normal red blood cell. Sickling is initiated by any event leading to hypoxic changes in tissue. In the liver, sickling is most prominent in the perivenular region where oxygen tension is lowest. Impediment of blood flow in this region enhances the hypoxic change, further increasing the sickling process.

Prognosis

1. Overall prognosis is dependent on treatment and possible prevention of complications such as infection, cerebrovascular accident, and renal and cardiac diseases.

References

Bauer TW, Moore GW, Hutchins GM. The liver in sickle cell disease: A clinicopathologic study of 70 patients. Am J Med 1980;69:833–837.

Mills LR, Mwakyusa D, Milner PF. Histopathologic features of liver biopsy specimens in sickle cell disease. Arch Pathol Lab Med 1988;112:290–294.

Omata M, Johnson CS, Tong M, et al. Pathological spectrum of liver diseases in sickle cell disease. Dig Dis Sci 1986;31:247–256.

Schubert TT. Hepatobiliary system in sickle cell disease. Gastroenterology 1986;90:2013–2021.

General References

Balistreri WF, Schubert WK. Liver disease in infancy and childhood. In: Schiff L, Schiff ER, eds. Diseases of the Liver, 6th ed. Philadelphia: J.B. Lippincott, 1987:1337–1426.

Ishak KG, Sharp HL. Developmental abnormality and liver disease in childhood. In: MacSween RNM, Anthony PP, Scheuer PJ, eds. Pathology of the Liver, 2nd ed. Edinburgh: Churchill Livingstone, 1987:66–98.

Ishak KG, Sharp HL. Metabolic errors and liver disease. In: MacSween RNM, Anthony PP, Scheuer PJ, eds. Pathology of the Liver, 2nd ed. Edinburgh: Churchill Livingstone, 1987:99–180.

Portman BC, MacSween RNM. Diseases of the intrahepatic bile ducts. In: MacSween RNM, Anthony PP, Scheuer PJ, eds. Pathology of the Liver, 2nd ed. Edinburgh: Churchill Livingstone, 1987:424–463.

Ruebner BH, Cox KL. Liver disease in infancy. In: Peters RL, Craig JR, eds. Liver Pathology. New York: Churchill Livingstone, 1986:37–60.

Ruebner BH, Cox KL. Liver disease in childhood. In: Peters RL, Craig JR, eds. Liver Pathology. New York: Churchill Livingstone, 1986:61–72.

CHAPTER 9

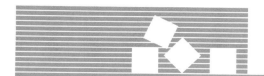

Neoplasms and Related Lesions

■ **Primary Benign Neoplasms**

Liver Cell Adenoma

Major Morphologic Features

1. Hepatocytes are uniform and generally hydropic, and appear cytologically benign.
2. Portal tracts, duct structures, and fibrous septa are absent.
3. There is a sharp border with nonneoplastic hepatocytes.
4. Fibrous capsule is present in 74% of cases, most commonly in the larger lesions.

Other Features

1. The cords are closely arranged, with the normal cord–sinusoid pattern at times not apparent; however, the cords are not more than two cells thick.
2. Cells are generally larger than the nonneoplastic hepatocytes.
3. Endothelial lining cells are present along the trabecular cords.
4. Thin-walled vasculature structures and small arterioles appear throughout the lesion.
5. Tumor cells may exhibit eosinophilic, granular cytoplasm and contain fat, glycogen, bile, and, in rare instances, various types of pigments (lipochrome, hemosiderin).
6. Mallory's hyalin and granulomas have been described but are rare.
7. Sinusoids may be focally dilated and congested, sometimes forming a peloid pattern.
8. Thick-walled arterioles are often present at the periphery of the tumor.

9. Areas of hemorrhage (30% when multiple lesions are present, 20% in solitary adenomas) and necrosis (60% in large adenomas) may occur; fibrous scars may be present in areas of previous necrosis.
10. Tumor is usually found beneath Glisson's capsule, but there is almost always a rim of normal liver (often compressed or atrophic) between the adenoma and the capsule.
11. Atypical, pleomorphic cells with distorted hyperchromatic nuclei and abundant cytoplasm may be seen, usually at the periphery of the lesion; transformation to hepatocellular carcinoma, with microinvasion into the adjacent nonneoplastic liver, has been described in these lesions but is rare.

Differential Diagnosis

1. *Well-differentiated hepatocellular carcinoma:* Liver cell adenoma and well-differentiated hepatocellular carcinoma may morphologically appear quite similar, especially in needle biopsy or aspiration specimens. The following features of hepatocellular carcinoma are used in distinguishing between the two lesions, since these changes are *not* seen in the adenoma:
   a. Trabecular cords greater than two to three cells thick
   b. Infiltration of cells through tumor capsule, or *irregular* growth pattern of tumor cells into nonneoplastic liver (e.g., tonguelike projections)
   c. Growth pattern of tumor cells in lymphatic and vascular channels
   d. Numerous or atypical mitoses
2. *Focal nodular hyperplasia:* This lesion, with fibrous septa radiating from a central scar, is grossly and in some areas morphologically quite distinctive; however, areas away from the scar appear similar to ade-

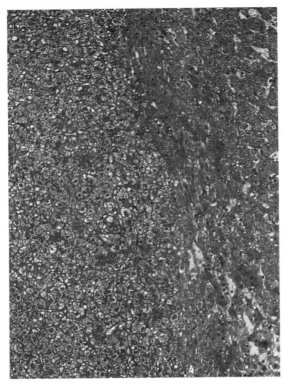

Figure 9–1. Liver cell adenoma. The neoplastic cells *(center and lower left)* are hydropic, without any distinct cord–sinusoid pattern. The normal liver cells *(upper right)* are approximately the same size as the neoplastic cells, but the cytoplasm is more eosinophilic. Although a fibrous septum between these two regions is not present, the nonneoplastic cells immediately adjacent to the lesion exhibit mild atrophy caused by compression.

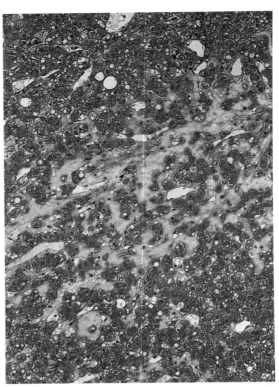

Figure 9–3. Liver cell adenoma. Sinusoidal dilatation is present; the sinusoids are filled with unusual staining plasma components.

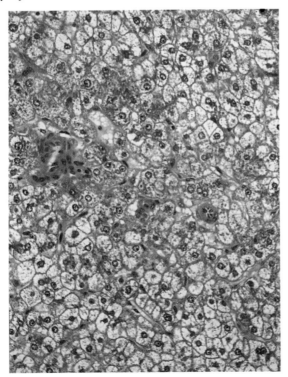

Figure 9–2. Liver cell adenoma. The cells are uniformly hydropic, with the cord–sinusoid pattern difficult to evaluate. Small arterioles are present; however, duct structures are absent.

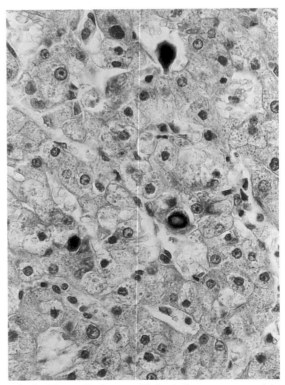

Figure 9–4. Liver cell adenoma. Hydropic hepatocytes containing bile plugs are present. The bile *(above)* has most likely been secreted into the adjacent sinusoid. Adenomas have also been shown to contain fat, lipochrome, and glycogen.

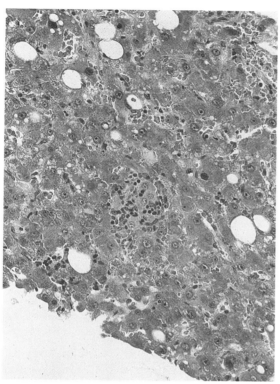

Figure 9–5. Liver cell adenoma. The eosinophilic hepatocytes contain variable degrees of predominantly macrovesicular fat. A small well-formed epithelioid granuloma containing lymphocytes *(center)* is present. Giant cells within granulomas have also been described.

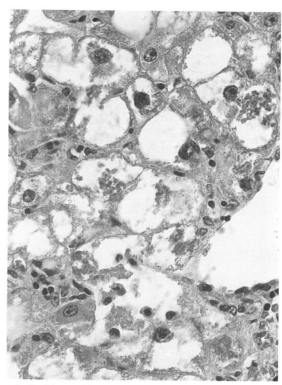

Figure 9–7. Liver cell adenoma. These hydropic hepatocytes contain macrovesicular fat. Eosinophilic material is present in numerous cells and represents alcoholic hyalin, confirmed by immunoperoxidase stain.

noma. Comparison of the morphologic and radiologic features of the two lesions is shown below:

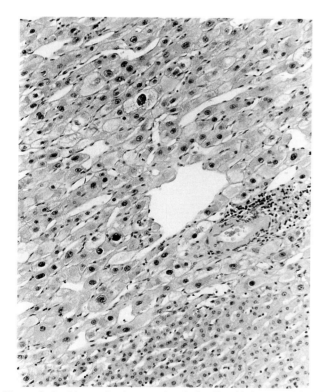

Figure 9–6. Liver cell adenoma. Atypical cells with large nuclei and abundant cytoplasm are present; however, the basic cord–sinusoid pattern is maintained without formation of thickened cords. Smaller nonneoplastic hepatocytes are seen *(lower right).*

	Liver Cell Adenoma	Focal Nodular Hyperplasia
Morphology		
Capsule	Common	Absent
Portal tracts	Absent	Absent
Fibrous septa	Very rare	Common
Bile duct proliferation	Absent	Common
Lymphocytic infiltration	Absent	Common
Bile	Variable	Rare
Fat	Frequent	Rare
Glycogen	Variable	Variable
Lipochrome	Variable	Rare
Endothelial lining cells	Present	Present
Radiology		
Technetium sulfur-colloid scan	No isotope uptake, "cold defect"	Takes up technetium
Angiography	Looping centripetal blood flow	Centrifugal blood flow
	Hypervascular or hypovascular	Hypervascularity with dense capillary blushing
Computed tomography	Absence of scar	Stellate central scar, hypodense arterial phase, then hyperdense

3. *Nodular regenerative hyperplasia:* This rare entity consists of a liver partially or diffusely replaced by small well-delineated nodules less than or equal to 1 cm in diameter that morphologically resemble liver cell adenoma as well as regenerative nodules seen in cirrhosis. This entity has been described in Felty's syndrome, congestive heart failure, and subacute bacterial endocarditis. Portal hypertension may also accompany this lesion. Distinguishing between the two lesions on the biopsy specimen alone may not be possible.

4. *Partial nodular transformation:* In this very rare lesion the *hilum* of the liver consists of well-defined nodules surrounded by fibrous tissue and resembling cirrhotic nodules, responsible for presinusoidal portal hypertension with splenomegaly and esophageal varices formation. It is distinctive because of its hilar location; the rest of the liver is uninvolved.

Clinical and Biologic Behavior

1. Liver cell adenoma was an exceptionally rare hepatic tumor before the advent of oral contraceptives in 1960; since then, however, this lesion has significantly increased in frequency, although it is still uncommon (3–4/100,000 new cases per year in long-term users of oral contraceptives).
2. Ninety per cent of cases present in women, 75% between ages 20 and 39 and 85% in those on oral contraceptives.
3. Approximately one third of patients present with abdominal pain (tumor necrosis) and a third with an abdominal mass. Rupture and intraperitoneal hemorrhage are complications that consequently may occur.
4. Slight elevation of serum aminotransferases levels occurs in 50% of cases, and less than 20% of patients have elevated alkaline phosphatase levels; the alpha-fetoprotein is *not* elevated.
5. The tumors tend to occur several years after ingestion of either mestranol or ethinyl estradiol, with the risk markedly increasing after 5 years.
6. Classification:
   a. Estrogenic origin (oral contraceptives, steroid therapy)
   b. Androgenic origin
   c. Spontaneous
   d. Associated with other conditions—glycogen storage disease type 1A, galactosemia, tyrosinemia, diabetes mellitus, hemosiderosis, cirrhosis
7. Androgenic related tumors are seen in association with 17-alpha alkylated compounds used in the treatment of Fanconi's anemia.
8. The spontaneous type occurs at any age, with the incidence equal for men and women.
9. Gross features of resected tumors often aid in diagnosis:
   a. Usually solitary (80%)
   b. Well-circumscribed and encapsulated (74%)

c. Yellow-brown to red in areas of hemorrhage and pelioid changes
   d. 5 to 20 cm in diameter
   e. Predominantly in the right lobe
   f. Located just beneath Glisson's capsule and a thin rim of normal liver.
10. During pregnancy the incidence of hemorrhage and necrosis is markedly increased in adenomas related to oral contraceptives.
11. Regression of lesions may occur on discontinuance of oral contraceptives; spontaneous regression may also occur.
12. An adenoma can rarely progress to hepatocellular carcinoma; however, this malignancy is observed more frequently in adolescents with untreated glycogen storage disease type 1A.

Aspiration Cytology

1. Cells are generally larger than normal hepatocytes, and the cytoplasm is somewhat hydropic.
2. Nuclei are relatively small with uniform nuclear chromatin.
3. Nucleoli are not prominent.
4. Mitoses are exceptionally rare, and cytoplasmic inclusion bodies are absent.
5. Nuclear pleomorphism rarely may be seen and is usually associated with abundant cytoplasm.

Treatment and Prognosis

1. Withdrawal of oral contraceptives is advised, with close follow-up using a scanning modality to assess regression.
2. In asymptomatic cases, the decision to resect the tumor depends on its size and location. The rare possibility of progression to hepatocellular carcinoma also favors resection.
3. Surgery is the treatment of choice for symptomatic tumors. Rupture and intraperitoneal hemorrhage are likely with large tumors; thus resection, and even lobectomy, should be considered. Hepatic artery ligation or embolization may be considered in large, unresectable hemorrhagic tumors.
4. Prognosis is excellent when resection is complete.

References

Edmondson HA, Henderson B, Benton B. Liver-cell adenomas associated with use of oral contraceptives. N Engl J Med 1976;294:470–472.

Foster JH, Berman MM. The benign lesions: Adenoma and focal nodular hyperplasia. In: Major Problems in Clinical Surgery, Vol XXIII, Solid Liver Tumors. Philadelphia: W. B. Saunders, 1977:138–178.

Kerlin P, Davis GL, McGill DB, et al. Hepatic adenoma and focal nodular hyperplasia: Clinical, pathologic, and radiologic features. Gastroenterology 1983;84:994–1002.

Poe R, Snover DC. Adenomas in glycogen storage disease type 1: Two cases with unusual histologic features. Am J Surg Pathol 1988;12:477–483.

Wheeler DA, Edmondson HA, Reynolds TB. Spontaneous liver cell adenoma in children. Am J Clin Pathol 1986;85:6–12.

Bile Duct Adenoma

Major Morphologic Features

1. Proliferation of well-differentiated duct elements is contained within a thin fibroconnective stroma; the ducts are sharply demarcated from the adjacent parenchyma.
2. Epithelial cells are cytologically benign, with absence of pleomorphism and mitoses.

Other Features

1. Duct structures are tubular, sometimes branching with small to absent lumina that do not contain bile.
2. A mild mononuclear inflammatory infiltrate with occasional scattered neutrophils may be seen within the fibroconnective stroma and is characteristically present at the border of the lesion.
3. A fibrous capsule is not present.
4. Portal tracts may be present within the adenoma, with the interlobular duct composed of slightly smaller epithelial cells having more intensely straining nuclei than the tumor cells.

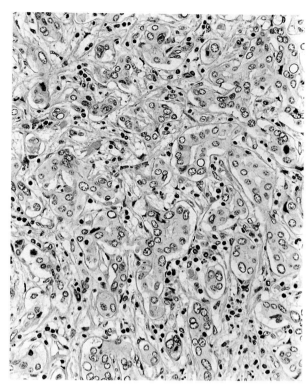

Figure 9–9. Bile duct adenoma. The neoplasm is composed of well-differentiated duct structures. Mitosis is not present. Collagen and scattered lymphocytes are present between the ducts.

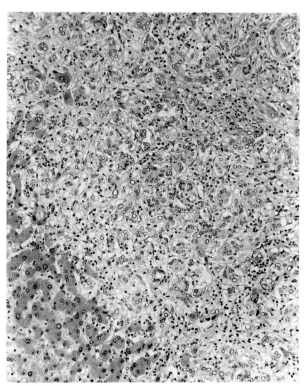

Figure 9–8. Bile duct adenoma. A well-demarcated border between the tumor and noninvolved liver is evident. A mild lymphocytic infiltrate is present within the neoplasm.

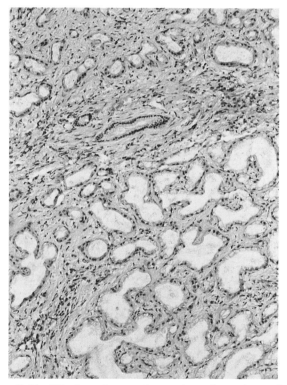

Figure 9–10. Bile duct adenoma. A normal portal tract is completely surrounded by enlarged and somewhat dilated neoplastic duct structures. The normal duct is composed of cells that are smaller than the neoplastic cells.

5. Adenomas are located immediately beneath Glisson's capsule.
6. In rare instances the epithelium and lumen may contain mucin; microcalcifications have also been noted.

Differential Diagnosis

1. *Well-differentiated cholangiocarcinoma, metastatic adenocarcinoma:* Both of these lesions may resemble bile duct adenoma; however, there are a number of morphologic features that may distinguish these malignant lesions from the adenoma:

	Bile Duct Adenoma	Cholangio-carcinoma	Metastatic Adenocarcinoma
Growth pattern	Noninvasive	Invasive into trabeculae	Invasive into sinusoids
Compression of adjacent liver	No	No	Yes
Necrosis	No	Occasional	Often
Fibrous stroma	Variable	Abundant	Variable
Pleomorphism, mitoses	No	Yes	Yes

2. *Von Meyenburg complexes:* These structures consist of moderately dilated ducts, with the lumina often containing bile, and usually located in portal tracts; these features are not present in bile duct adenomas. These complexes may be multiple, and unlike adenomas are associated with congenital and developmental disorders such as choledochal cyst, Caroli's syndrome, polycystic disease, and congenital hepatic fibrosis.

Immunohistochemistry

1. *Keratin, epithelial membrane antigen:* Positive staining is characteristic of bile duct adenomas and may be helpful in differentiating from metastatic adenocarcinomas that stain negatively.

Clinical and Biologic Behavior

1. Bile duct adenomas are rare (6/97,000 consecutive autopsies at University of Southern California), asymptomatic, firm gray-white lesions found incidentally at surgery or autopsy.
2. They are usually solitary (83%), well demarcated, and present immediately beneath Glisson's capsule (95%); they range from 1 to 10 mm (93%) and rarely up to 2.0 cm in diameter.
3. There are no definite reports of malignant transfor-

mation to cholangiocarcinoma; small lesions rarely exhibit enough atypia for concern, especially since in virtually all cases the entire lesion had been surgically resected.
4. Although some group these adenomas with von Meyenberg complexes, the latter are not true neoplasms but are hamartomatous lesions consisting of aggregations of dilated cystic ducts in portal areas.
5. Bile duct adenomas may represent a reactive process to focal hepatic injury rather than a neoplasm or developmental anomaly.

Treatment and Prognosis

1. If diagnosis is established by an adequate ultrasound or CT-guided needle biopsy, no treatment is necessary. If malignancy cannot be excluded in larger lesions, surgical resection may be indicated.

References

Allaire GS, Rabin L, Ishak KG, et al. Bile duct adenoma: A study of 152 cases. Am J Surg Pathol 1988; 12:708–715.
Govindarajan S, Peters RL. The bile duct adenoma: A lesion distinct from Meyenburg complex. Arch Pathol Lab Med 1984;108:922–924.

Cystadenoma

Major Morphologic Changes

1. Multiloculated cystic structure is characterized by the following:
   a. Lining by columnar to cuboidal nonciliated epithelial cells, with eosinophilic or mucinous cytoplasm
   b. Adjacent layer of mesenchymal stroma
   c. Outer layer of dense collagen sharply delineating the cyst from the adjacent hepatic parenchyma

Other Features

1. Epithelial lining cells may be flattened and occasionally sloughed from the cyst wall.
2. Lining may be smooth or exhibit undulations of the wall, with projections or infoldings of the epithelial lining into the underlying stroma.
3. The mesenchymal stroma may contain variable amounts of collagen, smooth muscle, fat, benign glandular structures, and acute and chronic inflammatory cells.
4. Stromal hemorrhage and calcification may be present.
5. The mesenchymal stroma may be absent in a minority of cases.
6. The outer layer may exhibit large vessels, nerves, small glands, and rare small islands of hepatocytes.

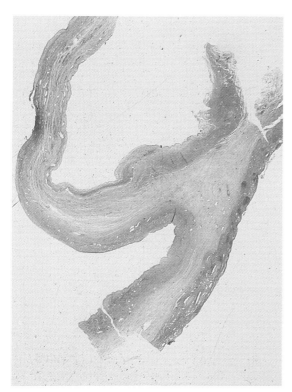

Figure 9–11. Cystadenoma. A low-power photomicrograph shows a cystic structure that appears smooth and well defined. The inner protrustion and proliferation of the wall causes the cyst to grossly appear multiloculated.

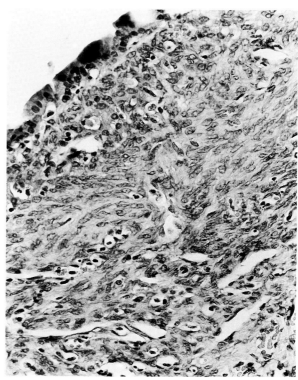

Figure 9–13. Cystadenoma with mesenchymal stroma. The subepithelial stromal component is hypercellular and composed of round to spindle-shaped cells. An overlying simple cuboidal epithelium lines the cyst wall.

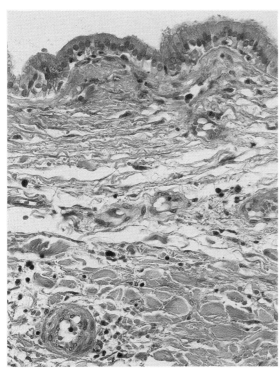

Figure 9–12. Cystadenoma. High power shows the cyst lining to be composed of cuboidal to slightly columnar epithelium. The underlying fibrous stroma exhibits little cellularity. Dense collagen with a single arteriole is present. A mesenchymal stroma is absent.

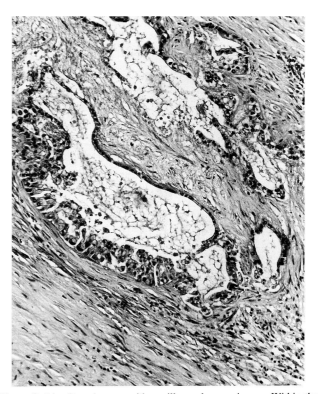

Figure 9–14. Cystadenoma with papillary adenocarcinoma. Within the fibrous wall are cystic structures partially lined by pseudostratified cuboidal to columnar epithelium with hyperchromatic nuclei. A mucinous secretory substance is present within the cysts.

7. The adjacent liver shows atrophic change due to compression by the cyst; cholestasis can be seen in obstructive lesions from larger cysts or cysts that originate from the large intrahepatic ducts (*intraductal cystadenoma*).

Differential Diagnosis

1. *Simple cysts:* These lesions are lined by simple cuboidal or columnar epithelium and surrounded by fibroconnective tissue. Mesenchymal stroma, seen in most cases of cystadenoma, is not present surrounding the simple cyst. In addition, the majority of cystadenomas are multiloculated, while simple cysts are unilocular.
2. *Cystadenocarcinoma:* These adenocarcinomas arise within choledochal cysts and from malignant transformation of the cystadenoma. This neoplasm exhibits a papillary growth into the cyst lumen and direct infiltration into the hepatic stroma.

Special Stains

1. *Masson:* Collagen is demonstrated (blue) within the stroma, with counterstain (red) identifying smooth muscle elements.
2. *Periodic acid–Schiff after diastase, mucicarmine:* Mucin can often be identified within the lumen of the cyst as well as the cytoplasm of the epithelial lining cells.

Clinical and Biologic Behavior

1. Cystadenomas are benign intrahepatic multiloculated cystic tumors categorized as *with* (CMS) or *without* (COMS) mesenchymal stroma:

	CMS	COMS
Percent of total cystadenomas	78%	22%
Sex	Only female	75% male
Age, benign (mean)	43	53
Age, malignant transformation	59	Male: 54
		Female: 35
Probability of malignant transformation	Extremely rare	23% of cases

2. Patients present with an abdominal mass; 50% have accompanying abdominal pain.
3. Laboratory tests are nonspecific, occasionally with mild elevations of serum aminotransferase levels; serum alkaline phosphatase and bilirubin may become elevated when large lesions obstruct the biliary tract.
4. Typical gross findings include multilocularity in 71%, 7 to 25 cm in diameter, 65% in left lobe, mucinous contents, and smooth or trabeculated inner lining.

5. COMS has been experimentally produced in rats treated with aflatoxin.
6. Malignant transformation, characterized grossly by solid inner protruding masses, may occur in up to one fourth of cases of COMS, with some tumors exhibiting transition zones between benign and malignant regions.

Aspiration Cytology

1. The cysts contain mucinous, rarely serous gelatinous fluid with benign columnar to cuboidal mucin-containing epithelial cells.
2. Nuclear atypia and proliferation of papillary projections suggest possible malignancy.

Treatment and Prognosis

1. Surgical resection when complete is curative.
2. In large nonresectable tumors, marsupialization can be performed, especially in CMS in which risk of malignant transformation is extremely low.
3. Involvement of large intrahepatic or extrahepatic ducts may make surgical resection difficult; relief of obstruction with stenting (endoscopic, surgical) may be considered.

References

Ishak KG, Willis GW, Cummings SD, et al. Biliary cystadenoma and cystadenocarcinoma: Report of 14 cases and review of the literature. Cancer 1977;38:322–338.

Marsh JL, Dahms B, Longmire WP. Cystadenoma and cystadenocarcinoma of the biliary system. Arch Surg 1974;109:41–43.

Van Roekel V, Marx WJ, Baskin W, et al. Cystadenoma of the liver. J Clin Gastroenterol 1982;4:167–172.

Wheeler DA, Edmondson HA. Cystadenoma with mesenchymal stroma (CMS) in the liver and bile ducts. Cancer 1985;56:1434–1445.

Vascular Neoplasms

CAVERNOUS HEMANGIOMA

Major Morphologic Features

1. Large dilated communicating blood-filled spaces are lined by endothelial cells.
2. Relatively thick and poorly cellular fibrous septa are present between the vascular channels.

Other Features

1. The hemangioma is well demarcated from the rest of the liver and often located immediately beneath Glisson's capsule.

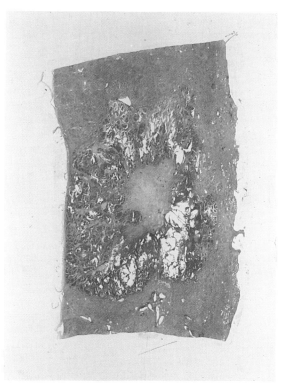

Figure 9–15. Cavernous hemangioma. Low power exhibits numerous small and medium-sized dilated vascular channels, often containing red blood cells. In the center a somewhat ill-defined hyalinized stroma without obvious vascular structures is present.

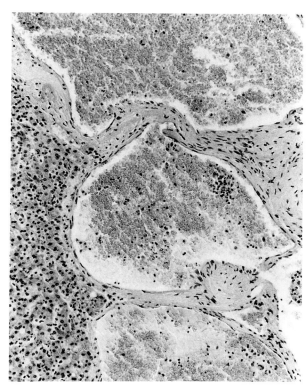

Figure 9–17. Cavernous hemangioma. The large vascular structures are filled with red blood cells and lined by flattened endothelial cells.

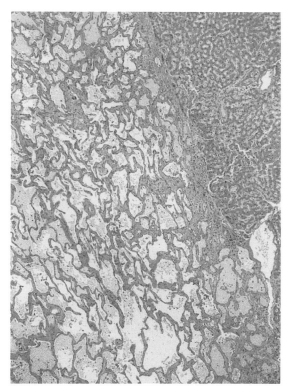

Figure 9–16. Cavernous hemangioma. A sharp border is present between the numerous dilated vascular structures and the adjacent hepatic parenchyma.

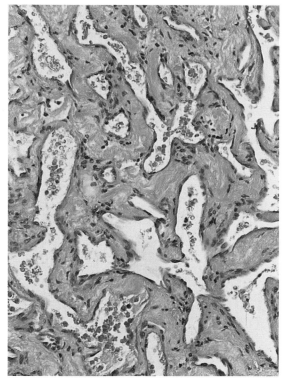

Figure 9–18. Cavernous hemangioma. The fibrous septa are thickened and relatively acellular. Eventually there is total replacement of the hemangioma by a hyalinized stroma that may undergo calcification.

2. Large "feeding" vessels are present at the edge of the lesion.
3. Large thick-walled vessels are often identified between the vascular spaces, representing hepatic venous outflow; thrombosis of these vessels may lead to fibrous obliteration of the vascular spaces.
4. The septa may exhibit duct structures and myxoid changes.
5. The vascular spaces may have fibrin deposited along the endothelial lining, and are often sites of thrombosis.
6. Older lesions may exhibit hyalinization of the septa, with calcification.
7. Chronic liver disease is not present in nontumor liver; however, features such as von Meyenberg complexes, benign cysts, and focal nodular hyperplasia have been described.

Differential Diagnosis

1. *Angiosarcoma:* Angiosarcoma may present as a solitary lesion. The majority of these patients are ill, while patients with cavernous hemangioma are generally asymptomatic or may have mild or vague abdominal discomfort. Biopsies are generally not recommended in either lesion because of risk of hemorrhage. Thin-needle aspiration may be performed, with demonstration of overtly malignant endothelial cells in angiosarcoma. Cavernous hemangioma has a typical arteriographic appearance where opacification and slow filling of the dilated vascular spaces from the peripheral "feeder" vessels result in peripheral enhancement of contrast medium, a phenomenon also seen on computed tomography with contrast medium. Delayed enhancement of isotope within the lesion is also seen on blood pool scans.
2. *Peliosis hepatis:* These lesions are multiple, quite small (from less than 1 mm to 1 cm in diameter), and filled with blood; they do not exhibit septa and often do not have lining of the spaces by endothelial cells.
3. *Hereditary hemorrhagic telangiectasis:* Multiple dilated small portal and periportal vascular channels are present, a feature not seen in cavernous hemangioma.
4. *Hemangioendothelioma:* This infantile morphologically benign neoplasm is capillary in nature and not found in adults.

Immunohistochemistry

1. *Factor VIII–related antigen:* Endothelial cells are identified by positive cytoplasmic staining.

Clinical and Biologic Behavior

1. Cavernous hemangioma is the most common benign hepatic neoplasm; its overall incidence is 0.4% to 19.0% (1% in University of Southern California experience of 91,000 autopsies); it is also the most common site for hemangioma formation in the abdomen.
2. There is a female predominance (6:1) in patients younger than 40; hormonal stimulation plays a role in their development, since the lesions may enlarge during pregnancy, with hemangiomas also forming in the skin and gingiva. In the elderly, the lesion is more common in men (2:1).
3. The majority of patients are asymptomatic (86%); the lesion in these instances is usually less than 4 cm in diameter. Symptomatic hemangiomas present as abdominal discomfort and sometimes pain caused by compression of adjacent viscera. Sudden pain is usually secondary to tumor thrombosis or spontaneous rupture and hemorrhage into the abdominal cavity (larger lesions).
4. Liver test results are usually normal.
5. Ninety per cent are solitary, and most are less than 5 cm (may be a few millimeters); however, exceptionally large tumors may occur (30 cm).
6. The lesions may occur in either lobe; although the usual location is immediately beneath Glisson's capsule, they may occur anywhere within the parenchyma.
7. The lesions are termed *giant* when they attain sizes greater than 10 cm; in addition, the entire liver very rarely may be replaced by very small lesions (angiosarcoma has been reported in this variant).
8. The tumors are usually red to red purple, with dilated "cavernous" vascular features; the older lesions often become gray-white and firm owing to fibrosis that begins centrally. Involution may occur, and focal calcification may become apparent on radiographs.
9. The neonate may develop severe complications of heart failure secondary to arteriovenous shunting, as well as rupture and coagulopathy, and must therefore be promptly diagnosed and treated.

Aspiration Cytology

1. Although aspiration is contraindicated, the lesion may not be suspected when sclerotic; it may be confused then with a primary or metastatic solid tumor.
2. Aspiration of these lesions reveals considerable blood, benign spindle (endothelial) cells, fibroconnective tissue with minimal to absent inflammatory infiltration, and rare calcium deposits.

Treatment and Prognosis

1. Majority of lesions are asymptomatic and incidentally discovered on ultrasound or computed tomography performed for workup of other disorders or during surgery; no treatment is necessary for small lesions.
2. Although larger lesions are at risk of rupture, it is not clear if surgery is necessary. Large symptomatic lesions should be resected if they are accessible to the surgeon.
3. When the lesion is not resectable because of its location, size, and number, radiation therapy has been tried but is not generally recommended.
4. Prognosis is excellent after resection, without recurrence after long-term follow up.

References

Adam YG, Huvos AG, Fortner JG. Giant hemangiomas of the liver. Ann Surg 1972;172:239–245.

Caturelli E, Rapaccini GL, Sabelli C, et al. Ultrasound-guided fine-needle aspiration biopsy in the diagnosis of hepatic hemangioma. Liver 1986;6:326–330.

Schwartz SI, Husser WC. Cavernous hemangioma of the liver: A single institution report of 16 resections. Ann Surg 1987;205:456–465.

Zafrani ES. Update on vascular tumors of the liver. J Hepatol 1989;8:125–130.

INFANTILE HEMANGIOENDOTHELIOMA

Major Morphologic Features

1. Proliferation of multiple small vascular channels lined by endothelial cells is subcategorized into two types:
   a. I—cytologically benign-appearing endothelial cells forming a single layer around the vascular channels
   b. II—pleomorphic, hyperchromatic, and multilayered endothelial cells exhibiting intravascular budding and branching

Other Features

1. The center of the lesions may have cavernous-type changes, with the periphery exhibiting more typical small vascular spaces.
2. Thrombosis and tumor infarction may occur, usually within the center of the lesion, with resultant scar formation and occasionally calcification.
3. The endothelial cells tend to infiltrate the sinusoids at the periphery and surround liver cell trabeculae; these hepatocytes may undergo duct transformation.
4. Extramedullary hematopoiesis may be present within the vascular spaces.

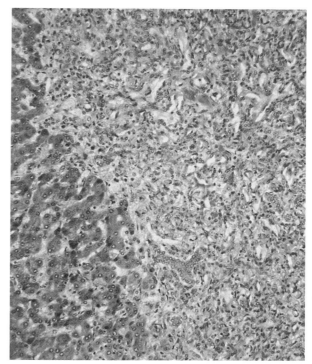

Figure 9–19. Infantile hemangioendothelioma. The neoplasm is well demarcated from the adjacent hepatic parenchyma. Small vascular spaces can be identified within the tumor.

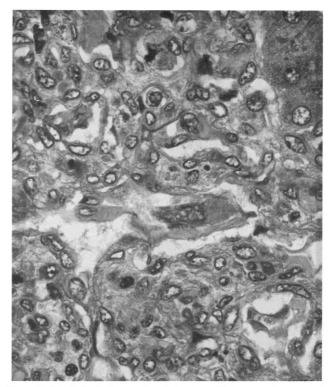

Figure 9–20. Infantile hemangioendothelioma. High power shows proliferation of numerous small vascular channels lined by a single layer of endothelial cells having plump clear nuclei.

5. Rare instances of malignant transformation to angiosarcoma may occur; these cases may represent, however, some of the more aggressively growing type II lesions.

Differential Diagnosis

1. *Cavernous hemangioma:* The central portion of both lesions may have virtually identical cavernous changes, but the peripheral capillary vascular spaces are not features of cavernous hemangiomas.
2. *Angiosarcoma:* Infiltration of benign-appearing endothelial cells within sinusoids at the periphery of the lesion is a worrisome feature of hemangioendothelioma, since this growth pattern characteristically occurs in angiosarcoma. Differentiation will depend on the cytologically malignant features of angiosarcoma. Type II hemangioendothelioma may be difficult to distinguish from angiosarcoma.

Immunohistochemistry

1. *Factor VIII–related antigen:* Endothelial cells are identified by positive cytoplasmic staining.

Clinical and Biologic Behavior

1. Infantile hemangioendothelioma resembles the capillary hemangioma of the skin and represents 12% of all primary hepatic neoplasms in the infant.
2. The tumors are twice as common in females; approximately 50% are discovered incidentally at surgery or autopsy.
3. Symptomatic patients present during the first 6 months of life with hepatomegaly, often as an abdominal mass, with 25% having severe high-outflow congestive heart failure (arteriovenous hepatic shunting); cutaneous hemangiomas are present in 19% to 87% of cases.
4. The tumor mass may be solitary or consist of multiple red-purple nodules involving both lobes; the nodules appear gray in areas of fibrosis.
5. Spontaneous involution is common; however, malignant transformation with metastasis has been described.

Aspiration Cytology

1. Aspiration is contraindicated; however, in unsuspected lesions, the presence of abundant red cells and numerous cytologically benign (type I) or atypical (type II) endothelial cells in an infant is suggestive of the lesion.

Treatment and Prognosis

1. When the tumor is solitary, or when multiple but confined to a focal segment, surgical resection is recommended, since probability of cure is very high.
2. Hepatic artery ligation and radiation are considered for large, nonresectable lesions.
3. Mortality is 70% owing to high-output heart failure, although a recent series suggests a lower mortality; other complications include hepatic failure and hemorrhage.

References

Dachman AH, Lichtenstein JE, Friedman AC, et al. Infantile hemangioendothelioma of the liver: A radiologic-pathologic-clinical correlation. AJR 1983;140:1091–1096.
Dehner LP, Ishak KG. Vascular tumors of the liver in infants and children: A study of 30 cases and review of the literature. Arch Pathol 1971;92:101–111.
Vorse HB, Smith I, Luckstead EF, et al. Hepatic hemangioendotheliomatosis of infancy. Am J Dis Child 1983;13⁻:672–673.

■ Primary Malignant Neoplasms

Hepatocellular Carcinoma

COMMON PATTERNS (TRABECULAR, ACINAR, DUCTULAR)

Major Morphologic Features

1. Trabecular cords are more than two to three cells thick, composed of well to moderately differentiated neoplastic liver cells, and lined by thin endothelial cells (*microtrabecular*).
2. Radial *acinar* and *pseudoglandular* arrangement of neoplastic hepatocytes is seen around a centrally maintained canaliculus (12% cases); the lumen frequently contains bile.
3. *Ductlike* structures are focally present (5%–10% cases), often within a fibrous stroma.

Other Features

1. Tumor cells exhibit variable degrees of differentiation, but morphologic features of typical hepatocytes are generally maintained:
   a. Round to oval nuclei have prominent nucleoli.
   b. Eosinophilic, granular, or hydropic cytoplasm may be relatively abundant; however, the nuclear/cytoplasmic ratio is generally increased.
2. Other features characteristic of hepatocytes may be present:
   a. Bile, fat, and glycogen
   b. Cytoplasmic eosinophilic material, inclusion bodies, and rarely ground-glass–like cells

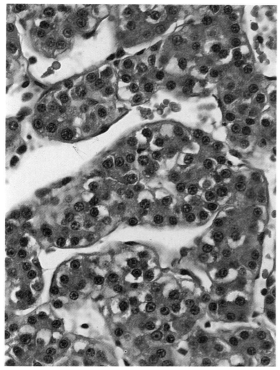

Figure 9–21. Hepatocellular carcinoma. The thickened hepatic cords are four to six cells thick and composed of liver cells having an increased nuclear/cytoplasmic ratio. The cords are lined by thin endothelial cells.

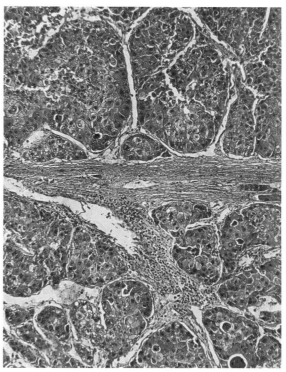

Figure 9–23. Hepatocellular carcinoma. The macrotrabecular pattern exhibits fibrous septa with a mild lymphocytic infiltrate. Occasional groups of hepatocytes form a radial arrangement around dilated biliary canaliculi containing bile plugs.

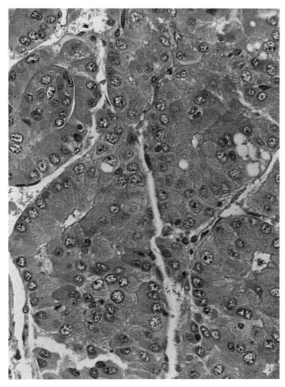

Figure 9–22. Hepatocellular carcinoma. The thickened cords are composed of hepatocytes having abundant eosinophilic cytoplasm. An occasional neoplastic cell contains fat.

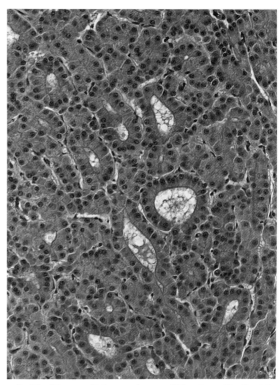

Figure 9–24. Hepatocellular carcinoma. Dilated canaliculi with acinar formation of neoplastic hepatocytes are prominent.

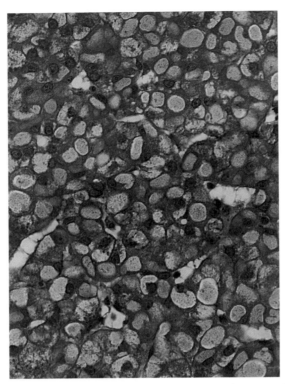

Figure 9–25. Hepatocellular carcinoma. The neoplastic hepatocytes have formed cytoplasmic inclusions and resemble ground-glass cells. Although tumor cells may contain the hepatitis B virus, the ground-glass inclusions seen in this photomicrograph are *not* due to the virus.

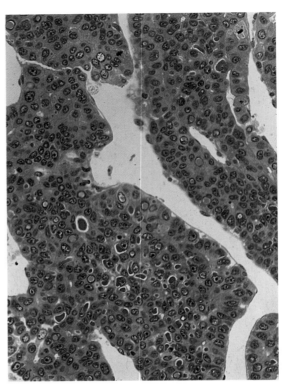

Figure 9–27. Hepatocellular carcinoma. The macrotrabecular pattern is composed of small hepatocytes, many containing oval to round eosinophilic inclusions often surrounded by a thin clear space. These types of inclusions have been shown to stain positively for alpha-1-antitrypsin, alpha-fetoprotein, and fibrinogen.

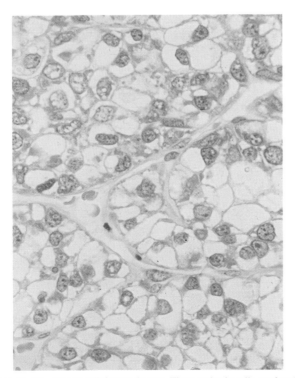

Figure 9–26. Hepatocellular carcinoma. The neoplastic cells are forming thickened trabeculae lined by endothelial cells; however, all the hepatocytes have a completely empty-appearing cytoplasm (*clear cell* type).

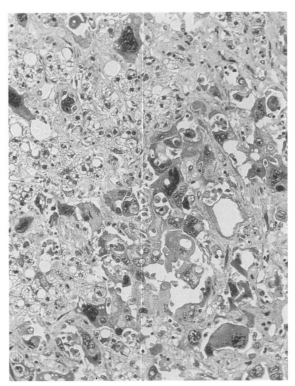

Figure 9–28. Hepatocellular carcinoma. The majority of cells contain abundant cytoplasm and single or multiple nuclei that are markedly enlarged, often distorted, and hyperchromatic (*giant cell* type).

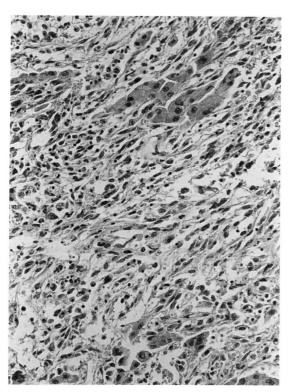

Figure 9–29. Hepatocellular carcinoma. The cells contain small hyperchromatic nuclei with spindle-shaped cytoplasm often running parallel to adjacent tumor cells. Residual nonneoplastic hepatocytes *(above)* are surrounded by tumor cells. This spindle cell variant of hepatocellular carcinoma may be difficult to differentiate from a sarcoma.

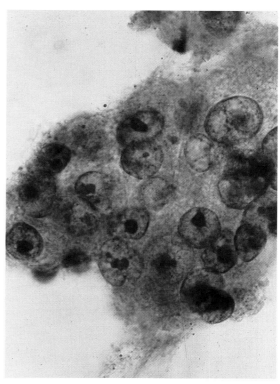

Figure 9–31. Hepatocellular carcinoma. The aspirate cytology reveals round to oval nuclei with prominent nucleoli. The cytoplasm is moderate in size and slightly granular.

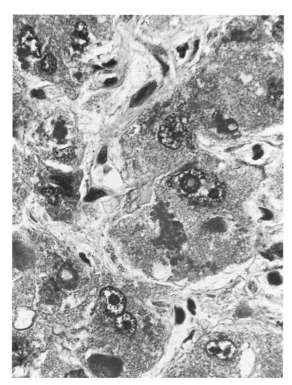

Figure 9–30. Hepatocellular carcinoma. The enlarged tumor cells contain abundant alcoholic hyalin, confirmed by immunoperoxidase stain.

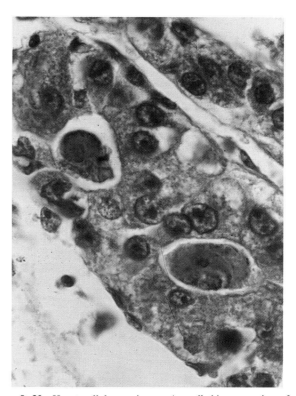

Figure 9–32. Hepatocellular carcinoma. A needle biopsy specimen from the same neoplasm (see Figure 9–31) shows typical hepatocellular carcinoma with dilated canaliculi containing bile.

(HBsAg negative) composed of proteins normally synthesized in the hepatocytes (alpha-1-antitrypsin, alpha-fetoprotein, fibrinogen, albumin)

   c. Mallory's hyalin in tumor cells (4%–12% cases) in the presence or absence of coexisting alcoholic liver disease

3. Mitoses are often present and occasionally atypical (tripolar); they may be uncommon in well-differentiated tumors.
4. Exceptionally thickened trabeculae more than 10 cells thick may be formed *(macrotrabecular)*.
5. Solid growth pattern may resemble *cobblestoning.*
6. Marked accumulation of eosinophilic secretory material in dilated acinar structures produces an *adenoid* pattern.
7. Abundant small vascular channels are often present; larger vessels may exhibit thrombosis, with resultant ischemic necrosis and hemorrhage of tumor.
8. Highly vascularized lesions may have a spongy hemorrhagic appearance (*pelioid* pattern).
9. Larger lesions may exhibit *pseudocapsules* (compresed reticulin fibers) or true fibrous capsules.
10. Inflammatory infiltration is scanty to absent in most cases.
11. Growth of tumor merges into adjacent nonneoplastic trabeculae, *not* sinusoids; larger lesions tend to bulge into adjacent liver with resultant compression and atrophy of nonneoplastic hepatocytes, sinusoidal dilatation and congestion.
12. Liver cell dysplasia (nuclear anisocytosis, hyperchromasia, pleomorphism) of nonneoplastic hepatocytes is seen frequently when tumor is also present.
13. Tumor thrombi may be present in portal (34%) and hepatic (22%) venous radicles, as well as in lymphatic channels within portal tracts and fibrous septa; intra-arterial and intraductal growth patterns have been described but are rare.
14. Cirrhosis is present in 60% to 90% of cases.
15. *Less common variants:*
   a. *Clear cell carcinoma:* Clear cytoplasm, either hydropic or containing abundant amounts of glycogen and/or fat
   b. *Spindle cell carcinoma:* Sarcomatous type of growth pattern
   c. *Giant cell carcinoma:* Multinucleated large and often markedly anaplastic cells

NOTE: Neoplasms are usually complex, and may be composed of a variety of individual growth patterns.

Differential Diagnosis

1. *Benign neoplasms and hyperplastic lesions (liver cell adenoma, focal nodular hyperplasia, nodular regenerative hyperplasia, regenerative cirrhotic nodule):* Well-differentiated hepatocellular carcinoma may be difficult to differentiate from these lesions on morphologic grounds alone, especially on needle biopsy or aspiration. Careful examination for thickened trabecular cords, individual cell atypia, presence of mitoses, tumor within vascular structures, and infiltration of tumor into adjacent liver are important features for the diagnosis of hepatocellular carcinoma. Clinical history (women taking oral contraceptives for adenoma, presence of chronic liver disease in hepatocelular carcinoma), radiologic and laboratory data (HBsAg positive, elevation of alpha-fetoprotein in hepatocellular carcinoma) are often necessary for correct diagnosis.
2. *Cholangiocarcinoma:* Duct transformation with or without a fibrous stroma is present in 5% to 10% of patients with hepatocellular carcinoma; cholangiocarcinoma should be strongly considered if the biopsy specimen does not additionally identify areas of more typical changes of hepatocellular carcinoma. The presence of round to oval nuclei with prominent nucleoli and granular eosinophilic cytoplasm in some of the ductlike cells suggests hepatocellular carcinoma. Fibrosis is not typically seen in most cases of trabecular hepatocellular carcinoma. Additional biopsy may be necessary to distinguish between the two lesions, since ductal changes in hepatocellular carcinoma usually comprise only a small volume of the tumor, whereas cholangiocarcinoma is entirely composed of malignant duct epithelium.
3. *Metastatic tumor:* Metastatic neoplasms with round nuclei, prominent nucleoli, and eosinophilic cytoplasm may easily resemble hepatocellular carcinoma. Gland formation of metastatic adenocarcinoma may resemble hepatocellular carcinoma with acinar, pseudoglandular, and/or ductal growth patterns. Important features of hepatocellular carcinoma useful for differentiation include a merging of tumor into the trabeculae and *not* sinusoids of nontumor liver, endothelial lining around groups of tumor cells, and substances such as bile, fat, glycogen, albumin, alpha-1-antitrypsin, and Mallory bodies within the tumor cytoplasm.

Special Stains

1. *Periodic acid–Schiff:* Glycogen is present in cytoplasm of clear cell type.
2. *Periodic acid–Schiff after diastase:* Intracytoplasmic globules identify alpha-1-antitrypsin and other inclusions.
3. *Van Gieson:* Bile in tumor cells or acini is identified by variable degrees of green staining (dependent on amount of biliverdin).

Immunohistochemistry

1. *Alpha-fetoprotein* (AFP): Thirty-three to 80% of cases of hepatocellular carcinoma are associated with

elevated serum AFP. These cases generally have some degree of cytoplasmic staining of this protein in tumor cells; however, AFP may also be identified in tumor cells when the serum AFP level is not elevated.

2. *Cytokeratins:* Monoclonal antikeratin antibodies with different specificities exhibit immunoreactive staining patterns (positive Cam 5.2, negative AE1) characteristic for hepatocellular carcinoma but usually negative for cholangiocarcinoma and metastatic tumors.

3. *Other proteins (alpha-1-antitrypsin, albumin, fibrinogen):* These proteins identify cytoplasmic globules or diffuse staining and are useful in differentiating hepatic (positive staining) from nonhepatic origin of neoplasms.

4. *HBsAg:* Positive cytoplasmic staining within tumor cells has been described. Free and integrated HBV-DNA is well documented with hepatocellular carcinoma; however, the true incidence of positively staining tumor cells by immunoperoxidase method is low.

Clinical and Biologic Behavior

1. Hepatocellular carcinoma is the most common primary hepatic malignancy in the world; its incidence varies considerably with race, sex, and geographic location (Table 9–1).

2. The tumor is two to eight times more frequent in men; the average age at clinical presentation is 52 years in the United States and 37 years in Asia.

3. The majority of patients have chronic liver disease and are usually cirrhotic (84% of all cases in the United States); 62% of patients present with epigastric discomfort, fullness, or an abdominal mass, while 21% present with ascites, variceal bleeding, and decompensation. Rarely, intraperitoneal hemorrhage from tumor on the hepatic surface may be a presenting feature.

4. Liver tests reflect abnormalities related to the underlying chronic liver disease; however, a disproportionate elevation of alkaline phosphatase may be noted.

5. Serum alpha-fetoprotein is the single most useful laboratory test; the tumor is associated with levels greater than 400 ng/mL (normal, 5–10 ng/mL) in 61% of patients with underlying alcoholic cirrhosis, 79% with B-viral cirrhosis, and 33% of "normal" livers. Values may achieve levels as high as 1 million ng/mL.

6. Other conditions associated with elevated alpha-fetoprotein levels include acute fulminant viral hepatitis B (in those most likely to survive), pregnancy, fetal distress, gastric carcinoma with or without hepatic metastases, pancreatic carcinoma, embryonal tumors (yolk sac, teratocarcinoma, endodermal sinus tumors), cholangiocarcinoma (reported in Japanese series), and chronic active hepatitis (occa-

Table 9–1

AGE-ADJUSTED INCIDENCE RATE OF HEPATOCELLULAR CARCINOMA PER 100,000 (MALE) POPULATION

Geographic Area/Race	Rate
United States	
Chinese	7.8–18.1
White	1.8–2.9
Black	3.9–4.2
Japanese	2.7–5.7
Hispanic	4.1
Europe	
England	1.1–2.1
Germany	3.6
Sweden	3.4
Switzerland	6.3–9.7
Africa	
Mozambique	112.9
Zimbabwe	64.6
South Africa:	
Black (native)	28.4
White	1.2
Senegal	25.6
Algeria	1.6
Asia	
Hong Kong	34.4
Japan	2.5–11.9
Peoples Republic of China	31.7
India	1.3–4.7
Latin America	
Argentina	6.0–9.9
Costa Rica	5.0
Brazil	1.2–3.8
Panama	2.3

Modified from Munoz N, Bosch X. Epidemiology of hepatocellular carcinoma. In Okuda K, Ishak KG, eds. Neoplasms of the Liver. Tokyo: Springer-Verlag, 1987:3–19.

sionally elevated to values of greater than 400 ng/mL and tend to fluctuate but are never sustained or progressive). Over 70% of alpha-fetoprotein in hepatocellular carcinoma binds to the lectin concanavalin A, while the nonhepatic neoplasms with alpha-fetoprotein have a much lower affinity (useful in differential diagnosis).

7. Patients with hepatocellular carcinoma may have other metabolic abnormalities ("paraneoplastic" conditions): amyloidosis, carcinoid syndrome, dysfibrinogenemia, hypercalcemia, hypoglycemia, polycythemia, increased gonadotropins.

8. The most important predisposing condition associated with hepatocellular carcinoma is chronic hepatitis B; throughout the world the incidence of hepatocellular carcinoma parallels the incidence of chronic hepatitis B in that region. In Taiwan, approximately 80% of patients with hepatocellular carcinoma have chronic HBV infection; hepatocellular carcinoma is present between 44% and 52% of patients with B-viral cirrhosis in Japan, Hong Kong, and Africa.

9. There is exceptionally strong evidence that HBV DNA integration into the host genome will result in malignant transformation; the association has been

noted in patients with chronic active but not persistent viral hepatitis.

10. Other predisposing conditions include the following:
   a. Alcoholic cirrhosis (6%–10% of alcoholics who have stopped drinking, but rare in the active alcoholic)
   b. Cirrhosis secondary to chronic active hepatitis C (estimated at 10%, but some reports suggest the incidence to be much higher)
   c. Hemochromatosis (3%–27%)
   d. Estrogens (oral contraceptives and liver cell adenoma with malignant transformation, rare)
   e. Anabolic steroids
   f. Toxins (vinyl chloride, thorotrast associated with both angiosarcoma and hepatocellular carcinoma)
   g. Aflatoxins (mycotoxin found in many foodstuffs such as peanuts, corn, rice, wheat, soybeans, produced by the fungus *Aspergillus flavus*)

11. Most common sites of metastatic spread in cirrhotics:

Lung	38.8%
Portal vein	37.2%
Hepatic vein	22.9%
Regional lymph nodes	16.5%
Bone marrow	8.0%
Serosa of peritoneum	7.4%

In noncirrhotics, metastases are more common in lymph nodes (43.6%) and peritoneum (23.1%); in addition, approximately one half of cirrhotics but two thirds of noncirrhotics will develop metastatic disease (noncirrhotics are healthier and survive longer for chance of spread).

12. Theories of multicentric versus unicentric origin of the tumor have been postulated.

13. Needle biopsy is diagnostic in approximately 80% of the cases.

Aspiration Cytology

1. Polygonal cells have moderate granular cytoplasm that is more basophilic than the normal hepatocyte.
2. Round nuclei have prominent nucleoli and variable degrees of hyperchromasia.
3. Less well-differentiated tumors have scanty cytoplasm and higher nuclear-cytoplasmic ratios.
4. Trabecular formation with thin endothelial lining is seen.
5. Acinar or pseudoglandular formation, sometimes containing bile, is present.
6. Present within the cytoplasm are fat, bile, alcoholic hyalin, glycogen, and globular eosinophilic inclusions.

Note: Severe dysplasia of cells in an aspirate is not necessarily indicative of hepatocellular carcinoma, since this change is commonly seen as a feature of chronic active hepatitis B.

Treatment and Prognosis

1. Resection of tumors is the only hope for cure. Ultrasonographic screening is used in high-risk patients to identify small tumors (~2 cm).
2. Survival and postoperative morbidity are influenced by the presence of cirrhosis. Noncirrhotics generally do better, especially if the tumor is small, encapsulated, or confined to a segment or lobe.
3. Chemotherapy with intra-arterial infusion is of temporary benefit. Palliative radiation is of little value.
4. Injection of absolute alcohol into tumors identified on ultrasound or computed tomography has shown promise.
5. Hepatic transplantation is not recommended, since tumor recurrence from metastatic sites almost always develops after transplantation.
6. The average survival overall is 6 months after diagnosis, with the 5-year survival after surgery being only 10%.

References

Anthony PP, Vogel CL, Barker LF. Liver cell dysplasia: A premalignant condition. J Clin Pathol 1973;26:217–223.

Bedrossian CWM, Davila RM, Merenda G. Immunocytochemical evaluation of liver fine-needle aspirations. Arch Pathol Lab Med 1989;113:1225–1230.

Brechot C. Hepatitis B virus (HBV) and hepatocellular carcinoma: HBV-DNA status and its implications. J Hepatol 1987;4:269–279.

Edmondson HA, Steiner PE. Primary carcinoma of the liver: A study of 100 cases among 48,900 necropsies. Cancer 1954;7:462–503.

Kishi K, Shikata T, Hirohashi S, et al. Hepatocellular carcinoma: A clinical and pathologic analysis of 57 hepatectomy cases. Cancer 1983;51:542–548.

Liver cancer study group of Japan. Primary liver cancer in Japan, 6th report. Cancer 1987;60:1400–1411.

Munoz N, Bosch X. Epidemiology of hepatocellular carcinoma. In: Okuda K, Ishak KG, eds. Neoplasma of the Liver. Tokyo: Springer-Verlag, 1987:3–19.

Nakashima T, Kojiro M. Pathologic characteristics of hepatocellular carcinoma. Semin Liver Dis 1986;6:259–266.

Noguchi S, Yamamoto R, Tatsuta M, et al. Cell features and patterns in fine-needle aspirates of hepatocellular carcinoma. Cancer 1986;58:321–328.

Okuda K. Early recognition of hepatocellular carcinoma. Hepatology 1986;6:729–738.

FIBROLAMELLAR HEPATOCELLULAR CARCINOMA

Major Morphologic Features

1. Large polygonal hepatocytes with granular eosinophilic cytoplasm (*oncocytic*) are seen.
2. Collagen is laid down in a parallel (*lamellar*) fashion around columns and nests of tumor cells.
3. Large distinct lightly staining eosinophilic intracytoplasmic globules (*pale bodies*) occur in 50% of cases.

Other Features

1. Nuclei are round, with single prominent nucleoli.
2. Small cytoplasmic hyaline droplets are present in 72% of cases.
3. Cholestasis may be present, often within the lumen formed by groups of neoplastic cells having an acinar or pelioid growth pattern.
4. Mitoses are relatively scanty.
5. Alcoholic hyalin and multinucleated tumor cells may be seen but are rare.
6. Cirrhosis and chronic active hepatitis in nontumor liver are typically absent, with the liver completely "normal" in 75% of cases.
7. Copper and copper-binding protein are in some instances increased (feature unusual for more typical variants of hepatocellular carcinoma).

Differential Diagnosis

1. *Focal nodular hyperplasia:* The presence of fibrous strands within the tumor mass occurs in both focal nodular hyperplasia and fibrolamellar hepatocellular carcinoma. However, in focal nodular hyperplasia there is variable chronic inflammatory infiltration as well as atypical duct structures in the septa; these

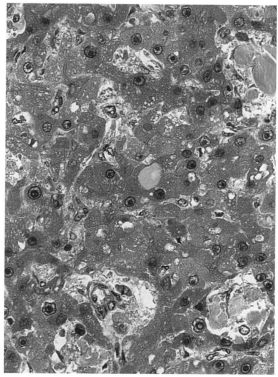

Figure 9–34. Fibrolamellar hepatocellular carcinoma. The enlarged tumor cells have abundant eosinophilic cytoplasm. A tumor cell *(center)* contains a well-defined eosinophilic staining cytoplasmic inclusion (pale body).

features are not seen in fibrolamellar hepatocellular carcinoma. In addition, the distinct cytoplasmic pale bodies and hyaline droplets are not a feature of focal nodular hyperplasia.
2. *Liver cell adenoma:* The hepatocytes in adenomas are usually hydropic, not eosinophilic, and without distinct inclusions. A fibrous stroma is characteristically absent in the adenoma.
3. *Sclerosing hepatic carcinoma:* The collagen is quite dense and acellular in sclerosing hepatic carcinoma and is not present surrounding tumor cells in a fibrillar, lamellar fashion. The hepatocytes are also smaller, without the prominent eosinophilic cytoplasm and inclusions typical for fibrolamellar hepatocellular carcinoma.
4. *Metastatic tumor initiating a fibrotic reaction:* Neoplasms such as breast, pancreas, and gallbladder metastatic to the liver may initiate a prominent sclerotic reaction. The type of collagen is relatively dense and not arranged in a lamellar fashion. Although primary (rare) and metastatic squamous cell carcinomas may have abundant eosinophilic cytoplasm, the presence of hyaline droplets and "pale bodies" in fibrolamellar hepatocellular carcinoma and of intercellular bridges and keratin pearl formation in squamous cell carcinoma will help distinguish between the two lesions.

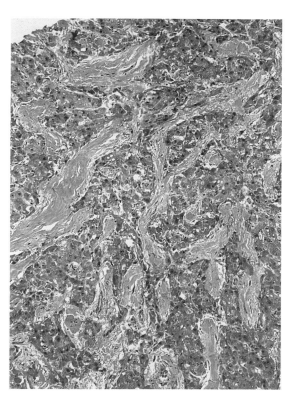

Figure 9–33. Fibrolamellar hepatocellular carcinoma. The tumor is composed of large eosinophilic hepatocytes arranged in nests and columns, separated by collagen laid down in a parallel fashion.

Special Stains

1. *Periodic acid–Schiff after diastase:* The pale bodies stain negatively. Granular cytoplasmic staining may be present and is suggestive of alpha-1-antitrypsin globules.
2. *Orcein:* Results are negative for pale bodies; positive brown-black granular staining is indicative of copper-binding protein.

Immunohistochemistry

1. *Alpha-fetoprotein:* This protein may be present as granular staining in occasional cells but is most often absent.
2. *Alpha-1-antitrypsin, fibrinogen, C-reactive protein:* These proteins are seen as diffuse cytoplasmic staining. The hyaline droplets frequently stain positively.

Clinical and Biologic Behavior

1. Fibrolamellar hepatocellular carcinoma differs from the typical form of liver cell carcinoma by the following:
   a. It arises predominantly in noncirrhotic livers (75%).
   b. It occurs in a younger population.
   c. Morphologic features are distinct.
   d. The overall prognosis is better than in typical trabecular hepatocellular carcinoma.
2. The tumor represents 1% to 7% of all types of liver cell carcinoma; in patients younger than 35 years of age, the incidence is 14% to 40%.
3. Mean age of presentation is 25 years of age (5 months to 69 years), compared with typical trabecular hepatocellular carcinoma (52 years).
4. Sex distribution is equal to a slight male predominance, with trabecular hepatocellular carcinoma exhibiting a male predominance of 4:1.
5. It clinically presents as abdominal pain (74%) and malaise (32%) and is associated with hepatomegaly or an abdominal mass.
6. Two thirds of the patients have tumor confined to the liver at time of diagnosis.
7. Laboratory tests demonstrate slight to moderate increases in serum aminotransferase levels and alkaline phosphatase activity; bilirubin is normal and HBsAg is negative. Alpha-fetoprotein is seldom elevated above 250 ng/mL. A high serum unsaturated vitamin B_{12} binding capacity (unique for this type of hepatocellular carcinoma) may be present.
8. The tumors are 4 to 17 cm in diameter, presenting as single mass lesions in 56% of cases and 12% of the time in the left lobe alone. In addition, a central scar is seen in 10% to 20% of cases, somewhat resembling focal nodular hyperplasia.
9. Autopsy studies have shown a difference in metastases from typical hepatocellular carcinoma (Table 9–2).

Table 9–2
METASTATIC SPREAD PATTERN OF HEPATOCELLULAR CARCINOMA (HCC)

	Fibrolamellar HCC (5 cases)	HCC, Noncirrhotic (39 cases)	HCC, cirrhotic (188 cases)
No metastases	40%	33.0%	54.8%
Abdominal lymph node	100%	43.6%	16.5%
Peritoneum	80%	23.1%	7.4%
Lung	40%	41.0%	38.0%
Spleen	40%	7.7%	2.1%

From Craig JR, Peters RL, Edmondson: HA, et al. Fibrolamellar carcinoma of the liver: A tumor of adolescent and young adults with distinctive clinicopathologic features. Cancer 1980; 46:372–379.

10. The tumor was first described in 1956 by Edmondson, with over 100 cases reported since then; retrospective studies at the University of Southern California did not find the lesion to be present before 1956, suggesting possibly a new etiologic agent (environmental, toxic) for hepatocellular carcinoma. Although seen in younger persons, the tumor is not believed to be associated with oral contraceptives (although 30% of women with this lesion were on birth control pills, the incidence in men and women is equal).
11. Fibrolamellar hepatocellular carcinoma has been postulated to represent the malignant counterpart of focal nodular hyperplasia. Some tumors grossly resemble focal nodular hyperplasia. True focal nodular hyperplasia lesions have been reported in livers with fibrolamellar hepatocellular carcinoma. However, transition zones have been demonstrated between the two lesions, and the majority of tumors do not have the gross features of focal nodular hyperplasia.

Aspiration Cytology

1. Large cells have prominent nucleoli and abundant eosinophilic granular cytoplasm.
2. The majority of cases contain hyaline droplets and/or pale inclusion bodies.

Treatment and Prognosis

1. Since two thirds of patients have tumor confined to the liver at diagnosis, and since 56% are single mass lesions, surgical resection has a high potential for cure. Overall, resection with cure occurs in 48% of cases, compared with 17% in hepatocellular carcinoma.
2. Nonresectable, multiple lesions are treated with vari-

ous regimens of chemotherapy or by using intra-arterial infusions and radiation but are of limited benefit.

3. Mean overall survival is 32 months (compared with 5.9 months for trabecular hepatocellular carcinoma).

References

Berman MA, Burnham JA, Sheahan DG. Fibrolamellar carcinoma of the liver: An immunohistochemical study of nineteen cases and a review of the literature. Hum Pathol 1988;19:784–794.

Craig JR, Peters RL, Edmondson HA, et al. Fibrolamellar carcinoma of the liver: A tumor of adolescent and young adults with distinctive clinicopathologic features. Cancer 1980;46:372–379.

Dodgson HJF. Fibrolamellar cancer of the liver. J Hepatol 1987;5:241–247.

Farhi DC, Shikes RH, Murari PJ, et al. Hepatocellular carcinoma in young people. Cancer 1983;52:1516–1525.

Lack EE, Neave C, Vawter GF. Hepatocellular carcinoma: Review of 32 cases in childhood and adolescence. Cancer 1983;52:1510–1515.

SCLEROSING HEPATIC CARCINOMA

Major Morphologic Features

1. Cords and nests of small to medium-sized neoplastic hepatocytes are surrounded by dense, hyalinized, and relatively avascular collagen.

Other Features

1. Ductlike structures may be found in smaller cells toward the center of the lesion; cells toward the periphery more closely resemble hepatocytes, with more abundant, granular eosinophilic cytoplasm and prominent nucleoli; these cells may also contain bile.
2. The ductlike cells have scanty granular, eosinophilic to clear cytoplasm, round hyperchromatic nuclei, and prominent nucleoli; these cells may stain positively for mucin.
3. Sinusoids are absent or very difficult to identify, with no discrete sinusoidal lining cells.
4. Tumor cells merge into nontumor trabeculae, *not* sinusoids, at the border of the lesion; fibrous capsules are not present.
5. Tumor cells do not typically exhibit cytoplasmic inclusions.
6. Focal necrosis and hemorrhage are not frequent.
7. Chronic liver disease is present in nontumor liver in approximately 47% of cases.

Differential Diagnosis

1. *Metastatic carcinoma:* The lesion has often been misdiagnosed as metastatic carcinoma (e.g., pancreatic). However, in metastatic tumor, the denseness of the collagen, especially toward the center of the lesion, is usually not as striking as in sclerosing

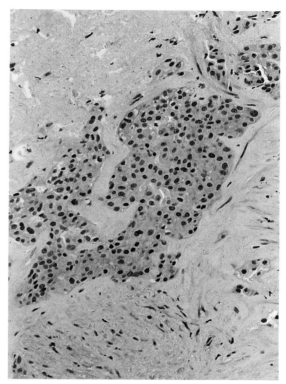

Figure 9–35. Sclerosing hepatic carcinoma. The neoplastic cells contain round nuclei and moderate eosinophilic cytoplasm. No distinct cords are formed. The cells are surrounded by dense relatively acellular collagen.

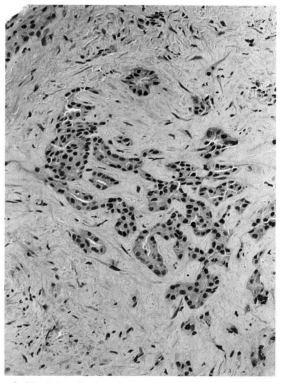

Figure 9–36. Sclerosing hepatic carcinoma. These groups of neoplastic hepatocytes have formed ductlike structures. This change is more characteristically seen in the center of the neoplasm, while tumor cells toward the periphery more closely resemble hepatocytes.

hepatic carcinoma. In addition, over one half of patients with metastatic pancreatic carcinoma are icteric owing to extrahepatic bile duct obstruction, while most patients with sclerosing hepatic carcinoma are anicteric.

2. *Cholangiocarcinoma:* The tumor cells at the peripheral aspects of sclerosing hepatic carcinoma have features more closely resembling hepatocytes (e.g., granular eosinophilic cytoplasm, distinct nucleoli). However, in biopsy specimens exhibiting extensive fibrosis and small tumor cells with or without ductlike features, it may be extremely difficult to distinguish between sclerosing hepatic carcinoma and cholangiocarcinoma. Proper evaluation may be possible only after tumor resection or at postmortem examination, when multiple tissue sections can be assessed.

Special Stains

1. *Periodic acid–Schiff after diastase, mucicarmine:* Clear cytoplasm in ductlike cells may stain positively for mucin.

Immunohistochemistry

1. *Alpha-fetoprotein:* Although serum alpha-fetoprotein levels are usually not elevated in sclerosing hepatic carcinoma, slight cytoplasmic staining may be present and helpful in distinguishing the tumor from cholangiocarcinoma and metastatic carcinoma.

Clinical and Biologic Behavior

1. Sclerosing hepatic carcinoma represents approximately 3.5% of all hepatocellular carcinomas and is often misdiagnosed as cholangiocarcinoma or metastatic carcinoma.
2. It is found equally in men and women between 40 and 65 years of age, with the average age at diagnosis of 62 years (7 1/2 years older than in typical hepatocellular carcinoma).
3. Presenting symptoms are abdominal pain, weight loss, and abdominal mass.
4. Laboratory tests show only mild increase in serum aminotransferase levels, usually with a normal bilirubin level.
5. HBsAg is negative and alpha-fetoprotein is elevated to levels greater than 400 ng/mL in only one third of cases.
6. Hypercalcemia is present in 69% of patients in the *absence* of bony metastasis (mean 12.1 mg/dL); values range from 8 to 17 mg/dL, associated with hypophosphatemia.
7. Chronic liver disease with cirrhosis is not present in the majority of cases (53% "normal" livers, 17% fibrosis, 30% cirrhosis), in contrast to typical hepa-

tocellular carcinoma in which cirrhosis is present in 84% of cases.
8. Metastatic pattern is similar to that of cholangiocarcinoma (regional lymph nodes in two thirds, lung, bone marrow, and serosa in one fourth); 82% of patients have metastases at time of diagnosis or autopsy.
9. The hypercalcemia (pseudohyperparathyroidism) may be due to production by tumor cells of a substance immunologically identical to parathormone and prostaglandin E (activates osteoclasts).
10. The neoplasm is called sclerosing "hepatic," not "hepatocellular," carcinoma, since there is some uncertainty of the cell of origin; the cell may be the same primordial stem cell of both hepatocyte and bile duct (63% of the cells in this tumor resemble hepatocytes, 20% ductules, 17% uncertain); the lesion most likely represents an extreme form of hepatocellular carcinoma with duct transformation.

Aspiration Cytology

1. Aspiration may be unrewarding owing to the intense nature of the fibrosis.
2. Small cells with hyperchromatic nuclei, scanty to moderate rather basophilic cytoplasm, and rather acellular collagen fibers may be identified.

Treatment and Prognosis

1. Surgical resection is usually not possible, since the majority (80%) of cases are diagnosed after metastasis has occurred. Advanced age at presentation may preclude surgery.
2. Survival from time of diagnosis is 4 1/2 months.

References

Craig JR, Peters RL, Edmondson HA. Tumors of the Liver and Intrahepatic Bile Ducts. Washington, DC: Armed Forces Institute of Pathology, 1989; 186–190.

Omata M, Peters RL, Tatter D. Sclerosing hepatic carcinoma: Relationship to hypercalcemia. Liver 1981;1:33–49.

Hepatoblastoma

Major Morphologic Features

1. The major cellular components include the following:
   a. *Epithelial:* Small cells with round to oval nuclei, prominent single nucleolus, and scanty eosinophilic, granular, or clear cytoplasm *(embryonal);* cells may also be arranged in a trabecular-cord fashion *(fetal).*

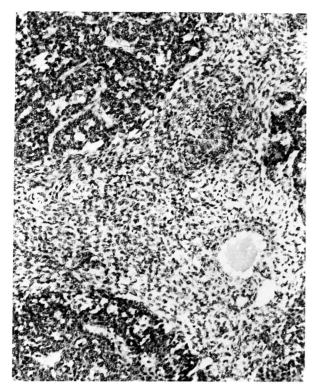

Figure 9–37. Hepatoblastoma. Two major cell types are present: *stromal (center)*, composed of solid spindle-shaped cells of mesenchymal origin, and *epithelial (upper and lower left)*, resembling small hepatocytes with formation of cords *(fetal* type).

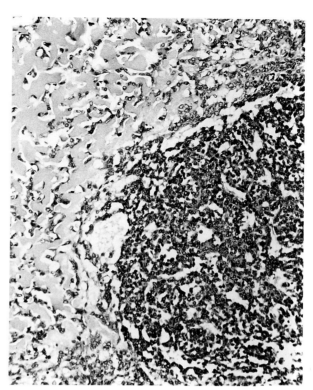

Figure 9–39. Hepatoblastoma. The mesenchymal element *(above and left)* is composed of osteoid cells. The adjacent epithelial component exhibits a distinct cord–sinusoid pattern.

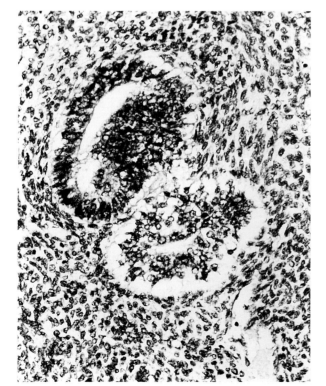

Figure 9–38. Hepatoblastoma. The stromal element exhibits centrally placed large neoplastic cells that are hyperchromatic with a basophilic cytoplasm. These cells tend to form ductlike elements *(embryonal* type).

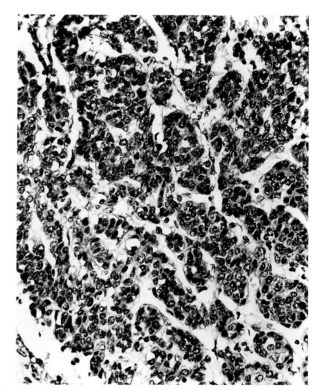

Figure 9–40. Hepatoblastoma. The fetal element is composed of small cells that form thickened cords lined by endothelial cells.

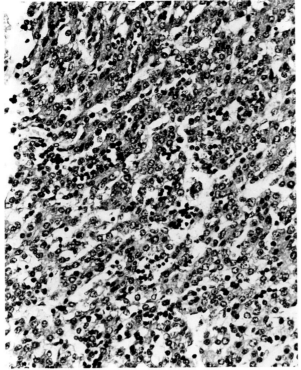

Figure 9–41. Hepatoblastoma. Small aggregates of dark-staining cells (normoblasts) are present within the sinusoids.

    b. *Stromal:* Immature mesenchymal elements composed of cellular spindle cells, with variable amounts of collagen, osteoid, and/or chondroid substances

    c. *Anaplastic:* Loosely cohesive poorly differentiated cells with scanty cytoplasm and variable mitotic activity

2. Tumor growth is either purely epithelial (62.2%), mixed (31.3%), or anaplastic (6.5%).

Other Features

1. Epithelial cells may grow as sheets with no distinct arrangement.
2. Acinar, rosette, ductlike growth patterns and cystic structures may be present.
3. Cells with clear cytoplasm often contain lipid or glycogen.
4. Trabeculae with adjacent sinusoids lined by endothelial cells are distinctive of mature tumor and resemble hepatocellular carcinoma.
5. Cytoplasmic inclusions are not present.
6. Mitotic activity is generally low.
7. Choletasis may be identified within cytoplasm or retained dilated canaliculi.
8. Calcification may occur within osteoid components.
9. Fibrous septa often divide the tumor into various sized nodules; necrosis and hemorrhage may be seen in larger tumors.

10. Extramedullary hematopoiesis is common.
11. Squamous differentiation and keratin formation have been identified.
12. An anaplastic subtype may produce abundant amounts of mucin.

Differential Diagnosis

1. *Hepatocellular carcinoma:* More mature sinusoid-trabecular structures with larger cells resemble hepatocellular carcinoma. Examination of multiple tissue sections is necessary for identification of smaller more characteristic fetal cells and stroma of hepatoblastoma.
2. *Other primitive tumors:* Rare immature or sarcomatous neoplasms (e.g., osteosarcoma) may exhibit some morphologic features of hepatoblastoma. Investigation of numerous tissue sections for characteristic immunohistochemical staining patterns may be necessary for diagnosis.

Special Stains

1. *Periodic acid–Schiff:* Glycogen can be identified in clear cells.
2. *Oil red O:* Frozen sections may demonstrate triglycerides in clear cells.
3. *Mucicarmine:* Mucus may be identified in anaplastic mucoid type of tumor.

Immunohistochemistry

1. *Alpha-fetoprotein, cytokeratin:* All tumors exhibit diffuse cytoplasmic staining of epithelial, and occasionally stromal, components. Embryonal cells tend to have a paranuclear pattern of cytokeratin staining.
2. *Epithelial membrane antigen, vimentin:* Positive staining is usually seen in osteoid components.
3. *Ferritin, alpha-1-antitrypsin:* Positive staining is seen in one half to two thirds of cases.

Clinical and Biologic Behavior

1. Hepatoblastoma is the most common hepatic tumor in neonates and young children, accounting for 43% of all hepatic neoplasms; however, it is one of the least common tumors in relation to other neoplasms (0.2%–5.8%), nephroblastoma 5 to 10 times more common. Hepatoblastoma represents less than 0.5% of hepatic neoplasms in older children and adolescents.
2. Age at onset is approximately 18 months (birth–40 months); there is a slight male predominance.
3. Clinical presentation is hepatomegaly and/or an

abdominal mass; failure to thrive, intermittent vomiting, and diarrhea can occur, but jaundice is rare.

4. Serum aminotransferase levels are usually normal, and the serum bilirubin value may be infrequently elevated.

5. Alpha-fetoprotein level is elevated in 80% to 90% of patients; although alpha-fetoprotein is elevated in the normal neonate (10,000–14,000 ng/mL), these values rapidly decrease to 5 to 10 ng/mL at age 1 year; the neonate with hepatoblastoma will exhibit a disproportionately marked increase.

6. Other associated conditions include osteopenia (18.5%), hemihypertrophy, fetal alcohol syndrome, maternal hormone use, macroglossia, sexual precocity secondary to ectopic gonadotropin production, and cardiac and renal malformations.

7. The tumor is usually a single (80%) well-circumscribed mass 5 to 25 cm in diameter that usually involves the right lobe; hemorrhage, cystic degeneration, and necrosis may be present.

8. Osteoid is seen in approximately 37% of cases and may represent a secondary lesion resulting from thrombosis. Osteoid is rarely identified in metastatic lesions.

9. Typical metastatic sites are the lungs, lymph nodes, and peritoneum, but metastases may be found almost anywhere within the abdominal cavity.

10. The tumor has been identified in siblings and in association with other tumors (nephroblastoma, adrenal cortical carcinoma).

11. The origin is believed to be from a primitive cell capable of diverse differentiation; developmental anomalies may play a part in pathogenesis, since anomalies are present in up to 30% of patients with this malignancy.

Aspiration Cytology

1. Small cells with eosinophilic to clear cytoplasm are present.
2. Hyperchromatic nuclei have prominent nucleoli.
3. Well-differentiated tumors may exhibit trabecular structures lined by endothelial cells.
4. Collagen and stroma elements such as osteoid may be present.
5. Different subtypes will exhibit anaplastic and embryonal cells and mucus.

Treatment and Prognosis

1. Tumor is rapidly progressive, with death due to liver failure, tumor rupture, hemorrhage, and metastatic disease.
2. Tumor is generally resistant to radiation and chemotherapy, with surgery being the only definitive treatment.

References

Abenoza P, Manivel JC, Wick MR, et al. Hepatoblastoma: An immunohistochemical and ultrastructural study. Hum Pathol 1987;18:1025–1035.

Haas JE, Muczynski KA, Krailo M, et al. Histopathology and prognosis in childhood hepatoblastoma and hepatocarcinoma. Cancer 1989;64:1082–1095.

Ishak KG, Glunz PR. Hepatoblastoma and hepatocarcinoma in infants and childhood: Report of 47 cases. Cancer 1967;20:396–422.

Kasai M, Wastanabe I. Histologic classification of liver cell carcinoma in infancy and childhood and its clinical evaluation: A study of 70 cases collected in Japan. Cancer 1970;25:551–563.

Stocker JT, Ishak KG. Hepatoblastoma. In: Okuda K, Ishak KG, eds. Neoplasms of the liver. Tokyo: Springer-Verlag, 1987:127–142.

Weinberg AG, Finegold MJ. Primary hepatic tumors of childhood. Hum Pathol 1983;14:512–537.

Vascular Neoplasms

ANGIOSARCOMA (MALIGNANT HEMANGIOENDOTHELIOMA)

Major Morphologic Features

1. Two major growth patterns include the following:
   a. Proliferation of plump, oval, and fusiform hyperchromatic endothelial cells multilayered along dilated sinusoids which often form a cavernous growth pattern
   b. Solid sheets of tumor cells with formation of small vascular spaces often containing red blood cells

Other Features

1. Solid growth pattern may consist of pleomorphic spindly cells with no definite formation of microvascular structures.
2. Tumor cells infiltrate into sinusoids with formation of neoplastic capillaries.
3. Infiltration of tumor cells into portal and sublobular veins is often seen.
4. Focal areas of hemorrhage are common.
5. Individual and small groups of tumor cells are often seen isolated in sinusoids away from the main tumor mass.
6. Neoplastic cells rarely are multinucleated.
7. Dilated sinusoids and cavernous regions are adjacent to tumor and are lined by hypertrophic and hyperplastic endothelial cells (preneoplastic).
8. Hepatocytes forming cords adjacent to both hyperplastic and neoplastic endothelial cells exhibit variable degrees of atrophic change; some areas may have total replacement of hepatocytes by collagen, fibrin, and tumor cells.
9. Cholestasis in parenchyma that is surrounded and infiltrated by tumor is often present.
10. Sinusoids adjacent to the tumor contain increased numbers of leukocytes, usually macrophages and neutrophils.

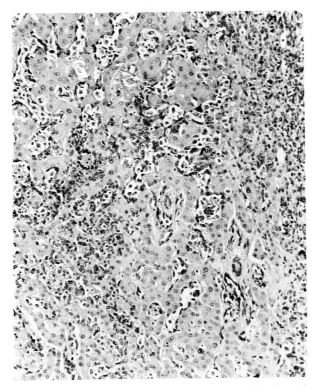

Figure 9–42. Angiosarcoma. The hepatocytes are lined by hyperchromatic plump endothelial cells laid down in single or multiple layers. The hepatocytes are normal in size to slightly small with adjacent dilated sinusoids.

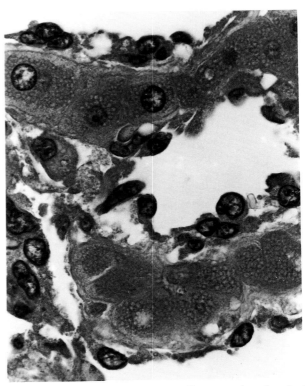

Figure 9–44. Angiosarcoma. The tumor cells are round, oval, and spindle shaped and closely packed along the hepatic cord. The hepatocytes contain microvesicular fat.

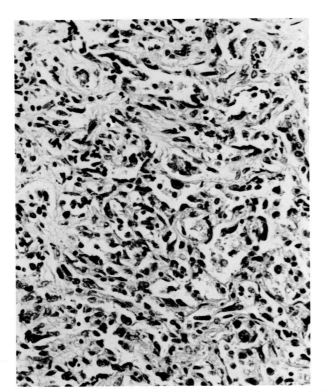

Figure 9–43. Angiosarcoma. This field is almost entirely composed of neoplastic endothelial cells with marked atrophy of the hepatic cords.

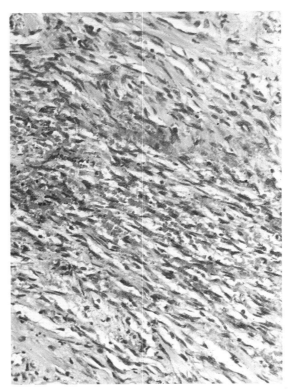

Figure 9–45. Angiosarcoma. The tumor is composed of sheets of thin spindle cells forming small vascular channels. Red blood cells are seen within these vessels and extravasated between tumor cells. This is an example of *Kaposi's sarcoma* in a patient with the acquired immunodeficiency syndrome.

11. Extramedullary erythropoiesis may be present in nonneoplastic regions.
12. Evidence of chronic liver disease in nontumor liver is often present; changes usually consist of fibrous portal tracts containing increased vascular channels (*"noncirrhotic portal fibrosis"*).
13. Sheets of spindle cells admixed with red blood cells and forming small vascular channels *(Kaposi's sarcoma)* are more commonly seen in immunodeficient patients (i.e., those with the acquired immunodeficiency syndrome).

Differential Diagnosis

1. *Cavernous hemangioma:* Angiosarcoma usually has cavernous features. The fibrosis seen in cavernous hemangiomas is composed of cytologically benign fibroblasts, and although endothelial hyperplasia lining the cystic areas is usually present, the degree of hyperplasia is not as striking as in cavernous changes adjacent to angiosarcoma. Cytologically anaplastic endothelial cells are a definitive differential feature.
2. *Sarcomas of other types:* Solid growth patterns of angiosarcoma without obvious neoplastic vessel formation may be difficult to differentiate from sarcomas of other etiologies (e.g., leiomyosarcoma). Demonstration of factor VIII–related antigen in tumor cells is diagnostic of angiosarcoma.
3. *Malignant reticuloendothelioses:* Malignant Kupffer cells may in some ways resemble the aggregates of markedly anaplastic cells often present in angiosarcoma. Solid tumor growth may occur in both types of malignancies. Erythrophagocytosis, a feature characteristic of malignant reticuloendothelioses, is not seen in angiosarcoma.
4. *Kupffer cell reaction in salmonellosis:* Typhoid fever *(Salmonella typhi* infection) is characterized by prominent Kupffer cell hyperplasia and hypertrophy. No mass lesions occur, and the change is diffuse throughout the liver without cavernous features.

Special Stains

1. *Masson:* Collagen fibers often present adjacent to atrophic hepatocytes are accentuated.
2. *Phosphotungstic acid hematoxylin:* Fibrin may be demonstrated along sinusoidal borders.

Immunohistochemistry

1. *Factor VIII–related antigen:* Positive staining of neoplastic cells is characteristic of angiosarcoma; however, not all tumors stain positively and the staining pattern is usually focal. Therefore, multiple sections from different areas of the tumor must be examined.

Clinical and Biologic Behavior

1. Primary angiosarcoma of the liver is extremely rare, its incidence ranging from 0.002% to 0.013% in various autopsy series.
2. The tumor represents only 0.4% of all primary hepatic neoplasms at the University of Southern California, with hepatocellular carcinoma 30 to 100 times more frequent.
3. The tumor occurs 85% of the time in men between 50 and 60 years of age (range, 24–93 years).
4. Two thirds of the patients present with hepatomegaly, often associated with right upper quadrant pain, weight loss, and jaundice; they may also present less often with anemia, thrombocytopenia, or disseminated intravascular coagulation *without* evidence of liver disease, or with asymptomatic elevations of liver tests.
5. Ascites is present in 70% of cases; esophageal varices may also be present, suggesting an underlying chronic liver disease.
6. Laboratory data exhibit leukocytosis in two thirds of patients, leukopenia in one fifth, anemia and thrombocytopenia in two thirds, usually an elevation of the bilirubin value (typically below 10 mg/dL), normal to moderate elevation in aminotransferase activities, normal alpha-fetoprotein level, and occasionally a profile of disseminated intravascular coagulation.
7. Liver is enlarged (may be greater than 3000 g at autopsy); multiple masses occur in over two thirds of cases, the individual lesions varying from large cavernous to smaller dark red to solid gray-white. Diffuse involvement of all lobes by cavernous features has been reported.
8. Metastatic pattern shows involvement of the spleen, lungs, lymph nodes, and bone.
9. The following risk factors are present in approximately 40% of patients:
   a. *Thorotrast:* This colloid solution containing 20% thorium dioxide (emits alpha, beta, and gamma radiation) was used extensively from 1930 to 1953 by radiologists as an arteriographic agent. It is phagocytized by Kupffer cells and macrophages, with a biologic half-life of approximately 400 years. Studies have shown that almost 1% of exposed patients may develop angiosarcoma; the latent period is 12 to 24 years. Hepatocellular carcinoma is also associated with thorotrast exposure (latent period approximately 19 years).
   b. *Vinyl chloride:* This substance is used in polymerization in the plastics industry; exposed workers have a 400 times greater incidence of angiosarcoma than the normal population.
   c. *Arsenicals:* Chronic exposure of vintners to arsenical insecticides, ingestion of arsenic-containing wine and water, and prolonged treatment with Fowler's solution (1% potassium arsenite) for psoriasis increase the risk of angiosarcoma (latent period, 13–25 years).

d. *Others:* Diethylstilbestrol, long-term oral contraceptives, androgenic-anabolic steroids, radium exposure, and hemachromatosis increase the risk of angiosarcoma.

Aspiration Cytology

1. Aspiration is generally contraindicated because of complications of hemorrhage; if performed, the aspirate will contain mostly red blood cells with scattered oval to fusiform atypical cells exhibiting hyperchromatic nuclei, prominent nucleoli, and variable amounts of cytoplasm.

Treatment and Prognosis

1. Patients with this highly malignant neoplasm have a mean survival of 5 1/2 months from the time of clinical presentation; the cause of death is usually hemoperitoneum and/or liver failure.
2. Radiation and chemotherapy are not known to be effective.

References

Ishak KG. Malignant mesenchymal tumors of the liver. In: Okuda K, Ishak KG, eds. Neoplasms of the Liver. Tokyo: Springer-Verlag, 1987:162–167.

Locker GY, Doroshow JH, Zwelling LA, et al. The clinical features of hepatic angiosarcoma: A report of four cases and a review of the English literature. Medicine 1979;58:48–64.

Ludwig J, Hoffman HN. Hemangiosarcoma of the liver: Spectrum of morphologic changes and clinical findings. Mayo Clin Proc 1975;50:255–263.

Popper H, Thomas LB, Telles NC. Development of hepatic angiosarcoma in man induced by vinyl chloride, thorotrast, arsenic. Am J Pathol 1978;92:349–376.

Zafrani ES. Update on vascular tumors of the liver. J Hepatol 1989;8:125–130.

EPITHELIOID HEMANGIOENDOTHELIOMA (VASOABLATIVE ENDOTHELIOSARCOMA)

Major Morphologic Features

1. Two predominant cell types:
   a. *Dendritic:* Elongated stellate eosinophilic processes containing well-defined cytoplasmic vacuoles, usually within a myxoid or pseudocartilaginous stroma
   b. *Epithelioid:* Rounded relatively abundant eosinophilic cytoplasm, hyperchromatic nuclei, and prominent nucleoli
2. Sinusoidal growth of tumor with atrophy of adjacent liver cells is present.
3. Growth within terminal hepatic and sublobular veins, often as sessile clusters, with eventual complete occlusion and recanalization of larger vessels is present.

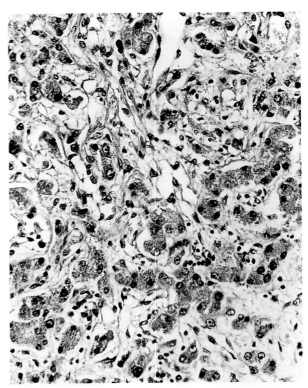

Figure 9–46. Epithelioid hemangioendothelioma. Oval to spindle-shaped cells line the sinusoids, with adjacent atrophy of the hepatocytes.

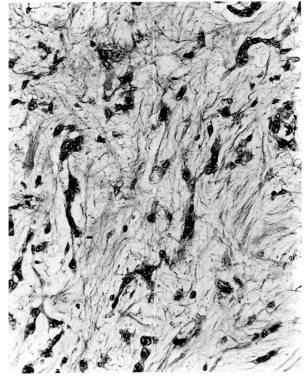

Figure 9–47. Epithelioid hemangioendothelioma. Enlongated dendritic cells are present within a myxoid stroma.

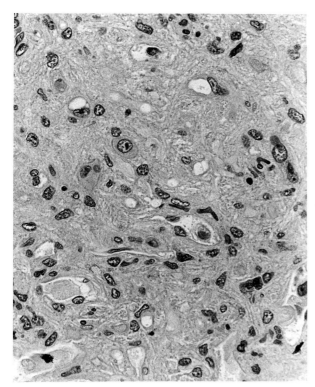

Figure 9–48. Epithelioid hemangioendothelioma. Plump epithelioid cells are present within an abundant fibrous stroma, often singly lining small vascular spaces.

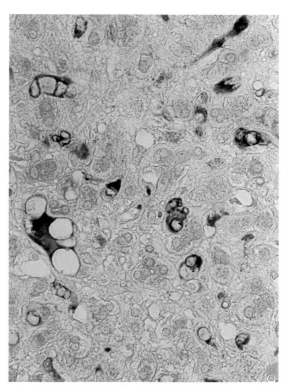

Figure 9–50. Epithelioid hemangioendothelioma (immunoperoxidase). Factor VIII–related antigen is strongly demonstrated within the cytoplasm of many of the tumor cells.

Other Features

1. Sinusoidal growth may occur as single or small aggregates of cells, often surrounding portal tracts, or as larger sheets of cells.
2. Hyalinization and fibrosis of stroma gradually occurs, with eventual dense sclerosis; tumor cells may then appear isolated and sometimes difficult to identify.
3. Cells exhibiting features intermediate between epithelioid and dendritic types are present.
4. Mitoses are more frequent in epithelioid cells.
5. Degenerative changes and ischemic necrosis may be seen in larger lesions and in areas exhibiting outflow obstruction caused by vascular tumor growth.
6. Approximately 50% of cases exhibit a stromal inflammatory reaction consisting of lymphocytes, plasma cells, neutrophils, and eosinophils.
7. Sclerotic regions demonstrate dystrophic calcification in approximately one third of cases; cartilage and bone are not present.

Differential Diagnosis

1. *Cholangiocarcinoma:* Malignant bile duct neoplasms typically exhibit prominent sclerosis, and the epithelioid cells in epithelioid hemangioendotheli-

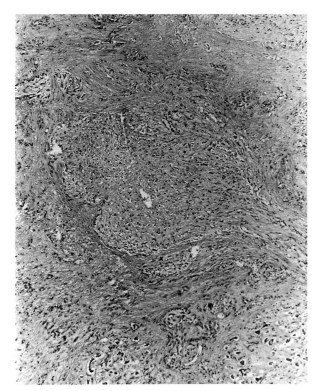

Figure 9–49. Epithelioid hemangioendothelioma. Tumor growth is present within a sublobular vein with complete occlusion and focal areas of recanalization.

oma may be mistaken for this neoplasm on needle biopsy. Positive factor VIII staining would demonstrate the vascular origin in epithelioid hemangioendothelioma.

2. *Sclerosing hepatic carcinoma:* This tumor also presents with a sclerotic and hyalinized stroma but exhibits hepatocellular differentiation at its periphery.

3. *Angiosarcoma:* Although angiosarcoma may have solid growth features, the cells are generally more spindly, with absence of both epithelioid and dendritic myxoid components.

4. *Metastatic carcinoma:* Prominent sclerosis with scattered tumor cells can be suggestive of infiltrating carcinoma (e.g., pancreas, breast, stomach). Negative cytoplasmic staining for mucin, carcinoembryonic antigen, and positive factor VIII staining is characteristic for epithelioid hemangioendothelioma.

Special Stains

1. *Periodic acid–Schiff, Alcian blue:* Positive staining of the mucopolysaccharides in the myxoid stroma is usually present.

2. *Masson:* Deep red cytoplasmic staining of tumor cells, compared with pale blue staining of normal endothelial cells and prominent blue staining of collagen, can be seen. This stain easily identifies vessels containing tumor (which are often difficult to identify on hematoxylin and eosin stain).

Immunohistochemistry

1. *Factor VIII–related antigen:* Positive diffuse cytoplasmic staining of both dendritic and epithelioid cells is characteristic of all tumors; in almost 50% of cases more than two thirds of the tumor cells stain positively.

Clinical and Biologic Behavior

1. Epithelioid hemangioendothelioma is a slow-growing variant of angiosarcoma characteristic not only for its morphologic features but also for its significantly better prognosis than classic angiosarcoma.

2. There is a slight predominance in women, with the mean age at onset of 50 years (range, 19–86 years).

3. Clinical presentation is hepatomegaly with right upper quadrant pain, weight loss, and anorexia; jaundice is present in approximately 10% of patients; underlying chronic liver disease is not present.

4. Laboratory tests show normal to slightly increased serum aminotransferase levels, and only rarely is the serum bilirubin value elevated; the alpha-fetoprotein is not elevated.

5. The tumor grossly is multifocal in distribution, with most cases presenting with a large mass and numer-

ous smaller nodules ranging in size from 3 to 11 cm in diameter; fibrosis is fairly prominent throughout the tumor.

6. Metastatic sites are lymph nodes, bone, spleen, and peritoneum; metastases occur usually after the tumor has become quite large.

7. The lesion has only recently been described, and etiologic agents have not been established (may be environmental, food additives, air pollutants); although oral contraceptives have been described in association with this tumor, the risk factors documented for typical angiosarcoma (e.g., thorotrast, vinyl chloride, arsenicals) have not been found with epithelioid hemangioendothelioma.

Aspiration Cytology

1. A dry tap may occur because of the significant amount of fibrosis.

2. Tumor cells may be quite difficult to identify and present as single hyperchromatic oval to somewhat spindly cells with prominent nucleoli.

3. A clear cytoplasmic vacuole resembling fat may be present.

Treatment and Prognosis

1. Because of its slow-growing nature, survival is better than in hepatocellular carcinoma, with over 30% of patients living longer than 5 years.

2. Hepatic transplantation has been curative.

References

Clements D, Hubscher S, West R, et al. Epithelioid hemangioendothelioma. J Hepatol 1986;2:441–449.

Ishak KG, Sesterhenn IA, Goodman MZD. Epithelioid hemangioendothelioma of the liver: A clinicopathologic and follow-up study of 32 cases. Hum Pathol 1984;15:839–852.

Kelleher MB, Iwatsuki S, Sheahan DG. Epithelioid hemangioendothelioma: Clinicopathological correlation of 10 cases treated by orthotopic liver transplantation. Am J Surg Pathol 1989;13:999–1008.

Scoazec JY, Lamy P, Degott C, et al. Epithelioid hemangioendothelioma of the liver: Diagnostic features and role of liver transplantation. Gastroenterology 1988;94:1447–1453.

Cholangiocarcinoma

Major Morphologic Features

1. Adenocarcinoma is characterized by glandular (tubular) ductlike structures associated with prominent fibrosis.

2. Cells are generally small and cuboidal, with oval to round nuclei without prominent nucleoli and moderate to scanty eosinophilic to clear cytoplasm.

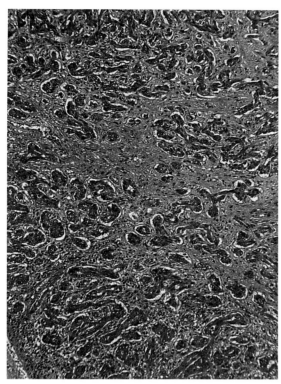

Figure 9–51. Cholangiocarcinoma. The tumor is composed of ductlike structures. An abundant fibrous stroma is present.

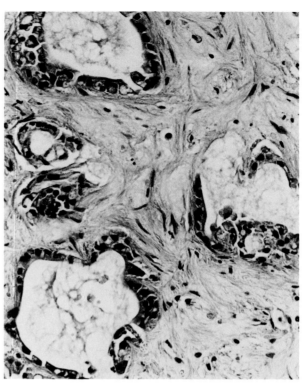

Figure 9–53. Cholangiocarcinoma. The dilated glandular structures are composed of cells often containing mucin that is secreted into the lumina.

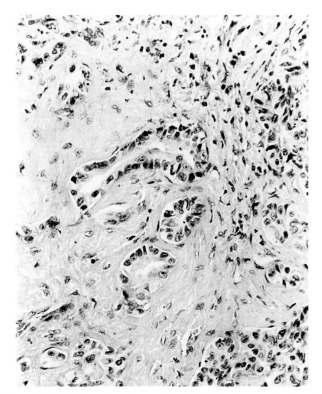

Figure 9–52. Cholangiocarcinoma. The epithelial cells are predominantly cuboidal. Most of the nuclei contain nucleoli, although this feature may be absent in cholangiocarcinoma. The fibrous stroma is rather dense.

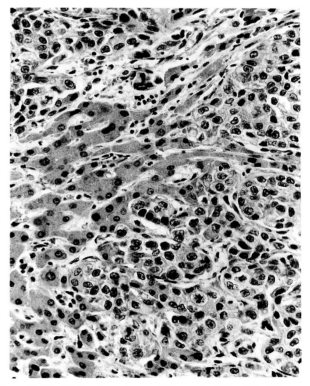

Figure 9–54. Cholangiocarcinoma. This poorly differentiated tumor exhibits a solid growth pattern of small to medium-sized cells. Infiltration occurs within sinusoids of the adjacent nonneoplastic liver, causing atrophic changes of the hepatic cords.

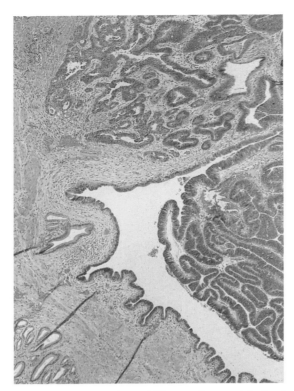

Figure 9–55. Cholangiocarcinoma. This tumor is seen originating from a major bile duct. The cells are composed of columnar epithelium forming a papillary-type configuration.

Other Features

1. Proteinaceous secretory material (*not* bile) may be present in duct lumen.
2. Neoplastic cells merge into sinusoids and not trabecular cords of nontumor liver at border of lesion; significant extension of this sinusoidal growth pattern, or compression of nontumor liver, does not occur.
3. Papillary growth patterns may occur; in rare instances *focal* or *diffuse papillomatosis* without significant parenchymal infiltration has been described.
4. Variants include the following:
   a. *Poorly differentiated* tumor with pleomorphic cells closely packed without associated fibrosis
   b. *Signet-ring* type
   c. *Mucinous* type with extensive extracellular mucin containing scattered tumor cells
   d. *Adenosquamous* type
   e. *Mucoepidermoid* type exhibiting mucous secretion as well as squamous differentiation
5. Patchy lymphocytic infiltration may be seen in fibrotic regions that is not oriented toward ducts and is more prominent at borders of tumor.
6. Tumor originating in large and major ducts tends to have a glandular growth pattern consisting of columnar cells often containing abundant mucin.

7. Large duct tumors may infiltrate along the submucosa and wall, with minimal parenchymal invasion; there may be prominent atrophy of nontumor liver distal to the major duct involved.
8. Hilar duct lesions may contain tumor cells that are difficult to identify within the dense fibrous tissue.
9. Hilar lesions are often associated with prominent intrahepatic cholestasis and changes of extrahepatic obstruction in nontumor liver.
10. Nontumor liver is usually noncirrhotic but may be involved in other types of liver diseases (e.g., primary sclerosing cholangitis, *Clonorchis sinensis* infection).

Differential Diagnosis

1. *Bile duct adenoma:* Peripheral well-differentiated cholangiocarcinoma less than 2 cm in greatest dimension may morphologically resemble a bile duct adenoma, a lesion usually found incidentally during surgical procedures and at autopsy. Cholangiocarcinomas, even well-differentiated types, usually exhibit some degree of atypicality. Because the adenomas are always small, any neoplastic ductular lesion greater than 2 cm in diameter is undoubtedly a cholangiocarcinoma or a metastatic lesion.
2. *Hepatocellular carcinoma with ductlike features:* Ductlike structures are present in 5% to 10% of cases of hepatocellular carcinoma. These features are only focal; further examination of multiple sections of tumor will disclose more typical features of hepatocellular carcinoma. In addition, demonstration of bile within the cytoplasm or lumen of duct structures is *not* a feature of cholangiocarcinoma.
3. *Sclerosing hepatic carcinoma:* Although cholangiocarcinoma may exhibit the marked degree of fibrosis seen in this hepatic neoplasm, the periphery of sclerosing carcinoma exhibits cytologic changes of hepatocellular origin not seen in cholangiocarcinoma.
4. *Metastatic adenocarcinoma:* Metastatic tumors eliciting a prominent desmoplastic reaction (e.g., pancreas, breast) may be morphologically indistinguishable from cholangiocarcinoma. Unlike the more common variants of bile duct carcinoma (peripheral location), pancreatic carcinoma often presents with jaundice and marked elevation of alkaline phosphatase activity at the time of metastasis. It may not be possible, however, to diagnose a tumor as cholangiocarcinoma until autopsy, when thorough examination fails to reveal a nonhepatic origin of the tumor.

Special Stains

1. *Mucicarmine:* Tumor cells and secretory material in duct lumen stain positive, most often in mucinous and large duct lesions.

Immunohistochemistry

1. *Tissue polypeptide antigen:* Strong positive cytoplasmic staining of tumors derived from duct epithelium is commonly seen; this staining is helpful in differentiating cholangiocarcinoma from negative to weak-staining hepatocellular carcinoma and metastatic adenocarcinoma.
2. *Carcinoembryonic antigen:* Positive staining is helpful in differentiation from hepatocellular carcinoma but *not* metastatic carcinoma.

Clinical and Biologic Behavior

1. Cholangiocarcinoma is a rare neoplasm with an overall incidence of 0.03% to 0.05% in autopsy series; the tumor represents approximately 8% to 12% of all hepatic primary malignancies (in some series up to 30%, but these series may also be including hepatocellular carcinoma with duct transformation and sclerosing hepatic carcinoma as subtypes of cholangiocarcinoma).
2. The tumor occurs predominantly in men 50 to 60 years of age.
3. Patients may present with painless jaundice; abdominal mass and hepatomegaly are not common except in widespread disease.
4. Laboratory test results may be nonspecific; however, alkaline phosphatase and bilirubin values may be moderately elevated when large duct obstruction or primary sclerosing cholangitis is present; carcinoembryonic antigen is occasionally increased, but alpha-fetoprotein is usually normal.
5. Four basic subtypes include the following:
   a. *Peripheral* (66%–75%)—white and firm with ill-defined borders; this subtype arises from duct epithelium at the lobular level.
   b. *Hilar* (18%–24%)—small, slow-growing; this subtype arises at the bifurcation of the right and left hepatic ducts.
   c. *Large duct* (6%–9%)—focally arise in a duct at a major tributary; intraductal growth pattern and prominent fibrosis with atrophy of lobe distal to the tumor may be seen.
   d. *Diffuse papillomatosis* (<1%)—intraductal growth spread throughout the liver, with minimal to absent parenchymal spread; this subtype seldom metastasizes, but complications of duct obstruction are severe.
6. Cirrhosis is not commonly seen in the nontumor liver.
7. Metastatic growth pattern is different from hepatocellular carcinoma (see Table below).
8. The overall incidence in patients with chronic ulcerative colitis is 0.4% to 1.4%; however, in patients with ulcerative colitis and primary sclerosing cholangitis, the incidence is as high as 7%. Some researchers therefore believe that the chronic inflammatory biliary lesion present in primary sclerosing cholangitis is a strong predisposing condition for the development of cholangiocarcinoma.
9. Other associated conditions include parasitic infestation (*Clonorchis sinensis* with secondary chronic inflammatory reaction, duct hyperplasia, and atypia: most of these cases are hilar), duct anomalies, cystic disease (16% of patients with cholangiocarcinoma, 0.6% with hepatocellular carcinoma), typhoid carriers (6.1% cholangiocarcinoma), and exposure to thorotrast and anabolic steroids (oxymetholone).
10. *Carcinoma of extrahepatic ducts:*
    a. Morphologically, the tumor is almost always cholangiocarcinoma (tubular), rarely papillary or squamous.
    b. Incidence is 0.012% to 0.46% in autopsy series.
    c. It usually occurs in patients 50 to 70 years, with men affected in 60% cases.
    d. Relative frequency in different sites is as follows:
       1) 8.5% bifurcation of common hepatic duct
       2) 31.4% common hepatic duct
       3) 7.6% cystic duct
       4) 18.6% bifurcation of common bile duct
       5) 33.9% common bile duct (including ampulla of Vater)

	Peripheral Cholangiocarcinoma (18 cases)	Hepatocellular Carcinoma, Cirrhotic (188 cases)	Hepatocellular Carcinoma, Noncirrhotic (39 cases)
No metastases	25.0%	54.8%	33.0%
Single metastases	18.8%	19.1%	25.0%
Lung	25.0%	38.8%	41.0%
Lymph node (portal)	68.8%	16.5%	43.6%
Portal vein	12.5%	37.2%	23.0%
Hepatic vein	18.8%	22.9%	18.0%
Bone marrow	25.0%	8.0%	7.7%
Peritoneum	25.0%	7.4%	23.1%
Gallbladder	0	5.3%	10.3%

Aspiration Cytology

1. Small cuboidal cells with pale eosinophilic or clear cytoplasm occasionally containing mucin are seen.
2. Nuclei are small and hyperchromatic without nucleoli.
3. Formation of tubular structures occurs.

Treatment and Prognosis

1. At clinical presentation the disease is usually too far advanced and nonresectable. Biliary tract obstruction can be stented palliatively using endoscopy, radiology (transhepatic), or surgery.
2. Overall survival ranges from a few weeks to 40 months, the longer survival most often seen in hilar carcinoma.
3. Hepatic transplantation is not offered because of recurrence of tumor in the graft in virtually all patients.

References

Klatskin G. Adenocarcinoma of the hepatic duct at its bifurcation within the porta hepatis: An unusual tumor with distinctive clinical and pathological features. Am J Med 1965;38:241–256.

Mori W, Nagasako K. Cholangiocarcinoma and related lesions. In: Okuda K, Peters RL, eds. Hepatocellular Carcinoma. New York: John Wiley and Sons, 1976:227–246.

Pastolero GC, Wakabayashi T, Oka T, et al. Tissue polypeptide antigen: A marker antigen differentiating cholangiolar tumors from other hepatic tumors. Am J Clin Pathol 1987;87:168–173.

Sugihara S, Masamichi K. Pathology of cholangiocarcinoma. In: Okuda K, Ishak KG, eds. Neoplasms of the Liver. Tokyo: Springer-Verlag, 1987:143–158.

Wee A, Ludwig J, Coffey RJ, et al. Hepatobiliary carcinoma associated with primary sclerosing carcinoma and chronic ulcerative colitis. Hum Pathol 1985;16:719–726.

Rare Primary Malignant Neoplasms

EMBRYONAL RHABDOMYOSARCOMA

1. Found almost exclusively in infants and children, this tumor clinically presents as jaundice and a right upper quadrant mass.
2. Spindle, stellate cells with plump cytoplasm and eccentric, often bizarre hyperchromatic nuclei are seen.
3. Multinucleation may be present.
4. The matrix of the tumor may contain Alcian blue–positive mucopolysaccharides; periodic acid–Schiff-positive cytoplasmic globules have been identified.
5. Cross striations in cells resembling rhabdomyoblasts are present but infrequent and stain positively with phosphotungstic acid hematoxylin.

Reference

Davis GL, Kissane JM, Ishak G. Embryonal rhabdomyosarcoma (sarcoma botyroides) of the liver. Cancer 1969;24:333–342.

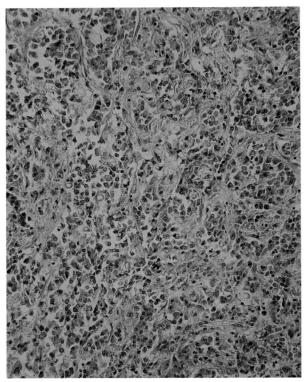

Figure 9–56. Embryonal rhabdomyosarcoma. The nuclei are round, oval, and often eccentric. No definite growth pattern is noted, and cohesiveness of the cells is minimal.

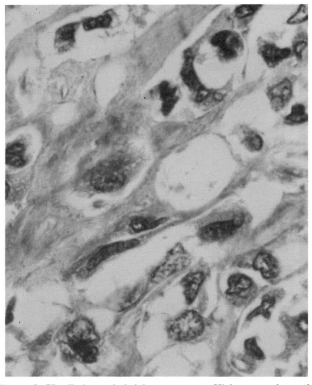

Figure 9–57. Embryonal rhabdomyosarcoma. High power shows the cells to have round, irregular to spindle-shaped nuclei. The cytoplasm is generally scanty with little cohesiveness of the cells. The thin elongated eosinophilic cytoplasm in occasional cells is slightly fibrillar, although no cross-striations are evident.

FIBROSARCOMA

1. Tumor is present predominantly in middle-aged men as a large abdominal mass and is occasionally associated with hypoglycemia.
2. Hypercellular spindly cells with interweaving fascicles held closely together by collagenous and reticulin fibers are present.
3. Mitoses are relatively uncommon.

Reference

Alrenga DP. Primary fibrosarcoma of the liver: Case report and review of the literature. Cancer 1975;36:446–449.

LEIOMYOSARCOMA

1. Tumor presents equally in men and women of all age groups as a right upper quadrant mass, with pain and occasionally ascites.
2. It is composed of spindle cells with interlacing bundles.
3. Eosinophilic cytoplasm is more abundant than in cells of fibrosarcoma and stains red with Masson trichrome.
4. Myofilaments are present, and the stromal collagenous and reticulin network is not as prominent as in fibrosarcoma.
5. Immunohistochemical staining with vimentin and desmin is often focally positive.

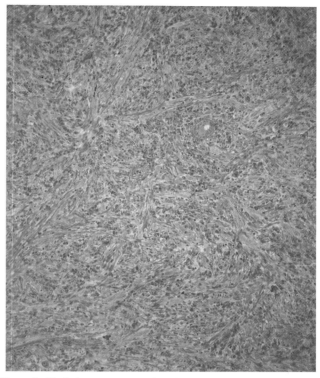

Figure 9–59. Leiomyosarcoma. The spindle cells have moderate eosinophilic cytoplasm and are arranged in whorls and bundles. On low power the tumor resembles fibrosarcoma.

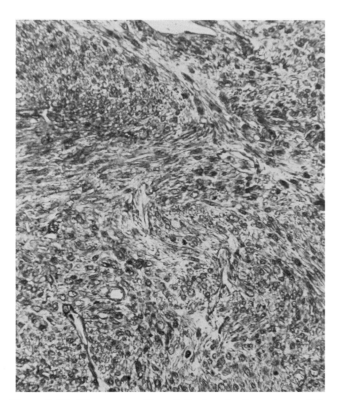

Figure 9–58. Fibrosarcoma. The spindle-shaped cells are hypercellular and form interweaving bundles and fascicles.

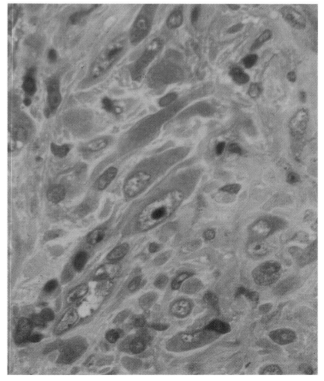

Figure 9–60. Leiomyosarcoma. High power shows the elliptical cells to contain moderate eosinophilic cytoplasm and round to spindle-shaped nuclei, occasionally with prominent nucleoli. Red cytoplasmic staining with Masson trichrome is helpful in differentiating these tumor cells from fibrosarcoma, which stains intensely blue.

Reference

Fong JA, Ruebner BH. Primary leiomyosarcoma of the liver. Hum Pathol 1974;5:115–119.

CHOLANGIOLOCELLULAR CARCINOMA

1. This primary carcinoma of the liver consists of cuboidal, round, or flattened tumor cells with eosinophilic cytoplasm resembling cholangioles within a dense fibrous stroma; a lumen is not present.
2. A similar morphologic feature may be focally seen in otherwise more typical variants of hepatocellular carcinoma with duct transformation and in cholangiocarcinoma.

Reference

Steiner PE, Higginson J. Cholangiolocellular carcinoma of the liver. Cancer 1959;12:753–759.

SQUAMOUS CELL CARCINOMA

1. Tumor arises predominantly in men having associated cystic or chronic inflammatory disorders involving the biliary system (e.g., Caroli's syndrome, chronic ulcerative colitis with primary sclerosing cholangitis, hepatolithiasis).

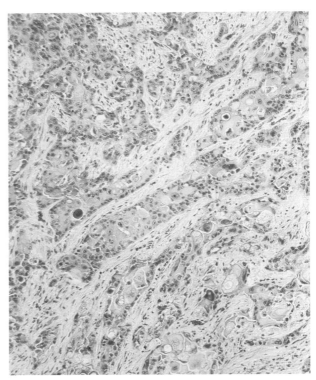

Figure 9–62. Squamous cell carcinoma. Large eosinophilic cells resembling neoplastic squamous cells are present, some undergoing necrosis with condensation of the keratin. Although the photomicrograph exhibits fibrosis and tumor formation, this type of neoplasm is often cystic.

2. Tumors may be solid but usually arise along a cyst wall, with the well-differentiated types exhibiting abundant eosinophilic cytoplasm with keratin formation.
3. This neoplasm may arise adjacent to malignant duct structures.

Reference

Song E, Kew MC, Grieve T, et al. Primary squamous cell carcinoma of the liver occurring in association with hepatolithiasis. Cancer 1984;53:542–546.

MESENCHYMAL SARCOMA

1. Also termed *malignant mesenchymoma* and "embryonal sarcoma," this tumor develops in children as large abdominal masses.
2. Cells are glandular, cystic, or markedly anaplastic with giant cell formation; spindle cells, osteoid, and cartilage, often with a myxomatous matrix, may be present.
3. Cytoplasmic periodic acid–Schiff after diastase–positive globules may be present.

Reference

Craig JR, Peters RL, Edmondson HA. Tumors of the liver and Intrahepatic Bile ducts. Washington, DC: Armed Forces Institute of Pathology, 1989:250–253.

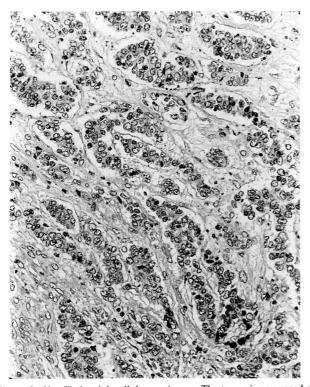

Figure 9–61. Cholangiolocellular carcinoma. The tumor is composed of small to cuboidal cells having round to oval nuclei rarely containing nucleoli. Formation of ductlike structures without lumina is present. Fibrosis between the glandular structures is somewhat variable and loose.

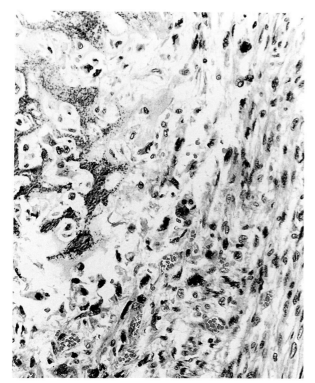

Figure 9–63. Mesenchymal sarcoma. The cells are round to elongated with no distinct organization. Cartilage and bone are present *(upper left)* within a loose framework.

■ Hematopoietic Neoplasms

Hodgkin's Lymphoma

Major Morphologic Features

1. Infiltration of portal tracts by lymphocytes, occasional eosinophils, and large mononuclear cells with scanty cytoplasm, large nuclei, and prominent nucleoli is seen; classic Reed-Sternberg cells are rare on biopsy although often abundant at autopsy.
2. Lymphocytic infiltration, with destruction and eventual effacement of duct structures, may be present.

Other Features

1. Variable degrees of portal fibrosis may be present, with disruption of the limiting plate.
2. Irregular involvement of different portal areas within the same biopsy specimen is often present, with some portal tracts appearing normal while others demonstrate more typical inflammatory changes.
3. Infiltration surrounding and invading large interlobular ducts near the hilum, with secondary biliary obstruction (perivenular cholestasis, bile duct proliferation in smaller portal tracts), occurs in approximately 3% of cases.

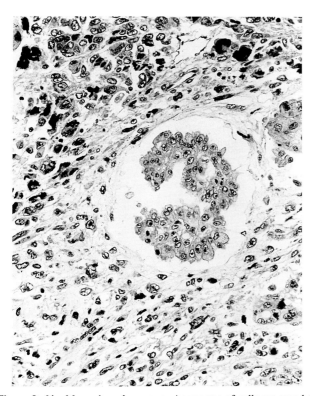

Figure 9–64. Mesenchymal sarcoma. Aggregates of cells are round to oval with prominent nucleoli. An adjacent clear space is present; overall the lesion resembles a renal glomerulus.

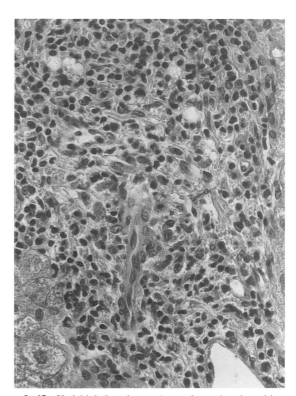

Figure 9–65. Hodgkin's lymphoma. A portal tract is enlarged by an inflammatory infiltrate consisting of lymphocytes, eosinophils, and occasional plasma cells.

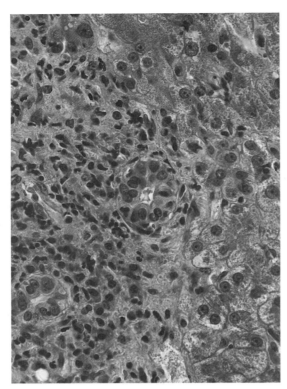

Figure 9–66. Hodgkin's lymphoma. The interlobular bile duct within this portal tract is slightly hyperplastic and infiltrated by lymphocytes and neutrophils. A bile duct *(lower left)* shows some hydropic change and atypia, with lymphocytes abutting the basement membrane.

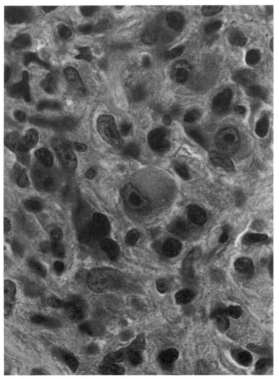

Figure 9–67. Hodgkin's lymphoma. Occasional large cells, some having abundant cytoplasm, are present in this portal tract. The nuclei are round to oval with large nucleoli and represent mononuclear Reed-Sternberg type cells.

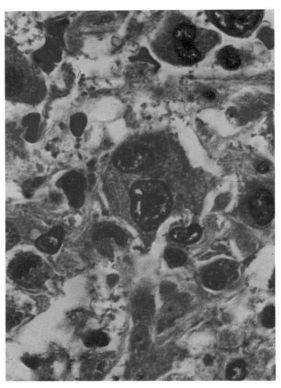

Figure 9–68. Hodgkin's lymphoma. A classic binucleated Reed-Sternberg cell with surrounding mononuclear cells and edema is present in this portal tract.

4. Involvement of the parenchyma with sparing of portal tracts is seldom seen.
5. Nonspecific changes that may occur *without* direct hepatic involvement by lymphoma include the following:
   a. Infiltration of portal tracts by lymphocytes, some of which are mildly atypical, as well as eosinophils and plasma cells (10%); mild cytologic atypia alone does not represent involvement by lymphoma.
   b. Noncaseating epithelioid granulomas, most commonly in portal regions (8% to 20%)
   c. Scattered macrovesicular fatty change with no zonal accentuation
   d. Perivenular cholestasis in absence of duct obstruction (2.2%)
   e. Hemosiderin in hyperplastic Kupffer cells or hepatocytes (secondary to hemolysis, transfusions, chronic anemia)
   f. Varying degrees of perivenular and midzonal sinusoidal dilatation (50%); peliosis hepatis has been described.

Differential Diagnosis

1. *Sarcoidosis:* Portal epithelioid granulomas seen in both sarcoidosis and Hodgkin's disease may morphologically appear similar. Sarcoid granulomas

tend to be quite numerous and often exhibit fibrosis with resultant subdivision into smaller granulomas.

2. *Infectious mononucleosis:* Atypical Reed-Sternberg–like cells in portal tracts may rarely be identified in patients with infectious mononucleosis. Considerable numbers of eosinophils, plasma cells, and destructive duct changes are not features of infectious mononucleosis. In addition, prominent numbers of atypical circulating sinusoidal lymphocytes characteristic of infectious mononucleosis are not present in Hodgkin's disease.

Clinical and Biologic Behavior

1. Hodgkin's lymphoma is responsible for approximately 2% of all malignancies (excluding hepatic primary lesions) that involve the liver in an autopsy study at the University of Southern California; 72% of all patients with Hodgkin's lymphoma (treated and nontreated) had hepatic involvement at autopsy.
2. Patients clinically present with fever and hepatomegaly; jaundice is present in 14% of cases.
3. Laboratory tests show variable elevations in serum aminotransferase levels, but moderate to marked increases in alkaline phosphatase and bilirubin values may be noted.
4. No cases of primary hepatic Hodgkin's lymphoma have been reported; the liver is involved only if the spleen and/or lymph nodes also have lymphoma.
5. The more common variants that involve the liver are the nodular sclerosing and mixed cellularity types.
6. The liver may be diffusely infiltrated, with most portal areas exhibiting infiltration, or may have irregularly distributed discrete, firm white nodules of varying size (usually not larger than a few centimeters in diameter).
7. Jaundice is secondary to the following:
   a. Widespread portal tract involvement (33%)
   b. Involvement of large hilar ducts producing obstructive change and mimicking hilar cholangiocarcinoma (3%)
   c. Perivenular cholestasis without identifiable duct obstruction (2.2%)
   d. Severe hemolysis with resultant bilirubin overload
8. Portal regions with atypical cells exhibiting prominent nucleoli, often admixed with lymphocytes, plasma cells, and eosinophils, strongly suggest Hodgkin's lymphoma, and in patients with known lymphoma these features are usually considered positive for hepatic involvement in staging procedures; in patients who do not have an established diagnosis, the presence of Reed-Sternberg cells in liver biopsy specimens is required for diagnosis.

Aspiration Cytology

1. Classic Reed-Sternberg cells and variants, with large single, binucleate or multilobed cells having prominent eosinophilic nucleoli, may be present but are relatively uncommon.
2. Mature lymphocytes, occasional eosinophils and plasma cells, and atypical large cells with moderate to scanty pale-pink cytoplasm and prominent nucleoli strongly suggest Hodgkin's lymphoma.
3. Similar cytologic patterns of lymphocytic atypicality may be seen in other conditions (e.g., infectious mononucleosis) and are therefore *not* diagnostic of Hodgkin's lymphoma on aspirate alone.

Treatment and Prognosis

1. Since primary Hodgkin's lymphoma has never been found in the liver alone, hepatic involvement represents an advanced stage of the disease.
2. Chemotherapy is offered but the prognosis is generally poor.

References

Abt AB, Kirschner RH, Belliveau RE, et al. Hepatic pathology associated with Hodgkin's disease. Cancer 1974;33:1564–1571.

Bruguera M, Caballero T, Carreras E, et al. Hepatic sinusoidal dilatation in Hodgkin's disease. Liver 1987;7:76–80.

Dich NH, Goodman ZD, Klein MA. Hepatic involvement in Hodgkin's disease: Clues to histologic diagnosis. Cancer 1989;64:2121–2126.

Lefkowitz JH, Falkow S, Whitlock RT. Hepatic Hodgkin's disease simulating cholestatic hepatitis with liver failure. Arch Pathol Lab Med 1985;109:424–426.

Leslie KO, Colby TV. Hepatic parenchymal lymphoid aggregates in Hodgkin's disease. Hum Pathol 1984;15:808–809.

Non-Hodgkin's Lymphoma

Major Morphologic Features

1. Marked expansion of portal tracts by lymphocytes is present, with only a mild degree of spillover into the adjacent parenchyma.
2. The infiltration is monomorphic, with no orientation toward any single portal structure.

Other Features

1. Most lymphocytic lymphomas are large cell cleaved and noncleaved types and exhibit a fairly uniform degree of portal infiltration throughout the liver *(diffuse);* however, mass lesions *(nodular)* may also occur, more often in poorly differentiated and T-cell types.
2. Portal tracts are usually sharply defined from the lob-

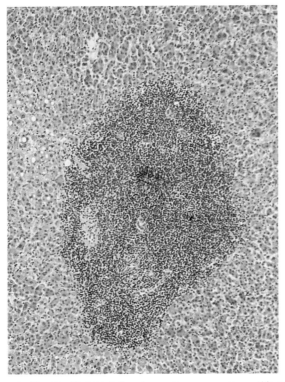

Figure 9–69. Non-Hodgkin's lymphoma. Low power shows this portal tract to be enlarged and expanded by a dense infiltrate of mononuclear cells.

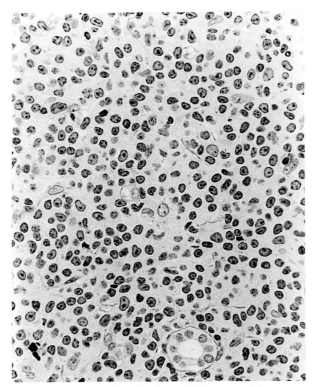

Figure 9–70. Non-Hodgkin's lymphoma. High power of the portal tract shows the cells to be monomorphic, large, and noncleaved. A bile duct *(below)* is surrounded but not infiltrated by these cells.

ule; however, involvement may be extensive, with variable degrees of replacement of adjacent hepatocytes by tumor cells.

3. The parenchyma shows a variable but minimal degree of sinusoidal infiltration by tumor cells, most prominent in the periportal zones; T-cell lymphomas have more of a tendency to extend into sinusoids in a chainlike fashion.

4. Portal enlargement is caused by the intense infiltrate, with fibrosis minimal to absent.

5. Focal hepatocytolysis, with occasional epithelioid granuloma formation, may be seen.

6. Hepatic cords are intact, with no significant inflammatory change; however, superimposed secondary infections may occur owing to immune deficiency.

7. Tumor necrosis may be identified in large nodular lesions; cholestasis is not typically present.

8. Hemosiderin may be identified within Kupffer cells and hepatocytes (secondary to hemolysis, transfusions, chronic anemia).

Differential Diagnosis

1. *Infectious mononucleosis:* Intense lymphocytic inflammatory infiltration is present in infectious mononucleosis; however, these cells are *polymorphic* (variability in size), with increased numbers of atypical large lymphocytes present within not only portal tracts but also sinusoids.

2. *Pseudolymphoma:* There may be fairly marked lymphocytic infiltration within the liver, usually distorting or even effacing the lobular architecture; features such as follicular hyperplasia and lymphocytic polymorphism are seen in pseudolymphoma.

3. *Nonspecific portal inflammatory changes:* Lymphocytic hyperplasia within the portal tracts is a nonspecific feature seen in many disorders (e.g., ulcerative colitis, rheumatoid arthritis, acute and chronic viral hepatitis). The lymphocytes in these conditions are always *polymorphic* in size and shape, unlike those seen in lymphoma. In addition, lymphoma generally exhibits a more prominent degree of infiltration.

4. *Poorly differentiated carcinoma:* Since primary lymphoma of the liver is rare, the diagnosis may often be misinterpreted because of frozen section artifact, giving the tumor a somewhat "carcinomatous" appearance. The presence of appropriate immunohistochemical markers (e.g., common leukocyte antigen) will rule out a nonhematologic origin of the tumor.

Special Stain

1. *Methyl green-pyronine:* Red to rose lavender cytoplasmic staining is an indicator of immunoglobulin synthesis by the tumor cell, suggesting B-cell origin.

Immunohistochemistry

1. Various representative markers in assessing cell type include the following:
   a. *Common leukocyte antigen (CLA):* B and T cell
   b. *Lambda and kappa light chains, heavy chains, B1:* B cell
   c. *Leu 2a, Leu 2b, OKT3, OKT4, OKT8, OKT11:* T cell

Clinical and Biologic Behavior

1. Non-Hodgkin's lymphoma constitutes 5.6% of all malignancies (excluding hepatic primary lesions) involving the liver in an autopsy study at the University of Southern California; 53% of all cases of lymphoma (treated and nontreated) show hepatic involvement at autopsy.
2. Liver biopsy may identify lymphoma 15% to 25% of the time in untreated patients with diffuse involvement; after treatment, or with partial remission, difficulty may occur in differentiating tumor cells from reactive portal lymphocytic infiltrates (the latter characteristically *polymorphic* in nature).
3. Approximately one fourth of cases have irregular solitary or multiple grossly identifiable lesions, while three fourths have diffuse portal involvement without mass lesions.
4. Spleen and/or abdominal lymph nodes are almost always affected when the liver is involved.
5. Primary hepatic lymphomas are very rare, only diagnosed after all other more common sites have been ruled out; these cases usually occur in middle-aged men and present as fever, malaise, and weight loss. Large solitary (8–16 cm in diameter) and/or smaller multifocal mass lesions (1–2 cm) are present, with approximately two thirds of cases representing a diffuse large cell type.
6. Primary hepatic lymphoma has been documented in acquired immunodeficiency syndrome.

Aspiration Cytology

1. Abundant numbers of monomorphic cells having large cleaved or noncleaved nuclei, often with prominent nucleoli, and scanty cytoplasm are highly suggestive of lymphoma.

Treatment and Prognosis

1. Malignant lymphoma with associated hepatic involvement is almost always indicative of advanced stage of the disease; the prognosis is generally poor.
2. Although primary hepatic lymphoma is quite rare,

results with both hepatic resection and combination chemotherapy have been encouraging.

References

Caccamo D, Pervez NF, Marchevshy A. Primary lymphoma of the liver in the acquired immunodeficiency syndrome. Arch Pathol Lab Med 1986;110:553–555.

DeMent SH, Mann RB, Staal SP, et al. Primary lymphomas of the liver: Report of six cases and review of the literature. Am J Clin Pathol 1987;88:255–263.

Edmondson HA, Craig JR. Neoplasms of the liver. In: Schiff L, Schiff ER, eds. Diseases of the Liver, 6th ed. Philadelphia: J.B. Lippincott, 1987:1116–1118.

Osborne BM, Butler JJ, Guarda LA. Primary lymphoma of the liver: Ten cases and a review of the literature. Cancer 1985;56:2902–2910.

Ryan J, Straus DJ, Lange C, et al. Primary lymphoma of the liver. Cancer 1988;61:370–375.

Leukemia

Major Morphologic Features

1. Sinusoids are filled with abundant numbers of circulating leukemic cells, with variable degrees of portal tract infiltration and expansion.
2. Hepatic cords are intact, with no significant inflammatory change or cell necrosis; however, superimposed secondary infections may occur (secondary to immune deficiency or chemotherapy).

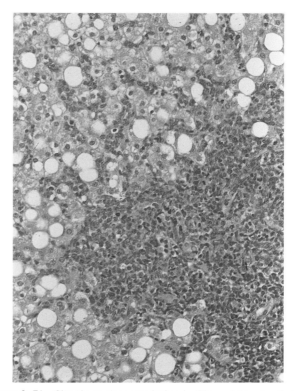

Figure 9–71. Chronic myelogenous leukemia. The portal tract and adjacent sinusoids show a marked infiltration by immature myeloid elements. The hepatocytes contain macrovesicular fat and appear normal.

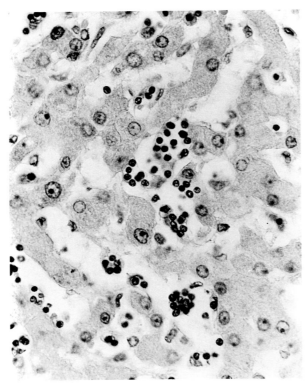

Figure 9–72. Chronic lymphocytic leukemia. The dilated sinusoids contain aggregates of small leukemic lymphocytes. The hepatic cords are unremarkable.

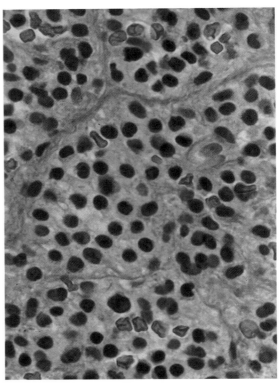

Figure 9–74. Hairy cell leukemia. High power shows the cells to have round nuclei without nucleoli and a moderate degree of eosinophilic cytoplasm. Positive cytoplasmic staining (frozen sections or touch preparations) with tartrate-resistant acid phosphatase is characteristic for these leukemic cells.

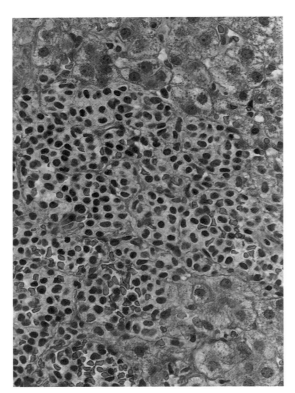

Figure 9–73. Hairy cell leukemia. The parenchyma is infiltrated by a well-defined aggregate of monomorphic mononuclear cells.

Other Features

1. Extramedullary hematopoiesis (aggregates of normoblasts, immature granulocytes, and/or megakaryocytes scattered in small clusters throughout the lobules) may be present in cases associated with myelofibrosis.
2. Hemosiderin deposition may be seen in Kupffer cells and hepatocytes (secondary to hemolysis, transfusions, chronic anemia).
3. Cholestasis and bile duct changes are not typically present.
4. *Hairy cell leukemia* exhibits cells with characteristic features:
   a. Mononuclear, moderate cytoplasm, slight indentation of nuclei, rare nucleoli, minute cytoplasmic processes
   b. Loose aggregation within sinusoids and portal tracts
   c. Adherence to sinusoidal walls, insinuation of cytoplasmic processes between endothelial pores, eventual infiltration into the space of Disse with marked displacement of endothelial cells
   d. Formation of randomly distributed *"pseudopeliotic"* lesions: parenchymal cavities lined and filled by leukemic cells and red blood cells

Differential Diagnosis

1. *Acute sclerosing hyaline necrosis:* Leukocytosis with white blood cell counts of 40,000/mm^3 to over 100,000/mm^3 may be found in this form of acute alcoholic liver disease, with the sinusoids filled with immature forms of polymorphonuclear leukocytes. These cases are always associated with hyaline necrosis of the hepatocytes and prominent perivenular sinusoidal collagen deposition. The white blood cell count returns to normal when the hepatitis resolves.
2. *Bacterial sepsis:* In bacterial infections with severe leukocytosis, distinction from leukemia on morphologic grounds alone may be quite difficult.
3. *Viral infections:* Marked portal and sinusoidal lymphocytosis typically occurs in infectious mononucleosis and cytomegalovirus infections. These cells are generally larger than leukemic lymphocytes, with rather abundant cytoplasm. The liver also exhibits focal necrosis, occasional ill-defined granulomas, and Kupffer cell hyperplasia, changes not seen in leukemia.

Special Stain

1. *Tartrate-resistant acid phosphatase:* Positive red cytoplasmic staining of cells prepared by frozen sections or touch preparations of biopsy specimens indicate hairy cell leukemia.

Clinical and Biologic Behavior

1. Leukemic infiltrates of all types are responsible for 6.9% of all neoplasms (excluding hepatic primary lesions) that involved the liver in an autopsy study at the University of Southern California (1960–1980); 79% of all cases of leukemia (treated and nontreated) showed hepatic involvement at autopsy.
2. Presence of extramedullary hematopoiesis should raise the possibility of myelofibrosis, massive replacement of bone marrow by tumor (leukemic as well as other types of malignancies), and severe anemia.
3. Certain types of lymphomas (i.e., small cell lymphocytic type) may enter a leukemic phase (chronic lymphocytic leukemia), with hepatic features of both circulating and portal infiltration by lymphocytes.
4. *Hairy cell leukemia* represents 2% to 5% of all leukemias and presents predominantly in middle-aged men (average age 50) with splenomegaly and signs of hypersplenism; the liver is commonly involved, although hepatomegaly develops in only 20% of patients. This form of leukemia may be overlooked on biopsy, since the cells infiltrate through the endothelial lining and replace endothelial cells. Tartrate-

resistant acid phosphatase activity can be demonstrated in these cells in frozen tissue sections for diagnosis.

Treatment and Prognosis

1. Leukemia does not significantly alter hepatic dysfunction; hence no treatment directed toward the liver is usually necessary.
2. Prognosis is generally related to the type of leukemia.

References

Edmondson HA, Craig JR. Neoplasms of the Liver. In: Schiff L, Schiff ER, eds. Diseases of the Liver, 6th ed. Philadelphia: J.B. Lippincott, 1987:1116–1118.

Yam LT, Janckila AJ, Chan CH, et al. Hepatic involvement in hairy cell leukemia. Cancer 1983;51:1497–1504.

Zafrani ES, Degos F, Guigui B, et al. The hepatic sinusoid in hairy cell leukemia: An ultrastructural study of 12 cases. Hum Pathol 1987;18:801–807.

Multiple Myeloma and Malignant Reticuloendotheliosis

MULTIPLE MYELOMA

1. Multiple myeloma comprises 5.6% of all malignancies (excluding hepatic primary lesions) in an autopsy study at the University of Southern California;

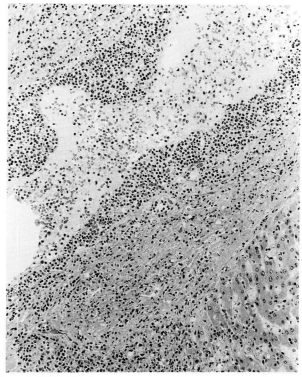

Figure 9–75. Multiple myeloma. A small hepatic vein wall is infiltrated by mononuclear cells, which appear accentuated along the vascular intima.

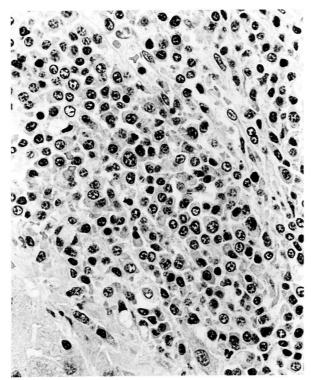

Figure 9–76. Multiple myeloma. High power shows the infiltrate to consist of immature plasma cells. The nuclei are round and often demonstrate clumped staining of the chromatin. Some cells have nuclei eccentrically placed within the cytoplasm.

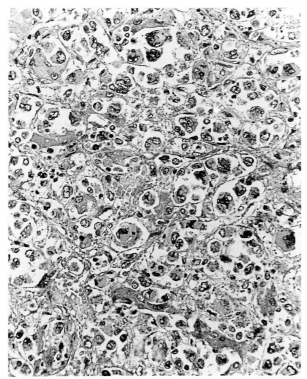

Figure 9–77. Malignant reticuloendotheliosis. The neoplasm consists of large pleomorphic Kupffer cells within dilated sinusoids. There is prominent atrophy of adjacent hepatocytes.

30% of cases of myeloma showed hepatic involvement at autopsy.
2. Hepatic changes may include the following:
   a. Plasma cell infiltration into portal regions
   b. Focal mass lesions and/or diffuse infiltration into sinusoids and veins
   c. Sinusoidal dilatation, rarely with changes resembling peliosis hepatis
   d. Eosinophilic, nonamyloid substance (light chains) within the space of Disse
   e. Amyloid deposits (Congo red positive) within sinusoids and/or portal structures; 6% to 15% of all cases of multiple myeloma are associated with systemic amyloidosis, with approximately 50% of these cases exhibiting hepatic involvement.
   f. Immunohistochemical demonstration of immunoglobulin or light chains in tumor cells

Malignant Reticuloendotheliosis

1. Very rare disorder characterized by the following:
   a. Large pleomorphic neoplastic Kupffer cells
   b. Prominent atrophy of the adjacent liver cell cords
   c. Erythrophagocytosis by tumor cells
2. The liver and spleen commonly are both enlarged and diffusely involved.

References

Glenner GG. Amyloid deposits and amyloidosis: The beta fibrilloses. N Engl J Med 1980;302:1283–1292, 1333–1343.
Randall RE, Williamson WC, Mullinax F, et al. Manifestations of systemic light chain deposition. Am J Med 1976;60:293–299.
Thomas FB, Clausen KP, Creenberger NJ. Liver disease in multiple myeloma. Arch Intern Med 1973;132:195–202.

■ Metastatic Neoplasms

Major Morphologic Features

1. Metastatic sites include both portal tracts (portal vein, lymphatics) and parenchyma (sinusoids, with compression and variable degrees of atrophy of adjacent hepatocytes).
2. Tumor cells generally retain the morphologic features of the primary site.

Other Features

1. Certain neoplasms (e.g., breast, pancreas, gallbladder) are often associated with prominent reactive fibrosis.
2. Tumor thrombi in hepatic veins are not common; however, in instances of large metastatic mass lesions, obstruction of hepatic venous outflow can occur, with perivenular congestion; perivenular hemorrhage, coagulative (anoxic) liver cell necrosis, and red blood cells within trabecular cords, replacing

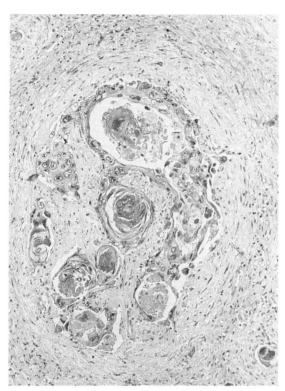

Figure 9–78. Squamous cell carcinoma, metastatic. The moderately differentiated squamous cells form large whorls with prominent keratin formation.

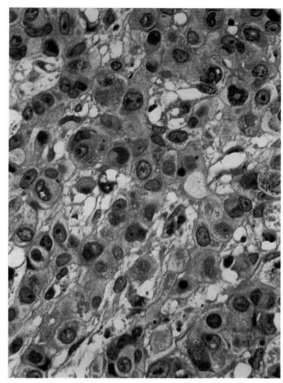

Figure 9–80. Malignant melanoma, metastatic. The tumor cells form nests and cords and contain a brown pigment representing melanin.

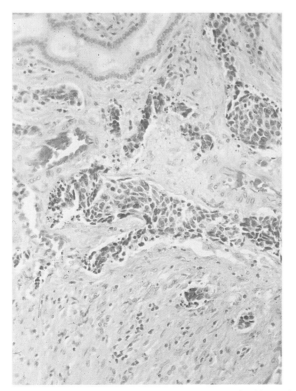

Figure 9–79. Oat cell carcinoma, metastatic. Medium-sized hyperchromatic cells with scanty cytoplasm fill these dilated lymphatic channels.

damaged liver cells (lesion seen in the acute Budd-Chiari syndrome), may be present.
3. Dilatation of interlobular bile ducts, acute cholangitis, and perivenular cholestasis may be present in adjacent nontumor liver caused by focal biliary obstruction; variable degrees of biliary fibrosis may also occur in long-term obstruction from slowly growing neoplasms.
4. A fibrous capsule adjacent to the tumor is seldom present.
5. Calcification may be seen (e.g., mucinous colonic carcinoma) but is rare.
6. Nontumor liver may exhibit foci of ischemic necrosis that is usually perivenular.
7. Reactive Kupffer cell hyperplasia is generally present; mild macrovesicular fatty change of hepatocytes can be seen.

Differential Diagnosis

1. *Hepatocellular carcinoma:* Certain neoplasms may exhibit some of the morphologic features seen in hepatocellular carcinoma (e.g., renal cell carcinoma with clear cells, malignant melanoma with trabecular-like structures). Distinguishing features of hepatocellular carcinoma that are *not* found in metastatic tumor:
   a. Bile within tumor cells or the lumen of acinar-type lesions

b. Alcoholic hyalin, alpha-1-antitrypsin inclusions within the cytoplasm

c. Lining of trabeculae by endothelial cells

d. Characteristic cytoplasmic features (e.g., enlarged eosinophilic cytoplasm with pale body in fibrolamellar hepatocellular carcinoma)

2. *Cholangiocarcinoma:* Adenocarcinomas eliciting a prominent stromal reaction may resemble cholangiocarcinoma. In many of these cases the only way a confident diagnosis of metastasis can be made is when there is a known primary extrahepatic site where the tumor has identical morphologic features as the hepatic lesion.

Special Stains

1. *Histochemical staining characteristics of the primary tumor:* Although helpful in identifying the type of neoplasm (e.g., *Fontana-Masson* for argentaffin granules in carcinoid; *mucicarmine* for mucin in colonic, pancreatic, gastric adenocarcinoma), distinction between primary (e.g., presence of mucin in cholangiocarcinoma) and metastatic may not be possible.

Immunohistochemistry

1. *Identification of tumor type:* Examples are *calcitonin* in medullary carcinoma of the thyroid, *S-100* in malignant melanoma, *carcinoembryonic antigen* in colonic, pulmonary adenocarcinoma. Positive staining for *alpha-fetoprotein* can assist in *ruling out* most types of metastatic disease (exceptions being gastric, testicular, yolk sac, embryonal).

Clinical and Biologic Behavior

1. Metastatic tumor is 16 times more frequent than primary neoplasm in the liver, present in approximately 8% of all cases at autopsy (incidence of hepatocellular carcinoma, 0.5%).

2. At autopsy, approximately one third of all tumors are metastatic to the liver.

3. Hepatomegaly is present in one third of patients with metastatic disease and sometimes is quite pronounced (liver weight >5000 g).

4. Ascites occurs in 18% of all cases of malignancy (in the presence or absence of hepatic metastases); however, 45% of patients with metastatic disease from the stomach, ovary, or gallbladder have ascites.

5. At autopsy, 14.5% of patients are jaundiced owing to large duct obstruction (pancreas, gallbladder, bile duct, and tumors metastatic to the hilum of the liver) or massive (>75%) hepatic replacement by tumor (colon, breast, melanoma).

6. Liver tests reveal normal or minimally increased serum aminotransferase levels; in contrast, marked increase in alkaline phosphatase and lactate dehydrogenase activities provide clues to metastatic liver involvement; increase in the serum bilirubin value occurs when the liver is diffusely infiltrated, or with obstruction of bile ducts.

7. Although alpha-fetoprotein values greater than 500 ng/mL in patients with mass lesions in the liver are virtually diagnostic of hepatocellular carcinoma, other metastatic tumors (gastric, testicular teratomas, yolk sac, embryonal) may rarely produce markedly elevated alpha-fetoprotein levels.

8. More common nonhematopoietic malignant tumors with percent metastasis to the liver at the time of death are shown below (2742 patients with malignancies at autopsy; Edmondson, 1987):

Primary Site	% Of Total No. of Malignancies	% With Hepatic Metastases
Bronchogenic	24.9	41.8
Prostate	12.1	12.6
Colon	11.8	56.0
Breast	8.0	53.2
Pancreas	6.5	70.4
Stomach	5.8	44.0
Kidney	5.2	23.9
Cervix	3.9	31.7

9. Multiple nodules in the liver are seen in 90% of cases; single massive nodules and infiltrative lesions can be present.

10. Of *all* liver biopsy specimens, 3.8% demonstrate metastatic disease. Unguided needle biopsy specimens of livers with mass lesions are positive for tumor 40% to 75% of the time; the yield is increased when the biopsy specimen or aspirate is ultrasound guided, multiple specimens are taken, or biopsies are performed during peritoneoscopy.

11. It was previously believed that cirrhotic livers were an unfavorable site for metastatic disease, but studies have shown this to be incorrect. In patients with extrahepatic malignancy, 39% of cirrhotic and 46% of noncirrhotic livers develop metastases (no statistical difference).

Aspiration Cytology

1. Characteristic features of primary lesions are identified.

Treatment and Prognosis

1. Localized metastatic lesions have been surgically resected in conjunction with removal of the primary tumor and absence of metastasis in other organs. In diffuse metastatic lesions surgery is not recommended. In a few cases of metastatic disease, hepatic transplantation has been performed.

2. Arterial ligation, embolism, and intra-arterial chemotherapy have not been effective.

3. When metastatic liver tumors produce bile duct obstruction, palliative stenting by endoscopy or by surgical choledochojejunostomy provides only temporary benefit.

4. The overall prognosis is generally poor, with death usually occurring 6 to 12 months after diagnosis; some tumors such as neuroblastoma and carcinoid carry a better prognosis.

References

Edmondson HA, Craig JR. Neoplasms of the Liver. In: Schiff L, Schiff ER, eds. Diseases of the Liver, 6th ed. Philadelphia: J.B. Lippincott, 1987;1109–1116.

Fisher ER, Hellstrom HR, Fisher B. Rarity of hepatic metastases in cirrhosis: A misconception. JAMA 1960;174:366–369.

Gerber MA, Thung SN, Bodenheimer HC Jr, et al. Characteristic histologic triad in liver adjacent to metastatic neoplasm. Liver 1988;6:85–88.

Strohmeyer T, Schultz W. The distribution of metastases of different primary tumors in the liver. Liver 1986;6:184–187.

■ Tumor-like Lesions

Focal Nodular Hyperplasia

Major Morphologic Features

1. Central scar exhibits radiating fibrous septa that subdivide the mass lesion into multiple segments.
2. Large vessels are seen in central portion of scar with irregular myointimal proliferation.
3. Radiating fibrous septa contain the following:
   a. Small vascular structures
   b. Atypical duct epithelium consisting of flattened cells, no distinct lumen, and serpentine growth pattern along the border of the septa
   c. Mild lymphocytic infiltration

Other Features

1. Hepatocytes are cytologically benign, often slightly hydropic and larger than the hepatocytes in the nontumor liver.
2. Hepatocytes may rarely contain fat, bile, glycogen, or lipochrome.
3. Endothelial lining cells and Kupffer cells are present along the trabecular cords.
4. No normal duct structures can be identified.
5. Fibrous capsules are not present.

Differential Diagnosis

1. *Liver cell adenoma:* Presence of radiating fibrous septa and atypical ducts is not seen in the liver cell adenoma. If the biopsy specimen only shows hepato-

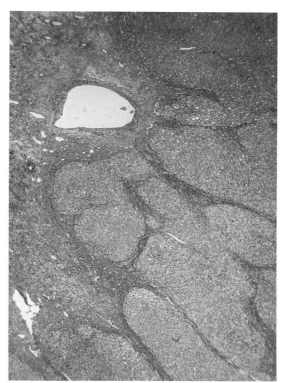

Figure 9–81. Focal nodular hyperplasia. Low power demonstrates a fibrous scar *(left)* containing variously sized vessels. The parenchyma tends to form nodules surrounded by thin fibrous septa.

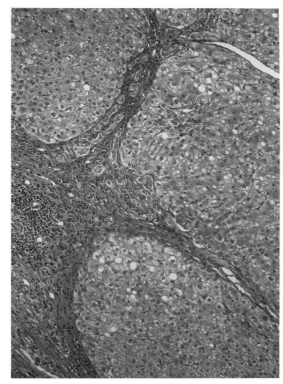

Figure 9–82. Focal nodular hyperplasia. High power shows the fibrous septa to contain lymphocytes. Ductlike structures line the fibrous bands.

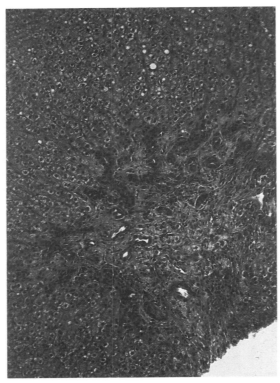

Figure 9–83. Focal nodular hyperplasia. A fibrous septum contains scattered lymphocytes, small vessels, and numerous atypical ducts having flattened epithelium and no good lumina. These ducts are located at the periphery of the septum.

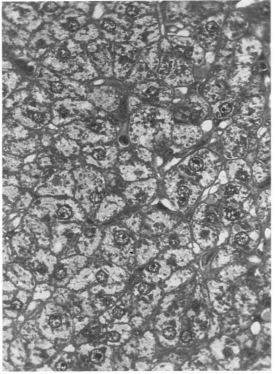

Figure 9–84. Focal nodular hyperplasia. The parenchyma is composed of hydropic liver cells. Endothelial lining and Kupffer cells are present.

cytes, however, distinction between the two entities may not be possible on morphologic grounds alone. Morphologic and radiologic features distinguishing between the two lesions are listed in the section on liver cell adenoma (see page 177).

2. *Well-differentiated hepatocellular carcinoma:* In a biopsy specimen exhibiting only hepatocytes without fibrous septa, features of well-differentiated hepatocellular carcinoma (prominent nucleoli, cords greater than two cells thick, mitoses, tumor cells within vascular channels, cells containing alcoholic hyalin) assist in differentiating between the two lesions.

3. *Fibrolamellar hepatocellular carcinoma:* Fibrous septa, and occasionally a central radiating scar, may be seen in fibrolamellar hepatocellular carcinoma. Atypical ducts are not present, however. Fibrolamellar hepatocellular carcinoma also has prominent eosinophilic cytoplasm with characteristic inclusions (''pale body'').

Clinical and Biologic Behavior

1. Focal nodular hyperplasia is a mass lesion that many believe is not a true neoplasm but rather a result of repeated vascular thrombosis with secondary myointimal proliferation and consequent hepatocellular regeneration.

2. Most patients (90%–95%) are women; although the majority of patients are between 20 and 39 years of age, case reports show an age range of between 14 months to 74 years.

3. The disorder is usually found incidentally at surgery for other causes, with only one fourth of patients having abdominal pain or a palpable mass.

4. Serum aminotransferase levels and alkaline phosphatase activity are normal in more than 80% of cases; the alpha-fetoprotein level is not elevated.

5. The lesion is usually solitary, light tan, and sometimes bulging from the surface and ranges in size from 2 to 15 cm; it is usually found immediately beneath Glisson's capsule.

6. There is no statistical relationship with the use of oral contraceptives.

7. Malignant transformation has not been reported.

Aspiration Cytology

1. Cells show round nuclei without prominent nucleoli and a relatively abundant clear cytoplasm.

2. Liver cell adenoma has identical features; a well-differentiated hepatocellular carcinoma cannot always be ruled out.

Treatment and Prognosis

1. Complications such as rupture are rare; treatment is relatively conservative.

2. Small lesions incidentally discovered at surgery may be totally resected, especially those that are pedunculated.

3. Some researchers believe oral contraceptives should be avoided owing to possible hemorrhage of focal nodular hyperplasia.

References

Foster JH, Berman MM. The benign lesions: Adenoma and focal nodular hyperplasia. In: Series Major Problems in Clinical Surgery, Vol XXIII, Solid Liver Tumors. Philadelphia: W.B. Saunders, 1977;138–178.

Kerlin P, Davis GL, McGill DB, et al. Hepatic adenoma and focal nodular hyperplasia: Clinical, pathologic, and radiologic features. Gastroenterology 1983;84:994–1002.

Knowles DM, Wolff M. Focal nodular hyperplasia of the liver: A clinicopathologic study and review of the literature. Hum Pathol 1976;7:533–545.

Wanless IR, Mawdsley C, Adams R. On the pathogenesis of focal nodular hyperplasia of the liver. Hepatology 1985;5:1194–1200.

Regenerative Lesions: Nodular Regenerative Hyperplasia and Partial Nodular Transformation

Major Morphologic Changes

1. Cytologically benign hydropic hepatocytes form small nodules composed of slightly thickened and irregularly aligned trabeculae.

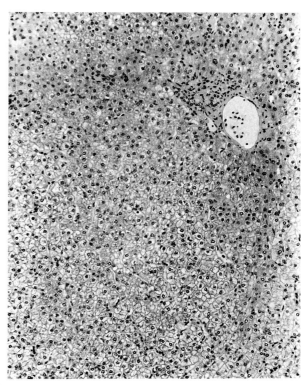

Figure 9–86. Nodular regenerative hyperplasia. The hepatocytes within the nodule are hydropic, with the sinusoids difficult to appreciate. Kupffer cell hyperplasia is not present. A portal tract *(upper right)* is normal in size. Adjacent liver cells are slightly atrophic *(lower right of portal tract).*

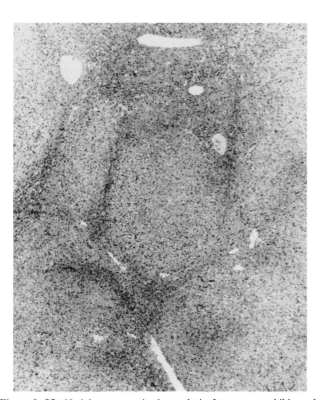

Figure 9–85. Nodular regenerative hyperplasia. Low power exhibits nodules formed by hyperplastic liver cells. The more heavily staining "septa" are not formed by fibrous septa but by atrophic liver cells. Small portal tracts are present at the periphery of the nodules.

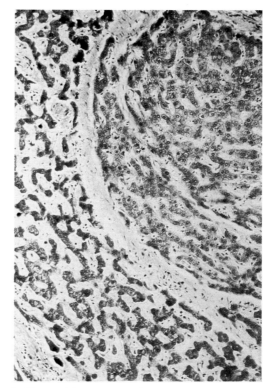

Figure 9–87. Partial nodular transformation (trichrome). True fibrous septa surround nodules of liver cells. The cord–sinusoid pattern within these nodules is preserved and dilated.

Other Features

Nodular Regenerative Hyperplasia

1. Although the nodules on low power exhibit rather sharp outlines, close examination shows the borders to be less defined, with compression of adjacent liver cells but without capsule formation.
2. Portal tracts are not fibrotic, with only minimal mononuclear inflammatory infiltration.
3. Bile ducts may be slightly increased or decreased.
4. Dilatation of the small portal venous radicles may be present.
5. The smaller nodules may predominate in periportal regions and surround individual portal tracts.
6. Thrombosis and recanalization of intrahepatic portal veins may occur.
7. Extramedullary hematopoiesis and cholestasis may rarely be seen.
8. A mild degree of Kupffer cell hyperplasia is often present.

Partial Nodular Transformation

1. Fibrosis occurs at the periphery of the larger nodules; sinusoidal dilatation of the nodules may occur.
2. Portal tracts are normal in size and may be located within a nodule.
3. Bile ducts are not increased in number.
4. Intrahepatic portal venous radicles may be decreased, but thrombosis does not occur.
5. Mild Kupffer cell hyperplasia is occasionally present.

Differential Diagnosis

1. *Multiple liver cell adenomas (hepatocellular adenomatosis):* Nodular regenerative hyperplasia uniformly involves the entire liver, while there is an irregular distribution with the adenomas. The nodules in nodular regenerative hyperplasia are less than 1 mm to 1 cm in diameter, while adenomas may reach 5 cm in greatest dimension.
2. *Cirrhosis:* Partial nodular transformation has nodules 3 to 40 mm in diameter, which resemble the regenerative nodules seen in many types of cirrhosis. Cirrhotic nodules uniformly affect the entire liver, while partial nodular transformation is focal and almost always limited to the perihilar region.

Clinical and Biologic Behavior

	Nodular Regenerative Hyperplasia	Partial Nodular Transformation
Age	Any age, usually adult	Never in children or adolescents
Clinical	Features of portal hypertension (ascites, recurrent esophageal variceal hemorrhage)	
Laboratory	Transaminase levels usually normal; bilirubin and alkaline phosphatase values normal or mildly elevated	
Associated Diseases	Hematologic (myeloproliferative disorders, leukemia, lymphoma) Neoplasms (kidney, pancreas, colon) Congestive heart failure Subacute bacterial endocarditis Autoimmune (Felty's, CRST syndrome, rheumatoid arthritis) Drugs (steroids, oral contraceptives)	No commonly associated conditions
Nodules *Size*	<1 to 3 mm, occasionally up to 10 mm	3–40 mm, sometimes up to 60 mm
Location	Diffusely scattered throughout liver	Usually perihilar, with remaining liver normal
Portal venous System	Intrahepatic thrombosis in small radicles, with normal extrahepatic portal vein	Extrahepatic thrombosis and thickening, sometimes calcification; cavernous transformation of extrahepatic portal vein
Pathophysiology	Obliteration of portal venous radicles (e.g., thrombosis in myeloproliferative disorders), recanalization with atrophy of hepatocytes (decreased blood flow) and compensatory hyperplasia of adjacent hepatocytes	Large vessel thrombosis, recanalization occurring in area of fastest blood flow (in veins that branch off a large vessel near the hilum), with atrophy of liver cells in hypoperfused regions and regeneration in adjacent hepatocytes
	Portal hypertension presinusoidal, secondary to thrombosis, recanalization of portal vein and nodule formation	Portal hypertension presinusoidal, most likely caused by combination of large portal vein thrombosis with recanalization and possible pressure of perihilar nodules on the portal vein itself

Treatment and Prognosis

1. Liver function is not significantly impaired, but consequences of portal hypertension such as ascites, bleeding esophageal varices, and encephalopathy may occur.
2. Management of bleeding esophagogastric varices initially is preferable by nonsurgical means such as endoscopic sclerotherapy; portal-systemic shunt surgery may be performed in cases of sclerotherapy failure.

References

Colina F, Alberti N, Solis JA, et al. Diffuse nodular regenerative hyperplasia of the liver (DNRH): A clinicopathologic study of 24 cases. Liver 1989;9:253–265.

Sherlock S, Feldman CA, Moran B, et al. Partial nodular transformation of the liver with portal hypertension. Am J Med 1966;40:195–203.

Steiner PE. Nodular regenerative hyperplasia of the liver. Am J Pathol 1959;35:943–953.

Stroymeyer FW, Ishak KG. Nodular transformation (NRH) of the liver: A clinicopathologic study of 30 cases. Hum Pathol 1981;12:60–71.

Wanless IR, Lentz JS, Roberts EA. Partial nodular transformation of the liver in an adult with persistent ductus venosus: Review with hypothesis on pathogenesis. Arch Pathol Lab Med 1985;109:427–432.

General References

Anthony PP. Tumours and tumour-like lesions of the liver and biliary tract. In: MacSween RNM, Anthony PP, Scheuer PJ, eds. Pathology of the Liver, 2nd ed. Edinburgh: Churchill Livingstone, 1987:574–645.

Craig JR, Peters RL, Edmondson HA. Tumors of the Liver and Intrahepatic Bile Ducts. Washington, DC: Armed Forces Institute of Pathology, 1989.

Edmondson HA, Craig JR. Neoplasms of the liver. In: Schiff L, Schiff ER, eds. Diseases of the Liver, 6th ed. Philadelphia: J.B. Lippincott, 1987:1109–1158.

Okuda K, Ishak KG, eds. Neoplasms of the Liver. Tokyo: Springer-Verlag, 1987.

Okuda K, Peters RL, eds. Hepatocellular Carcinoma. New York: John Wiley & Sons, 1976.

Peters RL. Neoplastic diseases. In: Peters RL, Craig JR, eds. Liver Pathology. New York: Churchill Livingstone, 1986:337–364.

CHAPTER 10

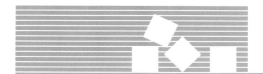

Miscellaneous Conditions

Neonatal Giant Cell Hepatitis

Major Morphologic Features

1. Syncytial giant cell transformation of hepatocytes is present; although typically accentuated in the perivenular zone, the cells may be present throughout the lobule in severe cases.
2. Portal tracts are normal in size, with mild to moderate predominantly lymphocytic infiltration and hyperplasia.

Other Features

1. Bile ducts may be normal in number to minimally increased.
2. Sinusoidal collagen is present to some degree around the larger multinucleated cells.
3. The number of nuclei in the giant cells ranges from 4 to more than 50.
4. Giant cells have hydropic to granular eosinophilic cytoplasm and may contain glycogen, bile, or hemosiderin; necrosis of giant cells is not usually seen.
5. Bile plugs in dilated canaliculi may be present.
6. Moderate degree of Kupffer cell hyperplasia is present, with focal areas of hepatocytolysis, usually more prominent in the perivenular zone.
7. Acidophil bodies may be present.
8. Extramedullary hematopoiesis of variable degrees is common.

Differential Diagnosis

1. *Other conditions that may exhibit syncytial giant cells include the following:*

   a. *Extrahepatic biliary atresia:* This is one of the more common disorders that elicit a syncytial giant cell transformation. Within the first 3 months of life there is marked bile duct proliferation. The portal tracts during this period are usually normal in size to mildly fibrotic; thereafter, the fibrosis becomes more prominent, with biliary cirrhosis described as early as 6 months after birth. Very early in this disorder, morphologic features differentiating these two entities may be quite minimal (Table 10–1).
   b. *Intrahepatic biliary atresia:* Bile ducts are decreased to absent in these cases but present to slightly increased in giant cell hepatitis.
   c. *Alpha-1-antitrypsin deficiency:* Ducts may be decreased in this disorder, and biliary fibrosis may be present, depending on the time of biopsy. Alpha-1-antitrypsin cytoplasmic inclusions in periportal hepatocytes are the key finding but may be quite small and exceptionally difficult to identify within the first 10 weeks of life. Serum alpha-1-antitrypsin levels with phenotyping are necessary for a definitive diagnosis, since hetero-

Table 10–1
DIFFERENTIAL FEATURES OF
EXTRAHEPATIC BILIARY ATRESIA AND
NEONATAL GIANT CELL HEPATITIS

Morphologic Change	Extrahepatic Biliary Atresia	Neonatal Hepatitis
Bile duct proliferation	+++	+
Portal fibrosis	+++	+
Sinusoidal fibrosis	−	+
Bile lakes	+	−
Giant cell, inflammatory changes	+	++
Persistent extramedullary hematopoiesis	+	++

Modified from Ruebner BH, Cox KL. Liver diseases in infancy. In: Peters RL, Craig JR, eds. Liver Pathology. New York: Churchill Livingstone, 1986:40–41.

227

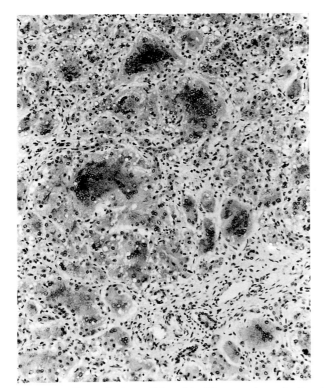

Figure 10–1. Neonatal giant cell hepatitis. The parenchyma is almost totally replaced by hepatocytes exhibiting syncytial giant cell transformation. A portal tract (*lower right*) is slightly enlarged with a mild lymphocytic infiltration and increase in bile ducts.

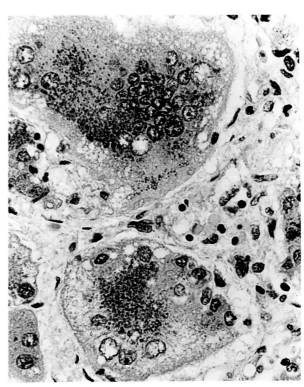

Figure 10–2. Neonatal giant cell hepatitis. The giant cells contain 30 to 50 nuclei. The granular cytoplasmic material represents hemosiderin. Microvesicular fat is present within the cytoplasm. The parenchyma exhibits an increased number of lymphocytes and a moderate Kupffer cell hyperplasia.

zygotes (PiMZ, overall incidence 3%) do *not* develop chronic liver disease.

Special Stain

1. *Diastase periodic acid–Schiff:* This stain is used to identify periportal alpha-1-antitrypsin globules or for diffuse cytoplasmic staining (patients younger than 10 weeks of age) of this protein to diagnose or rule out alpha-1-antitrypsin deficiency.

Immunohistochemistry

1. *Alpha-1-antitrypsin:* This confirms the etiology of the periodic acid–Schiff staining globules.

Clinical and Biologic Behavior

1. *Neonatal hepatitis* is generally defined as any condition in the neonate with conjugated hyperbilirubinemia, patent and normal extrahepatic biliary tree, and morphologic hepatic features of chronic inflammation and syncytial giant cell transformation of hepatocytes.

2. Numerous conditions are associated with this clinicopathologic disorder, the most common being alpha-1-antitrypsin deficiency (30% of all cases); however, approximately 50% of cases have no known cause.

3. Other etiologies include the following:
   a. *Biliary:* Intrahepatic atresia (Alagille's syndrome, paucity of duct syndrome), polycystic disease, congenital hepatic fibrosis
   b. *Metabolic:* Galactosemia, hereditary fructose intolerance, Indian childhood cirrhosis (copper), total parenteral nutrition, Niemann-Pick and Gaucher's diseases, iron storage disease (perinatal hemochromatosis)
   c. *Infectious:* Hepatitis viruses (types A, B, and non-A, non-B), cytomegalovirus, herpesvirus, rubella, coxsackievirus, *Toxoplasma, Treponema*

4. Although extrahepatic biliary atresia and choledochal cysts commonly produce giant cell change, many investigators omit these disorders when defining neonatal hepatitis. Nonetheless, they are almost always considered in the differential diagnosis.

5. Giant cell transformation is a result of mitotic inhibition and/or fusion of adjacent liver cells; this finding is rather nonspecific in the neonate with inflammatory, cholestatic, and numerous congenital and metabolic disorders. However, giant cell change is much rarer in children and adults; when seen in the older

age groups, the giant cells are relatively scanty and smaller, usually containing only four nuclei.

Prognosis

1. The overall prognosis is relatively good, with resolution of the hepatitis.
2. Careful follow-up is important to exclude homozygous alpha-1-antitrypsin deficiency (progression to cirrhosis with need for eventual hepatic transplantation), biliary atresia, or rare hepatic disorders such as intrahepatic familial cholestasis.

References

Ishak KG, Sharp HL. Developmental abnormality and liver disease in childhood. In: MacSween RNM, Anthony PP, Scheuer PJ, eds. Pathology of the Liver, 2nd ed. Edinburgh: Churchill Livingstone, 1987;73–74.

Montgomery CK, Reubner BH. Neonatal hepatocellular giant cell transformation: A review. In: Rosenberg HS, Bolande RP, eds. Perspectives in Pediatric Pathology. Year Book Medical Publishing Co, 1976;3:85–101.

Ruebner BH, Cox KL. Liver diseases in infancy. In: Peters RL, Craig JR, eds. Liver Pathology. New York: Churchill Livingstone, 1986;40–41.

■ Granulomatous Liver Disease

Description and Causes

1. *Granulomas* are defined as circumscribed collections of inflammatory cells, predominantly lymphocytes, histiocytes, and macrophages, associated with numerous disorders:
   a. *Infectious agents:* Brucellosis, tuberculosis, histoplasmosis, cytomegalovirus, leprosy
   b. *Hypersensitivity reactions:* Drugs such as sulfasalazine, phenytoin, thiabendazole
   c. *Neoplasms:* Hodgkin's lymphoma, liver cell adenoma
   d. *Foreign objects:* Talclike substances in intravenous drug users, thorotrast, mineral oil
   e. *Miscellaneous conditions:* Primary biliary cirrhosis, jejunoileal bypass, sarcoidosis
2. There are two morphologic classifications:
   a. *Epithelioid type:* Well demarcated, with macrophages transformed into rather large cells having oval to elliptical nuclei and prominent eosinophilic cytoplasm (epithelioid cell), often multinucleated, admixed and surrounded by predominantly lymphocytes and plasma cells (e.g., tuberculosis, sarcoid)
   b. *Inflammatory type:* Poorly defined, composed of lymphocytes, plasma cells, and occasionally eosinophils and neutrophils, without an epithelioid component (e.g., cytomegalovirus, drugs)
3. Granulomas may occur in from 3% to 10% of all liver biopsy specimens:

Systemic diseases	74%
Liver only	4%
Unknown etiology	22%

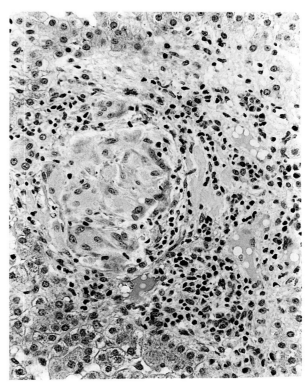

Figure 10–3. Sarcoidosis. A well-demarcated granuloma consisting of epithelioid cells and scattered lymphocytes is present at the edge of this portal tract. Necrosis and multinucleated giant cells are not present.

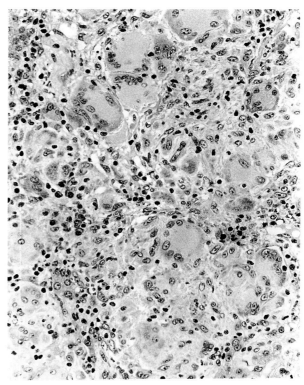

Figure 10–4. Sarcoidosis. Multiple epithelioid granulomas are present, each exhibiting numerous multinucleated giant cells.

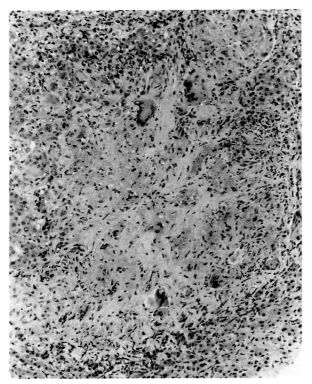

Figure 10–5. Sarcoidosis. A large epithelioid granuloma contains numerous multinucleated giant cells as well as collagen strands and bundles tending to divide the granuloma into smaller divisions.

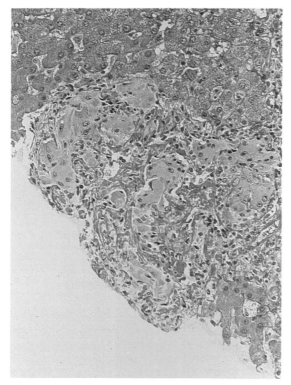

Figure 10–6. Sarcoidosis (trichrome). Dense collagen fibers produce septate divisions of the epithelioid granuloma.

4. Incidence in a series at the University of Southern California:

Disease	No. Patients (Total 173)	%
Sarcoidosis	49	28.3
Tuberculosis	46	26.6
Leprosy	9	5.2
Brucellosis	9	5.2
Hodgkin's disease	7	4.0
Q fever	6	3.5
Fungal infections	5	2.9
Syphilis	2	1.2
Miscellaneous (e.g., primary biliary cirrhosis)	15	8.7
Unknown etiology	25	14.4

5. Tuberculosis and sarcoidosis are the two most common causes of hepatic granuloma formation in most series; the incidence for tuberculosis ranges from 11% to 53% and that of sarcoidosis from 12% to 34%. Tuberculosis is discussed in detail in Chapter 7.

Sarcoidosis

Major Morphologic Features

1. Multiple noncaseating epithelioid granulomas are usually portal or periportal but may be found anywhere within the lobule.
2. Granulomas may exhibit segmentation into smaller units by fibrous septa, with fibrosis surrounding and eventually replacing the granuloma.

Other Features

1. Epithelioid cells are surrounded by abundant numbers of lymphocytes in active lesions.
2. Multinucleated giant cells may be seen but are uncommon.
3. Inclusions may be present and are characteristic of sarcoid granulomas:
   a. *Schaumann bodies:* Concentric basophilic laminations, rare in hepatic but more common in pulmonary granulomas
   b. *Asteroid bodies:* Spindly, radiating starlike structures within the epithelioid cells
4. Epithelioid granulomas may rarely show central fibrinoid necrosis with fragmentation of inflammatory cells.
5. Portal areas may exhibit variable degrees of fibrosis, with mild bile duct proliferation; progression to a biliary-type cirrhosis, with decreased ducts, has been reported.
6. Mononuclear inflammatory infiltration within the parenchyma as well as portal areas can be quite variable, with the more active lesions having prominent inflammatory features.

7. Kupffer cell hyperplasia is present and often quite prominent.
8. Hepatocytolysis is present to variable degrees.
9. Cholestasis is rare.

Differential Diagnosis

1. *Granulomas from other etiologies:* Segmentation of hepatic granulomas is a characteristic feature of sarcoidosis, rarely seen in granulomas of other etiologies. The epithelioid nature of the granuloma helps eliminate some infectious and most drug-induced granulomas. In some instances, special stains will aid in identifying acid-fast bacilli and fungi.
2. *Acute and chronic viral hepatitis:* In some instances the portal and parenchymal inflammatory changes in sarcoidosis may be quite prominent and suggestive of a viral hepatitis. Identification of granulomas may raise the possibility of viral hepatitis *superimposed* on a granulomatous disorder. These cases may be difficult to confidently evaluate on morphologic grounds alone.
3. *Primary biliary cirrhosis:* In the rare case of sarcoidosis with biliary fibrosis or cirrhosis and granuloma formation, the possibility of primary biliary cirrhosis from histology alone must be strongly considered; sarcoidosis with prolonged cholestasis has been reported to clinically resemble primary biliary cirrhosis. Antimitochondrial antibody, however, is negative and the serum IgM level is not elevated in sarcoidosis; in addition, hyalinization of granuloma and a positive Kveim test are not seen in primary biliary cirrhosis.

Special Stains

1. *Masson:* Septate granuloma, perigranulomatous fibrosis, and sclerosis are accentuated.
2. *Organism identification (acid-fast, periodic acid–Schiff, methenamine silver):* Possible infectious etiology of the granulomas can often be identified.

Clinical and Biologic Behavior

1. Sarcoidosis is a multisystemic granulomatous disease of unknown etiology; the major clinical manifestations are related to pulmonary involvement.
2. Patients present most commonly between the ages of 20 and 40 years; incidence within the United States is greatest in black women.
3. A small percentage present acutely with polyarthritis, iritis, and fever (Löfgren's syndrome); the majority (74%), however, exhibit nonspecific symptoms, with weakness, weight loss, anorexia, and low-grade fever; 16% are entirely asymptomatic on

diagnosis (abnormal chest radiograph on routine physical examination).
4. Pulmonary manifestations are most common, 60% at time of diagnosis and 90% as the disease progresses; the most common cause of death is attributable to complications of pulmonary fibrosis.
5. Systemic involvement includes the following:
   a. Liver (55%–90%)
   b. Ocular (20%–30%), possible blindness
   c. Neurologic (5%), encephalopathy, meningitis
   d. Myocardium, conduction defects
   e. Cutaneous (3%–25%), erythema nodosum
   f. Lacrimal, salivary glands (10%), enlargement, uveitis, fever (uveoparotid fever)
   g. Bone, cysts (rare)
   h. Muscles and synovium, arthritis
6. In the early stages of the disease, multiple hepatic granulomas are present; in latter stages, however, fibrosis, hyalinization, and occasionally total resolution of granulomas may occur.
7. Although hepatic granulomas are common, clinically significant liver disease is unusual (6.7%), manifesting with presinusoidal portal hypertension, esophagogastric varices, and, rarely, jaundice.
8. Laboratory tests reveal moderate elevations in serum alkaline phosphatase activity, mild to moderate increases in serum aminotransferase levels, and rarely hyperbilirubinemia; the angiotensin-converting enzyme is often elevated, and the Kveim skin test is positive in 80% of patients in the early stages of the disease.
9. The rare case of portal hypertension is secondary to significant portal fibrosis and granuloma formation in the portal tracts and consequent obstructive effects on the portal venous radicles (presinusoidal portal hypertension).
10. Helper T lymphocytes, markedly increased in sarcoidosis (normal helper/suppressor = 1.8/1, active sarcoidosis = 5–20/1), release lymphokines (interferon, migration inhibition factor, T-cell growth factor) that enhance inflammatory response and granuloma formation.
11. The etiology is unknown but believed to be related to a number of different factors, including genetic (predisposition of members of the same family, increased incidence of HLA-B8, HLA-B27), and autoimmune (decreased peripheral T lymphocytes, impairment of *in vitro* response of lymphocytes to many antigens and mitogens).

Treatment and Prognosis

1. Liver disease is seldom a clinical problem. When bleeding from esophageal varices develops in the rare case, management is similar to methods employed in cirrhosis of other etiologies.
2. Prognosis is generally good when pulmonary interstitial disease is absent or minimal, as seen in the majority of patients; with more systemic involve-

ment, prognosis becomes worse, with mortality rising to as high as 40% when significant pulmonary fibrosis is present.

References

Hercules HC, Bethlem NM. Value of liver biopsy in sarcoidosis. Arch Pathol Lab Med 1984;108:831–834.

Klatskin G. Hepatic granulomata: Problems in interpretation. Mount Sinai J Med 1977;44:798–812.

MacSween RNM. Liver pathology associated with diseases of other organs. In: MacSween RNM, Anthony PP, Scheuer PJ, eds. Pathology of the liver, 2nd ed. Edinburgh: Churchill Livingstone, 1987:651–653.

Mitchell DN, Scadding TG, Heard BE, et al. Sarcoidosis: Histopathological definition and clinical diagnosis. J Clin Pathol 1977;30:395–408.

Pereira-Lima J, Schaffner F. Chronic cholestasis in hepatic sarcoidosis with clinical features resembling primary biliary cirrhosis. Am J Med 1987;83:144–148.

■ Liver in Inflammatory Bowel Disease

Up to 50% of patients with ulcerative colitis and Crohn's disease have some degree of biochemical hepatic dysfunction, with 5% to 10% of these patients exhibiting clinically significant liver disease. A variety of hepatic changes may be present.

Nonspecific Reactive Changes (50%–75%)

1. Patients are clinically asymptomatic with regard to liver disease, with only mild elevations of serum aminotransferase and alkaline phosphatase levels.
2. Morphologic features include the following:

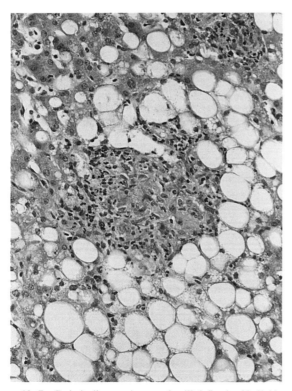

Figure 10–7. Crohn's disease. A somewhat ill-defined epithelioid granuloma is present. Most of the hepatocytes contain macrovesicular fat.

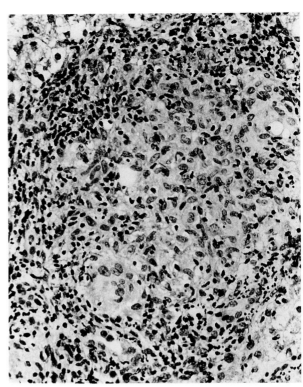

Figure 10–8. Crohn's disease. High power shows a granuloma composed of macrophages, epithelioid cells, lymphocytes, and a single multinucleated giant cell (*lower left*).

   a. Portal tract with variable degrees of lymphocytic infiltration and hyperplasia
   b. Mild bile duct proliferation
   c. Mild to moderate Kupffer cell hyperplasia with focal hepatocytolysis
   d. 1 to 2+ macrovesicular fatty change, with no distinct zonal distribution
   e. Epithelioid granuloma formation in 5% of cases (Crohn's disease)

Biliary Tract Disorders (5%)

PRIMARY SCLEROSING CHOLANGITIS (1%–5%)

1. Nonsuppurative fibrosing and obliterative lesions of interlobular bile ducts are present (see primary sclerosing cholangitis, page 45).
2. *Pericholangitis* was a term used in the past for portal tract lesions exhibiting ducts surrounded by lymphocytes. The term is actually a misnomer and represents either nonspecific portal lymphocytic infiltration (lymphocytes *not* oriented to duct structures) or primary sclerosing cholangitis involving small bile ducts.

CHOLANGIOCARCINOMA (0.4%–1.4%)

1. Cholangiocarcinoma is over 10 times more frequent in patients with ulcerative colitis, most often occurring in patients with long-standing inflammatory

bowel disease and associated primary sclerosing cholangitis.

2. These tumors occur in patients approximately 20 years younger than in those with typical cholangiocarcinoma.
3. The neoplasms are often multicentric, with intrahepatic and/or extrahepatic involvement of duct structures.
4. Morphologic features are those of typical cholangiocarcinoma (see cholangiocarcinoma, page 204).

Chronic Active Hepatitis (1%–2%)

1. Patients are HBsAg negative; the hepatitis may be autoimmune in etiology or secondary to chronic non-A, non-B infection.
2. Morphologic features are similar to those seen in chronic active hepatitis of viral etiology (see chronic active hepatitis, page 19).

Cirrhosis (1%–2%)

These cases are most likely a consequence of advanced primary sclerosing cholangitis (secondary biliary cirrhosis) or chronic active hepatitis.

References

Kern F. Hepatobiliary disorders in inflammatory bowel disease. In: Schiff L, Schiff ER, eds. Diseases of the Liver, 6th ed. Philadelphia: J.B. Lippincott, 1987:1450–1460.

MacSween RNM. Liver pathology associated with diseases of other organs. In: MacSween RNM, Anthony PP, Scheuer PJ, eds. Pathology of the Liver, 2nd ed. Edinburgh: Churchill Livingstone, 1987:653–655.

Perrett AD, Higgins G, Johnston HH, et al. The liver in Crohn's disease. Q J Med 1971;40:187–209.

Perrett AD, Higgins G, Johnston HH, et al. The liver in ulcerative colitis. Q J Med 1971;40:211–238.

Ritchie JK. Allan RN, MacCartney J, et al. Biliary tract carcinoma associated with ulcerative colitis. Q J Med 1974;43:263–279.

Wee A, Ludwig J, Coffey RJ, et al. Hepatobiliary carcinoma associated with primary sclerosing cholangitis and chronic ulcerative colitis. Hum Pathol 1985;16:719–726.

■ Autoimmune Hepatitis

Major Morphologic Features

1. Variable degrees of portal fibrosis are present, with increased lymphocytic and plasma cell infiltration in both portal tracts and parenchyma.

Other Features

1. Spillover of inflammatory cells from portal into periportal regions ("piecemeal necrosis") is usually seen.
2. Bile duct proliferation is mild to moderate.
3. Changes *irregularly* distributed from one lobule to another include the following:
   a. Parenchymal inflammatory infiltration

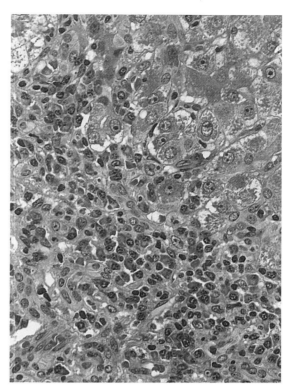

Figure 10–9. Autoimmune hepatitis. The fibrotic portal tract contains a prominent plasma cell infiltrate. Spillover of both lymphocytes and plasma cells into the periportal parenchyma is present.

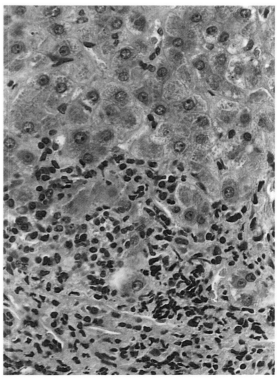

Figure 10–10. Autoimmune hepatitis. The portal and periportal inflammation in this example is entirely lymphocytic, with cuffing of lymphocytes around small groups of hepatocytes.

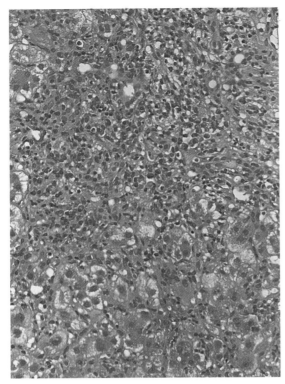

Figure 10–11. Autoimmune hepatitis. The lymphocytic and plasma cell infiltrates in the portal and periportal areas is extensive. Collapse of the reticulin framework can often be seen in autoimmune hepatitis.

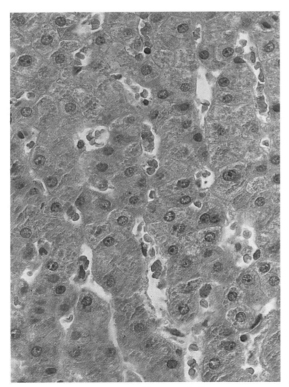

Figure 10–12. Autoimmune hepatitis. Necroinflammatory changes and Kupffer cell hyperplasia within the parenchyma are absent in a liver biopsy specimen from a patient receiving steroid therapy.

    b. Focal hepatocytolysis and prominent Kupffer cell hyperplasia
    c. Lymphocyte cuffing around single and small groups of hepatocytes
    d. Focal hydropic ''cobblestoning'' of hepatocytes (regeneration)

4. Variable degrees of dysplastic nuclear change of hepatocytes are occasionally present.
5. Inflammation and cell necrosis may rarely exhibit *uniform* changes throughout all lobules in the biopsy specimen.
6. Focal necrosis may be severe, in some instances confluent, with perivenular or multilobular collapse of the reticulin framework.
7. Plasma cell infiltration in many cases may be absent.
8. Inflammatory changes may be minimal in patients on steroid therapy.

Differential Diagnosis

1. *Chronic active hepatitis of other etiologies* (e.g., viral, drug): Although the basic morphologic features of all forms of chronic active hepatitis are generally the same, the presence of increased plasma cells and areas of confluent necrosis with parenchymal collapse hallmark chronic active hepatitis of the autoimmune type. These features, however, are not always present, especially in patients receiving steroid therapy. Absence of certain morphologic features characteristic of other etiologies (ground-glass cells in chronic hepatitis B, sinusoidal collagen, glycogen nuclei, and macrovesicular fat in chronic hepatitis non-A, non-B type), presence of appropriate autoimmune serologic markers (antinuclear, anti–smooth muscle antibodies), and rapid return of aminotransferase activities to normal with low-dose steroid therapy are characteristic for autoimmune chronic active liver disease.
2. *Acute viral hepatitis alone or superimposed on underlying chronic hepatitis:* Severe acute viral hepatitis alone, as well as acute delta infection in patients with acute or chronic hepatitis B, may in many ways resemble an extremely active autoimmune hepatitis with regard to marked inflammatory change and perivenular cell dropout. In addition, autoimmune hepatitis may in some cases exhibit uniform parenchymal changes from one lobule to another, simulating acute viral hepatitis. A feature of marked increase in plasma cells is helpful in diagnosing autoimmune hepatitis; however, minimal to moderate numbers of plasma cells can occasionally be seen in acute or chronic hepatitis of viral etiology. Immunoperoxidase staining for HBsAg, HBcAg, and delta antigen (the latter strongly positive in acute delta infection) as well as appropriate serum serologic markers (HBsAg, anti-HBc, anti-delta) may be necessary for diagnosis.

Special Stains

1. *Orcein:* Positive diffuse cytoplasmic staining suggests the presence of HBsAg, indicating a viral, not autoimmune, etiology.

Immunohistochemistry

1. *HBV markers (HBsAg, HBcAg, delta):* Positive staining pattern of *any* of these antigens will rule out an autoimmune etiology.

Clinical and Biologic Behavior

1. Autoimmune hepatitis, also termed *lupoid* hepatitis, is a liver disease first noted in the 1950s that primarily affects young women, often with hepatosplenomegaly, jaundice, and amenorrhea.
2. Females are affected almost nine times more frequently than males; the mean age is 47 years (range, 8 to 92 years). On physical examination stigmata of chronic liver disease may be seen.
3. Associated immunologic disorders are present in 50% of cases, including arthritis, vasculitis, ulcerative colitis, Hashimoto's thyroiditis, autoimmune hemolytic anemia, and glomerulonephritis.
4. In the typical case, serum globulin levels are elevated (predominantly IgG) sometimes to 8 to 10 g/dL. Serum aminotransferase levels are moderately elevated (500 IU/L) with hyperbilirubinemia (sometimes marked) and decrease in serum albumin and prothrombin activity. The presence of *autoantibodies* forms the basis for a number of positive serologic tests such as antinuclear, antismooth muscle, liver–kidney microsomal antibodies, liver-specific lipoprotein (LSP), and liver membrane antibody (LMA); antimitochondrial antibody (present in primary biliary cirrhosis) is *not* identified in autoimmune hepatitis.
5. The term *lupoid* hepatitis was initially used because patients often have a positive LE cell test (due to antinuclear antibody); however, systemic lupus erythematosus is not an associated disorder. Patients with systemic lupus erythematosus have livers that are normal or exhibit only mild nonspecific changes.
6. LSP and LMA are believed to be quite sensitive for autoimmune hepatitis but are not specific and can be seen in other liver diseases, including acute viral hepatitis; however, linear fluorescent membrane staining for LMA may be specific for autoimmune etiology.
7. Hepatocellular carcinoma is exceptionally rare but has been documented in the cirrhotic stage.
8. Pathophysiology involves a defect in T-lymphocyte suppressor cell function, forming increased levels of immunoglobulins and autoantibodies, which then attach to LSP and LMA, resulting in cell necrosis; genetic factors may be operative since autoantibodies may be seen in relatives of patients with autoimmune hepatitis (major histocompatibility complex on chromosome 6).

Treatment and Prognosis

1. Although early cirrhosis is often present at diagnosis, progression of the disease can be halted with steroid therapy. Even in advanced disease a trial with steroids is worthwhile. Management of complications of cirrhosis is the same regardless of the etiology.
2. Treatment duration is indefinite, and prognosis for responsive cases is good.
3. In advanced cases presenting with hepatic failure, or in nonresponsive disease, hepatic transplantation should be offered.

References

Hopf U, Meyer zum Buschenfelde KH, Arnold W. Detection of a liver-membrane autoantibody in HBsAg-negative chronic active hepatitis. N Engl J Med 1976;294:578–582.

Maddrey WC. Subdivisions of idiopathic autoimmune chronic active hepatitis. Hepatology 1987;7:1372–1375.

Montano L, Aranguibel F, Boffill M, et al. An analysis of the composition of the inflammatory infiltrate in autoimmune and hepatitis B virus-induced chronic liver disease. Hepatology 1983;3:292–296.

Peters RL. Viral inflammatory diseases. In: Peters RL, Craig JR, eds. Liver Pathology. New York: Churchill Livingstone, 1986:104–106.

Thomas HC. Immunologic aspects of liver disease. In: Schiff L, Schiff ER, eds. Diseases of the Liver, 6th ed. Philadelphia: J.B. Lippincott, 1987:170–172.

■ Conditions Occurring During Pregnancy

Acute Fatty Liver

Major Morphologic Features

1. Marked microvesicular fatty change in hepatocytes is most prominent in perivenular and midzonal regions.
2. Parenchyma has minimal mononuclear inflammatory infiltration and cell necrosis.

Other Features

1. Portal tracts are normal or may show a mild chronic inflammatory infiltrate; ducts are normal or exhibit mild reduplication.
2. Moderate to marked liver cell necrosis and inflammatory changes with cholestasis may rarely occur.
3. Fatty change may be panlobular in severe cases.
4. Hepatocytes exhibiting microvesicular change typically have somewhat smaller nuclei located toward the center of the cell.

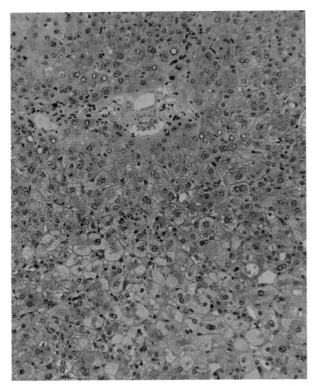

Figure 10–13. Acute fatty liver of pregnancy. The hepatocytes in the perivenular zone on low power appear swollen and hydropic. The midzonal and periportal liver cells are smaller, some exhibiting glycogen nuclei. The portal tract shows slight bile duct proliferation but is otherwise unremarkable.

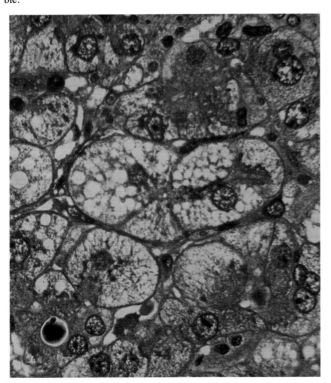

Figure 10–14. Acute fatty liver of pregnancy. High power shows that the perivenular hepatocytes are for the most part *not* hydropic but instead filled with microvesicular fat. Two bile plugs within dilated canaliculi are present.

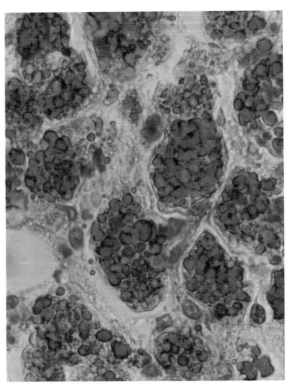

Figure 10–15. Acute fatty liver of pregnancy (oil red O). Fat stain (frozen section) shows the perivenular hepatocytes to be loaded with triglycerides. In severe cases this type of fatty change will also involve the midzonal and even periportal hepatocytes.

5. Variable degrees of macrovesicular fat are occasionally seen.
6. Megamitochondria have been described in hepatocytes.
7. Fibrin may be present within sinusoids in instances of concurrent disseminated intravascular coagulation.

■ **Differential Diagnosis**

1. *Drugs:*
   a. *Tetracycline:* Administration of intravenous tetracycline to pregnant women for urinary tract infections at first made recognition of acute fatty liver difficult, since tetracycline toxicity itself manifests a microvesicular fatty change. However, acute fatty liver does occur in the absence of tetracycline usage. Tetracycline toxicity is usually associated with moderate to marked degrees of nuclear anisocytosis. In addition, tetracycline exhibits a strong characteristic golden-brown autofluorescence on frozen section of fresh or formalin-fixed tissue.
   b. *Valproic acid:* This anticonvulsant may elicit a microvesicular fatty change indistinguishable from that seen in acute fatty liver. Discontinuation of the drug results in resolution of these hepatic changes.
2. *Reye's syndrome:* In acute fatty liver of pregnancy,

fatty change tends to spare periportal hepatocytes, while in Reye's syndrome panlobular fatty change is typical. Reye's syndrome is a disease of infants and children and is not found in pregnant women.

3. *Alcoholic foamy degeneration:* Microvesicular fat is present in perivenular hepatocytes in this form of acute alcoholic liver disease; however, variable degrees of sinusoidal collagen, portal arachnoid fibrosis, and occasionally hyaline necrosis are features of acute foamy change that are not seen in acute fatty liver.

Special Stains

1. *Oil red O:* Performed on frozen sections, this stain demonstrates fat in hepatocytes.
2. *Phosphotungstic acid hematoxylin:* Fibrin is demonstrated along sinusoids in cases associated with disseminated intravascular coagulation.

Clinical and Biologic Behavior

1. Acute fatty liver of pregnancy is a rare disorder (the incidence is 1/13,328 deliveries) and occurs in young primigravida women (mean age, 26 years) during the third trimester (usually around 35th week, although it may occur as early as 22 weeks).
2. Initial symptoms are vague and nonspecific, with headache and nausea followed by jaundice (93%), abdominal pain (58%), and encephalopathy (83%).
3. Laboratory tests show leukocytosis (83%); serum bilirubin is 5 to 6 mg/dL (93%), mild increase in alkaline phosphatase is seen, and aminotransferase levels are usually less than 500 IU/L (80%), although higher values have been reported; hypoglycemia is common; disseminated intravascular coagulation and renal failure may occur.
4. Prompt resolution of signs and symptoms is reported with termination of pregnancy; no progression to chronic liver disease has been documented.
5. Etiology is unknown, with environmental and/or toxic factors possibly playing a role; the disorder is not familial or infectious, and subsequent pregnancies are uncomplicated.

Treatment and Prognosis

1. Treatment is supportive with correction of hypovolemia, hypoglycemia, and aggressive management of encephalopathy, disseminated intravascular coagulation, renal failure, and pulmonary complications.
2. Pregnancy should be terminated promptly.
3. Early diagnosis (high index of suspicion in a pregnant woman with abnormal liver test results) is associated with better prognosis. Currently, maternal and fetal mortality rates are 18% and 23%, respectively.

References

Kaplan MM. Current concepts: Acute fatty liver of pregnancy. N Engl J Med 1985;313:367–370.
Pockros PJ, Peters RL, Reynolds TB. Idiopathic fatty liver of pregnancy: Findings in ten cases. Medicine 1984;63:1–11.
Riely C, Latham PS, Romero R, et al. Acute fatty liver of pregnancy: A reassessment based on observations in nine patients. Ann Intern Med 1987;106:703–706.
Rolfes DB, Ishak KG. Liver disease in pregnancy. Histopathology 1986;10:555–570.
Sherlock S. Acute fatty liver of pregnancy and the microvesicular fat diseases. Gut 1983;24:265–269.

Toxemia of Pregnancy

Major Morphologic Features

1. Fibrin deposition along sinusoids in periportal zones is often associated with coagulative (ischemic) liver cell necrosis and acute hemorrhage.

Other Features

1. Fibrin thrombi may also be present in portal veins.
2. In severe cases there may be multilobular necrosis, with large areas of infarction.

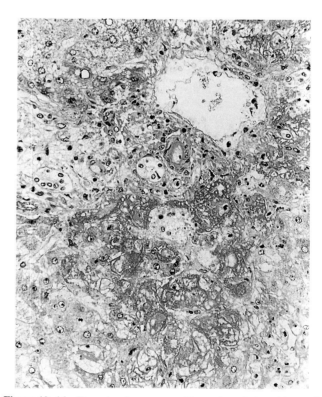

Figure 10–16. Toxemia of pregnancy. The periportal sinusoids are dilated and contain an eosinophilic fibrillar material that represents fibrin. Most of the hepatocytes in this region have dropped out or exhibit an eosinophilic ischemic-type necrosis. The adjacent portal tract shows minimal infiltration by lymphocytes and neutrophils.

3. Portal areas and parenchyma show minimal mononuclear inflammatory infiltration.
4. Liver biopsy results may be entirely normal.

Differential Diagnosis

1. *Other causes of fibrin thrombi:* Disseminated intravascular coagulation of any etiology may be responsible for portal vein and sinusoidal occlusion caused by fibrin thrombi.

Special Stain

1. *Phosphotungstic acid hematoxylin:* Fibrin lining the sinusoids is identified.

Clinical and Biologic Behavior

1. Toxemia of pregnancy (*preeclampsia*) is a systemic disease manifested by hypertension, proteinuria, and peripheral edema; the term *eclampsia* is used when the condition is complicated by seizures.
2. The disease is responsible for approximately 5% of all cases of jaundice in pregnancy and occurs in both young primiparous and older multiparous women during the third trimester.
3. Laboratory values show variable increases of serum aminotransferase levels, but marked elevations may be seen in severe cases; jaundice is rare, but when present the bilirubin does not exceed 6 mg/dL.
4. Pathogenesis of the liver lesion may be due to intravascular coagulation and/or segmental vasospasm of small hepatic arterioles with injury of endothelial cells in constricted regions. Prostaglandins are important in controlling blood pressure during pregnancy; in toxemia there may be a possible imbalance in synthesis of platelet-aggregation (thromboxane) and antiaggregation (prostaglandin I_2), factors responsible for disseminated intravascular coagulation.

Treatment and Prognosis

1. Treatment is supportive, with termination of pregnancy.

References

Antia FP, Bharadwaj TP, Watsa MC, et al. Liver in normal pregnancy, pre-eclampsia and eclampsia. Lancet 1958;2:776–778.
Arias F, Mancilla-Jimenez R. Hepatic fibrinogen deposits in pre-eclampsia. N Engl J Med 1976;295:578–582.
Long RG, Scheuer PJ, Sherlock S. Pre-eclampsia presenting with deep jaundice. J Clin Pathol 1977;30:212–215.
Rolfes DB, Ishak KG. Liver disease in pregnancy. Histopathology 1986;10:555–570.

Intrahepatic Cholestasis of Pregnancy
(See Chapter 3.)

■ Lesions Resembling Alcoholic Liver Disease

List of Disorders (Table 10–2)

Numerous disease entities in many ways may morphologically resemble, or even be identical to, changes seen in acute and chronic alcoholic liver disease. Mallory's hyalin, for example, has been described in over two dozen disorders. In small or fragmented biopsy specimens containing liver cells with hyalin, alcoholic liver disease is usually first in the differential diagnosis. History and laboratory data are then essential in making the correct diagnosis.

Reference

Kanel GC. Conditions resembling alcoholic liver disease. In: Peters RL, Craig JR, eds. Liver Pathology. New York: Churchill Livingstone, 1986:285–297.

Post Jejunoileal Bypass for Morbid Obesity

Major Morphologic Features

Acute Lesion
1. Perivenular sinusoidal collagen deposition is marked.
2. Macrovesicular fatty change is moderate to marked.
3. Variable degrees of hydropic change and hyaline necrosis occur and are most prominent in perivenular liver cells.

Chronic Lesion
1. Well-formed regenerative nodules are seen in a relatively quiescent cirrhotic stage; the septa are often thin.

Other Features

1. Portal tracts and fibrous septa exhibit a mixed inflammatory infiltrate consisting of both lymphocytes and neutrophils.
2. Collections of neutrophils are occasionally seen in the parenchyma, at times surrounding hepatocytes containing hyalin.
3. Macrovesicular fat does not have a distinct zonal distribution; the degree of fatty change is usually less in the cirrhotic stage.
4. Sinusoidal collagen is minimal to absent in the cirrhotic stage.
5. Noncaseating epithelioid granulomas may be present within the parenchyma in chronic disease in approximately 7% of cases.

Table 10–2
DISORDERS RESEMBLING ALCOHOLIC LIVER DISEASE

Disorder	Feature		
	Mallory Bodies (Hyalin)	*Sinusoidal Collagen*	*Fat*
Alcoholic liver disease	+++	+++	+++
Post jejunoileal bypass (or gastric stapling)	++	++	+++
Diabetes mellitus (adult onset)	+	+	+++
Obesity	+	+	+++
Vitamin A toxicity	+	++	+
Indian childhood cirrhosis	+++	++	
Wilson's disease	++	+	+
Chronic active hepatitis non-A, non-B		++	++
Chronic cholestasis:			
Extrahepatic biliary atresia	+		
Large duct obstruction	+		
Primary biliary cirrhosis	++		
Weber-Christian disease	+		
Abetalipoproteinemia	+		
Focal nodular hyperplasia	+		
Postintestinal resection	+		
Radiation	+	+	
Asbestosis	+		
Hepatocellular carcinoma	+		
Liver cell adenoma	+		
Drugs:			
Perhexiline maleate	+		
Diethylaminoethoxyhexestrol	+		
Glucocorticoids	+		++
Griseofulvin	+		
Methotrexate		++	+
Amiodarone	++	+	+
Estrogens	+		+
Hyperalimentation		++	+
Alpha-1-antitrypsin deficiency	+		

Frequency in liver biopsy: +++, common; ++, occasional; +, rare.

Differential Diagnosis

Table 10–2 lists numerous conditions that may have some features of post jejunoileal bypass. The following disorders histologically most closely mimic jejunoileal bypass:

1. *Acute sclerosing hyaline necrosis (acute alcoholic liver disease)*: This form of alcoholic hepatitis differs from acute post jejunoileal bypass by having more abundant hyalin and neutrophilic infiltration, perivenular and midzonal accentuation of the fatty change, and megamitochondria in the cytoplasm of the hepatocytes.

2. *Obesity and/or adult-onset diabetes mellitus*: Glycogen nuclei in periseptal hepatocytes are usually a prominent feature in the diabetic and not a feature of post jejunoileal bypass.

3. *Drugs (e.g., amiodarone)*: This antiarrhythmic agent may produce all the features of both acute sclerosing hyaline necrosis and post jejunoileal bypass.

Special Stain

1. *Masson trichrome:* The prominent perivenular sinusoidal collagen deposition is accentuated.

Immunohistochemistry

1. *Mallory's hyalin:* The antigenic staining pattern of hyalin in post jejunoileal bypass is identical to that seen in acute alcoholic liver disease.

Clinical and Biologic Behavior

1. Jejunoileal bypass is a surgical procedure for producing significant and rapid weight loss in the morbidly

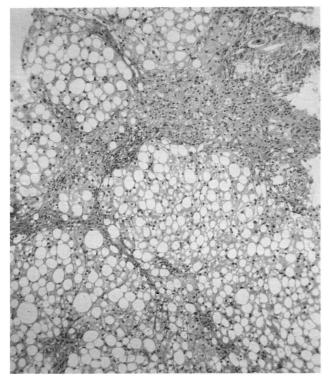

Figure 10–17. Postjejunoileal bypass. The portal tracts are fibrotic, with strands of collagen occasionally infiltrating into the parenchyma. The hepatocytes show extensive 4+ fatty change, predominantly macrovesicular.

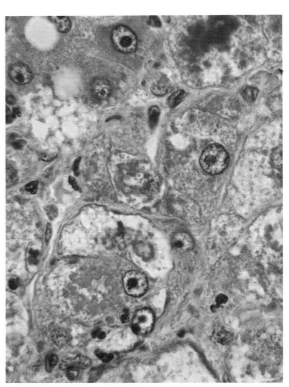

Figure 10–19. Postjejunoileal bypass. The hepatocytes are slightly swollen and hydropic, with some of the liver cells exhibiting macrovesicular and microvesicular fat. Numerous hepatocytes contain alcoholic hyalin, staining light pink to red. Neutrophils are seen infiltrating into a hepatocyte containing hyalin.

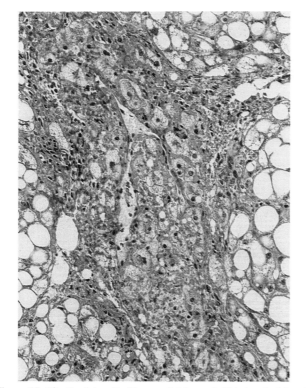

Figure 10–18. Postjejunoileal bypass (trichrome). This terminal hepatic vein shows extensive arachnoid fibrosis encasing individual hepatocytes. Macrovesicular fat is abundant in the surrounding liver cells.

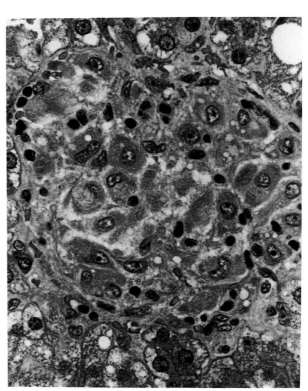

Figure 10–20. Postjejunoileal bypass. A well-defined granuloma consisting of epithelioid cells and lymphocytes is present within the parenchyma.

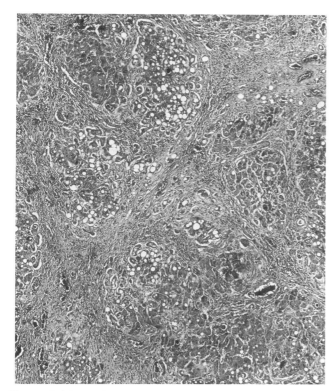

Figure 10–21. Postjejunoileal bypass. Cirrhosis with fibrous septa and poorly delineated regenerative nodules is present. Almost half of the hepatocytes contain macrovesicular fat.

obese patient. The gastrointestinal tract is shortened by anastomosing the proximal 14 inches of jejunum to the distal 4 inches of ileum.

2. Patients may lose anywhere from 65 to 127 pounds during the first 5 months after surgery.
3. Hepatic failure will develop in 2% to 7% of patients 2 to 9 months after surgery, with a high mortality unless normal continuity of the intestine is restored.
4. In acute disease, patients typically become jaundiced, with mild to moderate increase in serum aminotransferase levels; in some patients the aspartate aminotransferase–alanine aminotransferase ratio may be 2:1 or greater, mimicking acute alcoholic liver disease.
5. Patients who do survive this acute episode and do not have reversal of the bypass have a high risk of developing cirrhosis, sometimes within a few years after surgery.
6. Of all patients undergoing this procedure, 6.8% will develop severe fibrosis or cirrhosis 1 to 2 years following surgery.
7. Morphologically the acute changes resemble acute alcoholic liver disease (acute sclerosing hyaline necrosis) but occur after a latent period of at least 2 months post shunt; likewise, there is always a latent period (few years) in the alcoholic before acute liver disease occurs, suggesting that an indirect hepatotoxic effect of alcohol may be mediated by similar types of nutritional abnormalities as seen in post jejunoileal bypass.

8. Gastric bypass procedure for obesity will also result in similar hepatic abnormalities, although less frequently.
9. Pathophysiologic changes that may contribute to hepatic abnormalities include bacterial growth with toxin production within the excluded intestinal segment, decreased bile salt absorption and conversion to toxic metabolites, and relative malnutrition (similar to that seen in kwashiorkor).

Treatment and Prognosis

1. Reversal of bypass in acute disease is necessary.
2. If there is evidence for chronic liver disease, liver biopsy should be performed. If histopathologic changes typical for this lesion are noted and other etiologies excluded, early takedown of the bypass will prevent the development of cirrhosis.
3. Mortality ranges from 17% to 100% in acute disease.

References

Marubbio AT, Buchwald H, Schwartz MZ. Hepatic lesions of central pericellular fibrosis in morbid obesity, and after jejunoileal bypass. Am J Clin Pathol 1976;66:684–691.
Peters RL. Patterns of hepatic morphology in jejunoileal bypass patients. Am J Clin Nutr 1977;30:53–57.
Peters RL, Gay T, Reynolds TB. Post-jejunoileal-bypass hepatic disease: Its similarity to alcoholic hepatic disease. Am J Clin Pathol 1975;63:318–331.
Vyberg M, Ravn V, Andersen B. Pattern of progression in liver injury following jejunoileal bypass for morbid obesity. Liver 1987;7:271–276.

Obesity and Adult-Onset Diabetes Mellitus

Major Morphologic Changes

1. Moderate to marked macrovesicular fatty change with no distinct zonal distribution is present.
2. Increased numbers of glycogen nuclei in the diabetic, predominantly within periportal hepatocytes, are seen.

Other Features

1. Portal tracts exhibit mild bile duct proliferation and only minimal inflammatory changes.
2. Focal hepatocytolysis and mild mononuclear inflammatory infiltration may be present within the parenchyma.
3. Microvesicular as well as macrovesicular fatty change may both be present in the same biopsy specimen.
4. Although there is usually no zonal distribution of the fatty change, a minority of cases may exhibit perivenular accentuation.
5. Acute and chronic hepatic lesions are characterized by the following:

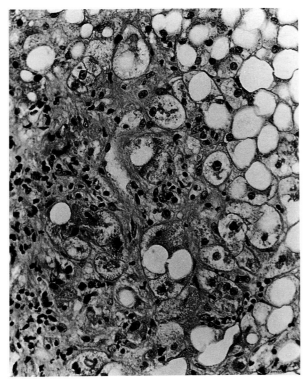

Figure 10–22. Obesity and adult-onset diabetes mellitus. The terminal hepatic venule is surrounded by extensive sinusoidal collagen that is infiltrated by both lymphocytes and neutrophils. Most of the hepatocytes contain macrovesicular fat. A rare cell contains alcoholic hyalin.

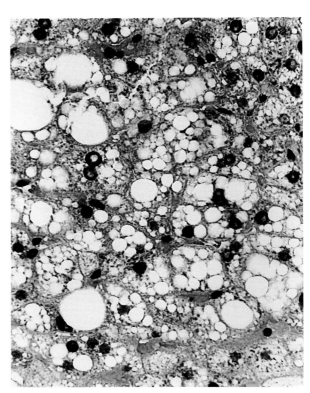

Figure 10–24. Obesity and adult-onset diabetes mellitus. The hepatocytes contain both macrovesicular and microvesicular fat. Thin strands of sinusoidal collagen are deposited between many of these cells.

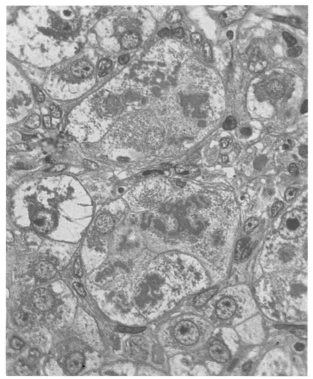

Figure 10–23. Obesity and adult-onset diabetes mellitus. Many of the swollen hepatocytes contain abundant alcoholic hyalin. A neutrophilic reaction to the hyalin is not present.

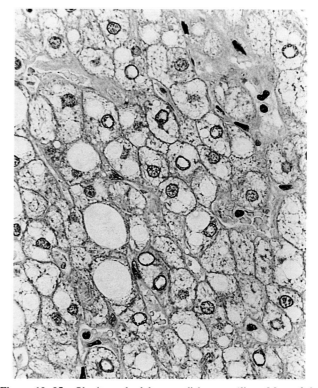

Figure 10–25. Obesity and adult-onset diabetes mellitus. Most of the hepatocytes contain glycogen nuclei. Both macrovesicular and microvesicular fat are present.

a. *Acute:* Hydropic hepatocytes containing alcoholic hyalin are most prominent in the perivenular zone; variable numbers of neutrophils are present within the lobule; sinusoidal collagen deposition is predominantly perivenular.

b. *Chronic:* Portal-perivenular fibrosis eventually leads to a micronodular cirrhosis. Arachnoid fibrosis is seen at edges of portal tracts and fibrous septa.

Differential Diagnosis

Table 10–2 lists numerous conditions that have morphologic features similar to those seen in obesity and adult-onset diabetes mellitus. The two disorders most difficult in differentiation include the following:

1. *Acute sclerosing hyaline necrosis (acute alcoholic liver disease):* Zonal distribution of fat (accentuation in zone 3), prominent sinusoidal collagen deposition, hyaline necrosis and neutrophilic infiltration, are typical features of acute sclerosing hyaline necrosis that are not usually seen in obesity and diabetes. Glycogen nuclei can be seen in all three conditions but are usually more abundant in diabetes.

2. *Post jejunoileal bypass:* As in alcoholic liver disease, jejunoileal bypass and acute changes of obesity and adult-onset diabetes are quite similar, with prominent glycogen nuclei again a feature most consistently seen in the diabetic.

Special Stain

1. *Masson trichrome:* Portal and perivenular sinusoidal collagen deposition is accentuated.

Clinical and Biologic Behavior

1. Twenty-eight to 39% of patients with diabetes mellitus, predominantly adult-onset type, have some degree of liver test abnormalities.

2. Patients generally are middle-aged women and are usually overweight; moderate elevations of serum aminotransferase levels and mild increase in alkaline phosphatase activity may also be seen in obesity in the absence of clinical diabetes; the exact incidence is difficult to evaluate, since fasting glucose levels may be normal, although glucose tolerance tests may confirm chemical diabetes. In addition, liver damage has been described a few years prior to clinical or biochemical manifestations of diabetes.

3. Cirrhosis is two to three times more frequent in diabetics than in nondiabetics, with cirrhosis presenting before the onset of diabetes in one third of these cases.

4. The degree of fat in the liver usually correlates with the degree of obesity but *not* to the duration or control of diabetes; fatty change generally is absent to mild in juvenile-onset diabetes.

5. Glycogen nuclei are present in over three fourths of cases of diabetes; the nuclei are quite abundant and are found in more than 20% of the hepatocytes.

6. Numerous glycogen nuclei may be seen in other conditions such as Wilson's disease, sepsis, and tuberculosis; however, usually the number of these nuclei is not as abundant as in diabetes.

7. The mechanism of liver damage is not known, but a number of features such as the fibrogenic potential of fat itself, precipitating factors such as viral hepatitis or chronic alcoholism in a fatty liver, and abnormal fat and carbohydrate metabolism in the diabetic may play some role.

Treatment and Prognosis

1. Weight loss is recommended.
2. It is uncertain whether adequate control of diabetes directly relates to improvement and prevention of liver disease in all patients.

References

Adler M, Schaffner F. Fatty liver hepatitis and cirrhosis in obese patients. Am J Med 1979;67:811.

Batman PA, Scheuer PJ. Diabetic hepatitis preceding the onset of glucose intolerance. Histopathology 1985;9:237–243.

Falchuk KR, Fiske SC, Haggitt RC, et al. Pericentral hepatic fibrosis and intracellular hyalin in diabetes mellitus. Gastroenterology 1980;78:535–541.

Itoh S, Tsukada Y, Motomura Y, et al. Five patients with nonalcoholic diabetic cirrhosis. Acta Hepatogastroenterol 1979;20:90–97.

Ludwig J, Viggiano TR, McGill DB, et al. Nonalcoholic steatohepatitis: Mayo Clinic experiences with a hitherto unnamed disease. Mayo Clin Proc 1980;55:434–438.

■ Hyperalimentation (Total Parenteral Nutrition)

Major Morphologic Feature

1. Perivenular cholestasis occurs in 16% to 90% of cases (directly related to duration of hyperalimentation).

Other Features

1. Variable degrees of macrovesicular, and occasionally microvesicular, fatty change are present but usually infrequent in the neonate; periportal macrovesicular fat is more common in the adult.

2. Portal tracts show mild bile duct proliferation.

3. Liver cells undergo hydropic change and may form pseudorosettes around dilated canaliculi containing bile.

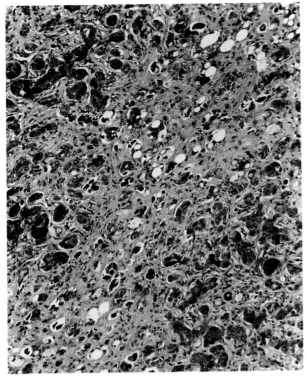

Figure 10–26. Hyperalimentation. Extensive diffuse sinusoidal collagen is present throughout the lobule. Macrovesicular fat is seen within occasional hepatocytes.

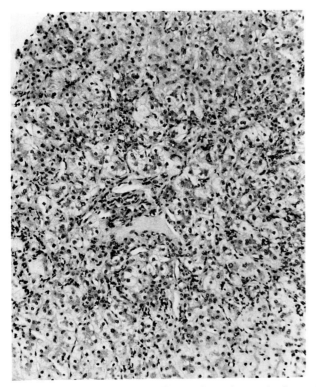

Figure 10–27. Hyperalimentation. The portal tract (*center*) is of normal size. The hepatocytes are hydropic. A lymphocytic infiltrate and Kupffer cell hyperplasia is seen in the surrounding parenchyma.

4. Syncytial giant cell transformation may occur in the neonate.
5. The lobule may exhibit variable degrees of lymphocytic infiltration and focal hepatocytolysis.
6. Portal and sinusoidal fibrosis, and very rarely cirrhosis of the biliary type, may occur with prolonged therapy.

Differential Diagnosis

1. *Neonatal giant cell hepatitis:* Both conditions elicit a syncytial giant cell transformation; pronounced cholestasis is more frequently seen associated with hyperalimentation.
2. *Extrahepatic biliary atresia, choledochal cyst:* Giant cell transformation, cholestasis, and biliary fibrosis may be seen in all of these disorders; however, bile duct proliferation is much less pronounced in hyperalimentation.

Clinical and Biologic Behavior

1. Liver disease associated with hyperalimentation (total parenteral nutrition [TPN]) may be seen in both the neonate and adult.
2. Jaundice occurs 4 to 47 days after onset of TPN due to cholestasis.
3. In the adult, serum aminotransferase levels are mild to moderately elevated in 93% of patients about 8 days after beginning TPN; these abnormalities then decrease and peak again to slightly higher levels 20 days after the start of therapy in 26% of cases; bilirubin rises to approximately 3 mg/dL.
4. In neonates, hyperbilirubinemia will be present in approximately 23% of cases; however, when TPN is prolonged, lasting 60 to 90 days, elevations of serum bilirubin will occur in 80% to 90% of patients.
5. With cessation of TPN, cholestasis resolves and the liver enzyme levels return to normal, sometimes rather slowly; in rare cases fibrosis may occur, and when TPN cannot be discontinued, cirrhosis may develop.
6. Gallstones and sludge are commonly present owing to bile stasis in the gallbladder.
7. Fatty change may be caused by imbalance of fatty acid and lipoprotein synthesis, with inability to properly secrete lipids.
8. Pathogenesis in the neonate may be related to a number of factors, including immaturity of intracellular enzymes; associated sepsis; absence of oral feeding causing inadequate gastric-duodenal stimulation of the gallbladder, decreased bile flow, and decreased clearance of bacterial (and other) toxins; abnormal carbohydrate; amino acid ratios; breakdown of tryptophan into hepatotoxic metabolites during storage of the intravenous solutions; relative amino acid and/or essential fatty acid deficiency; and hypersensitivity (eosinophilia has been rarely documented).

Treatment and Prognosis

1. Place patient on oral feeding and discontinue TPN, if possible.
2. The infusate and concentrations of amino acids should be modified.
3. Liver failure and death occur in 2% of infants.
4. The longer the duration of TPN, the more likely the development of biliary fibrosis and eventual cirrhosis.

References

Body JJ, Bleiberg H, Bron D, et al. Total parenteral nutrition-induced cholestasis mimicking large bile duct obstruction. Histopathology 1982;6:787–792.

Grant JP, Cox LE, Kleinman LM, et al. Serum hepatic enzyme and bilirubin elevations during parenteral nutrition. Surg Gynecol Obstet 1977;145:573–580.

Hughes CA, Talbot IC, Ducker DA, et al. Total parenteral nutrition in infancy: Effect on the liver and suggested pathogenesis. Gut 1983;24:241–248.

Postuma R, Trevene CL. Liver disease in infants receiving total parenteral nutrition. Pediatrics 1979;63:110–115.

Silk DBA. Parenteral nutrition in patients with liver disease. J Hepatol 1988;7:269–277.

■ Reye's Syndrome

Major Morphologic Features

1. Hepatocytes with microvesicular fatty change uniformly involve the entire lobule.
2. Minimal to absent inflammatory infiltrate occurs within the parenchyma.

Other Features

1. The size of the microvesicles is variable:
   a. Hepatocytes often appear swollen and hydropic on hematoxylin and eosin stain, with centrally located nuclei and no distinct fat vacuoles.
   b. The vacuoles may also be identifiable but small and seldom larger than the nucleus.
2. Portal tracts appear normal or exhibit only minimal lymphocytic infiltration.
3. Cholestasis is uncommon.
4. In exceptionally severe and fatal cases, focal mononuclear inflammatory infiltration and cell necrosis may be present.
5. Periportal ballooning degeneration and necrosis have been described but are rare.
6. In the recovery phase, microvesicular and macrovesicular fat is identified within Kupffer cells and portal macrophages.

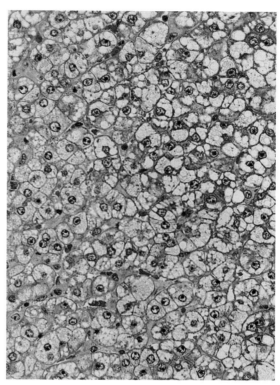

Figure 10–28. Reye's syndrome. Although the hepatocytes appear somewhat hydropic, the cytoplasm in fact is filled with microvesicular fat (confirmed by oil red O stain for fat on frozen section). Note that most of the liver cells have centrally placed nuclei, a feature commonly seen in cells containing extensive microvesicular fat.

Differential Diagnosis

1. Disorders that may cause microvesicular fatty change are listed below:
   a. *In pediatric age group:* Cholesterol ester storage disease, Wolman's disease, carnitine deficiency
   b. *Drugs, toxins:* Tetracycline, sodium valproate, hypoglycin (Jamaican vomiting sickness), margosa oil, aflatoxin
   c. *Miscellaneous conditions (not seen in children):* Fatty liver of pregnancy, acute alcoholic liver disease (foamy fatty change), obesity and adult-onset diabetes mellitus

Special Stain

1. *Oil red O:* Frozen sections of fresh or formalin-fixed tissue demonstrate cytoplasmic staining of fat.

Clinical and Biologic Behavior

1. Reye's syndrome is a rare disorder most often occurring in children before age 5 years, and almost exclu-

sively before age 18, consisting of acute encephalopathy and diffuse microvesicular fatty change of the liver; other organ systems also exhibit fatty change (kidney, heart, pancreatic islets). Cerebral edema is present without inflammatory changes.

2. The disease is seen worldwide, with an incidence of approximately 3.1/100,000; the overall incidence in the United States is 0.15 to 0.88 cases/100,000 children younger than age 18 years, with regional differences (2.8 to 4.7 in Ohio, the latter associated with an influenza B epidemic).

3. Both sexes are equally affected, with more frequent involvement of those living in suburban areas.

4. The disease most often follows an upper respiratory tract infection of viral etiology (90% of cases); the more common viruses are influenza B and varicella, but influenza A, reoviruses (1 and 2), echoviruses, and coxsackieviruses (A and B) have also been identified.

5. Approximately 1 week after the viral illness there typically is an acute onset of vomiting, delirium, and coma; seizures occur in 30% of cases.

6. Moderate elevations of serum aminotransferase levels (not greater than 500 IU/L) are reported, and bilirubin and alkaline phosphatase values are normal or only minimally elevated; hypoglycemia, acidosis, elevated serum ammonia levels, and decrease in prothrombin activity are often present.

7. Electron microscopy demonstrates enlarged and markedly distorted mitochondria that have a decreased matrix and contain dense bodies; glycogen depletion is common; these findings are found not only in hepatocytes but also in neurons within the cerebral cortex, suggesting that Reye's syndrome may be a generalized mitochondrial disorder.

8. Etiology is most likely related to viral illness; however, that alone cannot be a factor, since the disease occurs only in children and similar viral illnesses in other family members at the same time do not produce the disease. Concomitant environmental agents and toxins may also play a part.

9. Numerous investigations have implicated acetylsalicylate (aspirin) as a factor in the pathogenesis of Reye's syndrome; 93% to 97% of patients with this disorder had taken aspirin compared with 23% to 59% in control groups. In addition, there has been a decrease in incidence since 1982 after warning labels concerning Reye's syndrome were put on aspirin bottles. Many believe, however, that Reye's syndrome and aspirin toxicity are distinct entities presenting somewhat similar features.

Treatment and Prognosis

1. Treatment is supportive, with monitoring of blood glucose levels and aggressive management of complications seen in acute hepatic failure.

2. Monitoring intracranial pressure is important to en-

sure that permanent neurologic damage does not occur in a liver transplant candidate.

3. Exchange transfusions were previously tried and initially believed to show benefit; however, in severe disease and hepatic failure, hepatic transplantation should be offered.

4. Mortality, greater than 40% in the 1970s, has fallen to 26% in 1985, in part due to careful monitoring after prompt diagnosis and possible recognition of relationship to aspirin.

References

Bove KE, McAdams AJ, Partin JC, et al. The hepatic lesion in Reye's syndrome. Gastroenterology 1975;69:685–697.

Heubi JE, Partin JC, Partin JS, et al. Reye's syndrome: Current concepts. Hepatology 1987;7:155–164.

Hurwitz ES, Barrett MJ, Bregman D. Public health service study on Reye's syndrome and medication. N Engl J Med 1985;313:849–857.

Reye BDK, Morgan G, Baral J. Encephalopathy and fatty degeneration of the viscera: A disease entity in childhood. Lancet 1963;2:749–752.

Starko KM, Mullick FG. Hepatic and cerebral pathology findings in children with fatal salicylate intoxication: Further evidence for a causal relation between salicylate and Reye's syndrome. Lancet 1983;2:326–329.

■ Transplantation

Major Morphologic Features

1. *Early graft failure:*
   a. Perivenular and midzonal hepatocytes with marked hydropic change and/or coagulative-type necrosis are seen.

2. *Acute rejection:*
   a. Portal tracts show moderate to marked lymphocyte and plasma cell infiltration (96% of cases).
   b. Interlobular bile ducts with destructive changes are characterized by focal cytoplasmic vacuolization and infiltration by mononuclear cells and occasionally polymorphonuclear leukocytes (97%).
   c. *Endothelialitis:* Attachment of lymphocytes to the endothelium of portal and terminal hepatic veins occurs (40%).

3. *Chronic rejection:*
   a. Variable degrees of portal fibrosis are present.
   b. Arteriolar thickening, often with accumulation of foamy histiocytes in subintimal locations, is present.

Other Features

1. *Early graft failure:*
   a. Red blood cells may replace dying liver cells within hepatic cords in the perivenular zone.
   b. Arteriolar thickening with occasional thrombosis in portal tracts may occur.
   c. No significant portal inflammatory or duct changes are present.

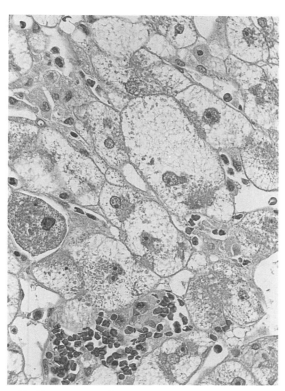

Figure 10–29. Transplantation, early graft failure. Perivenular hepatocytes are hydropic and swollen. A liver cell (*left*) is slightly small and undergoing ischemic necrosis.

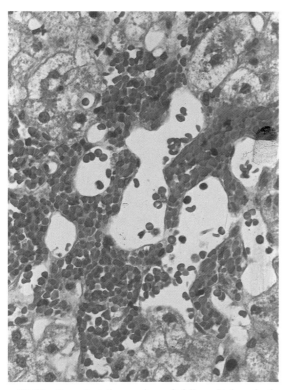

Figure 10–30. Transplantation, early graft failure. Perivenular hepatocytes have dropped out and are replaced by red blood cells. The adjacent sinusoids are dilated.

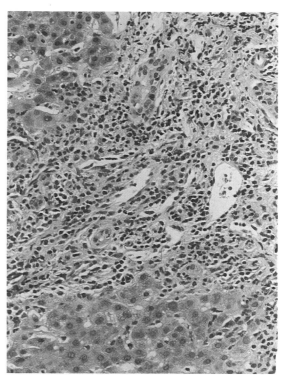

Figure 10–31. Transplantation, acute rejection. The portal tract exhibits fibrosis and a moderate lymphocytic infiltrate, which spills over into the periportal parenchyma. A bile duct is present but somewhat atypical in appearance. An increase in vascular channels is present.

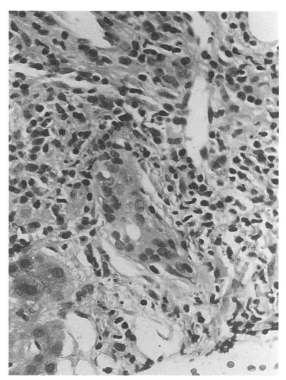

Figure 10–32. Transplantation, acute rejection. The interlobular bile duct is hypercellular, with some nuclei appearing piled on one another. Focal hydropic degeneration of the duct epithelium with infiltration of the basement membrane by lymphocytes can be seen. The surrounding portal tract exhibits a moderate lymphocytic infiltrate.

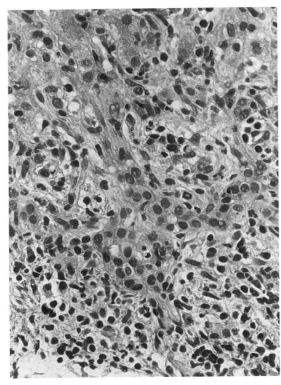

Figure 10–33. Transplantation, acute rejection. These atypical bile ducts rarely have a lumen, proliferate in a serpiginous pattern, and often gradually merge with cells differentiating into hepatocytes (*above*). Lymphocytes and occasional plasma cells are present within the portal tract.

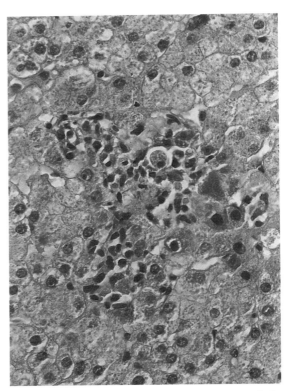

Figure 10–35. Transplantation, acute rejection. A cytomegalovirus nuclear inclusion (*lower right of inflammatory infiltrate*) is present within a hepatocyte. Focal necrosis with lymphocytic infiltration and acidophil body formation is seen. Although a neutrophilic reaction may occur, it is rare (see Figure 2–43).

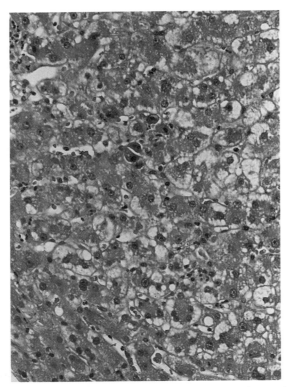

Figure 10–34. Transplantation, acute rejection. The parenchyma exhibits focal necrosis with formation of numerous acidophil bodies. Mild Kupffer cell hyperplasia is present. Most of the hepatocytes are hydropic.

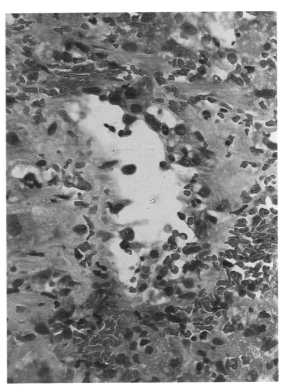

Figure 10–36. Transplantation, acute rejection. Lymphocytes are attached to the endothelium of the terminal hepatic vein (*endothelialitis*), with surrounding acute hemorrhage.

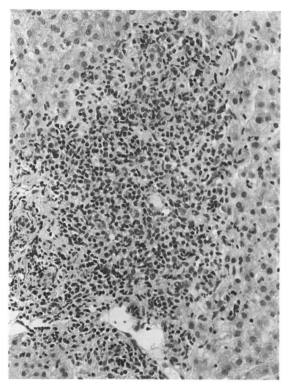

Figure 10–37. Transplantation, chronic rejection. The portal tract is slightly fibrotic and expanded by marked lymphocytic infiltration. Bile ducts are virtually absent.

d. The degree of ischemic change is quite variable, from slight (with eventual resolution and regenerative activity) to massive.
2. *Acute rejection:*
   a. Lymphocytic infiltration of portal areas may traverse the limiting plate with cuffing around single and small groups of periportal hepatocytes (resembling "piecemeal necrosis").
   b. Focal hepatocytolysis, mild to moderate Kupffer cell hyperplasia, and acidophil body formation within the parenchyma occur.
   c. Lymphocytes may be identified within the space of Disse.
   d. Neutrophils and occasional eosinophils are present within portal regions.
   e. Hepatocytes may be somewhat swollen.
   f. Variable degrees of perivenular cholestasis are occasionally present.
   g. Fibrin deposition may appear along endothelial borders or between the endothelium and muscular wall of inflamed vascular structures.
3. *Chronic rejection:*
   a. Parenchyma exhibits focal hepatocytolysis and rare acidophil body formation.
   b. Destructive duct features are ongoing, with eventual paucity of ducts.
   c. Endothelialitis is not usually present.

Differential Diagnosis

1. *Acute viral hepatitis:* Patients may clinically present with an acute hepatitis-like picture; biopsy specimen in acute rejection and graft failure does not exhibit the degree of hepatocytolysis, parenchymal lymphocytic infiltration, and Kupffer cell hyperplasia as seen in acute viral hepatitis. In addition, superimposed acute cytomegalovirus or Epstein-Barr virus infections are not uncommon in transplanted patients on immunosuppressive therapy.
2. *Drug toxicity:* Patients post transplant on immunosuppressive treatment (e.g., cyclosporine, azathioprine, cyclophosphamide) may exhibit variable degrees of liver cell necrosis and occasionally cholestasis. Destructive and inflammatory duct lesions and vascular injury, typically seen in rejection, are not present in drug-induced injury.
3. *Recurrence of chronic liver disease:* Transplanted livers develop inflammatory and bile duct injury that may resemble the morphology of the primary liver disease (e.g., primary biliary cirrhosis, chronic active hepatitis). Vascular injury is not a feature of these hepatic disorders, and granulomas, found in approximately 25% of patients with primary biliary cirrhosis, are not present in rejection.
Note: It is common, however, for morphologic changes of *coexisting* rejection to be present with the above disease entities as well.

Clinical and Biologic Behavior

1. Orthotopic transplantation, first performed in humans in 1963, has become a more common and successful surgical procedure for treatment of certain metabolic, biliary, inflammatory, and neoplastic liver diseases.
2. Indications for hepatic transplantation in a series of 140 adults and 104 children are shown in Table 10–3. Ten per cent of the patients had multiple diseases (e.g., hepatocellular carcinoma in a cirrhotic liver).
3. Some degree of acute rejection occurs in 20% to 80% of patients in spite of immunosuppressive therapy.
4. Rejection occurs within the first 2 months of surgery, usually within 5 to 15 days, and presents with fever, right upper quadrant tenderness and swelling, and often jaundice and ascites; patients with severe cases may develop disseminated intravascular coagulation, encephalopathy, and renal failure, necessitating immediate re-transplantation.
5. Laboratory values show an increase in serum aminotranferase levels, moderate increase in alkaline phosphatase activity, and hyperbilirubinemia.
6. Hypotension and inadequate preservation of the transplanted liver may predispose to immediate

Table 10–3
INDICATIONS FOR HEPATIC TRANSPLANTATION

Disease	Adults (%)	Pediatric (%)
Cirrhosis, nonalcoholic	32.9	9.6
Primary biliary cirrhosis	25.7	
Primary sclerosing cholangitis	13.6	1.0
Primary hepatic tumors	9.3	
Inborn errors of metabolism (e.g., alpha-1-antitrypsin deficiency, Wilson's disease, tyrosinemia)	7.9	22.1
Budd-Chiari syndrome	3.6	1.0
Secondary biliary cirrhosis	3.6	1.0
Acute hepatic necrosis	2.1	
Extrahepatic biliary atresia		53.8
Familial cholestasis		6.7
Neonatal hepatitis		2.9
Other	1.4	1.6

From Starzl TE, Iwatsuki S, Gordon RD, et al. Transplantation of the liver. In: Schiff L, Schiff ER, eds. Diseases of the Liver, 6th ed. Philadelphia: J.B. Lippincott, 1987:1255–1266.

graft failure; liver biopsy at the time of surgery in these patients will demonstrate features of severe ischemic necrosis.

7. The "vanishing bile duct syndrome," occurring in approximately 10% of patients, is an irreversible type of acute rejection presenting within the first 100 days of transplant, characterized by spiking fever, lethargy, jaundice, pruritus, dark urine, light stools, and ascites; the patient's condition rapidly deteriorates, necessitating re-transplantation. The speed of deterioration is somewhat unique for this type of rejection, with the morphologic changes revealing marked destructive changes of the ducts.

8. Chronic rejection is secondary to repeated clinical and/or subclinical bouts of acute rejection and may occur years after transplant.

9. Extrahepatic complications serious enough to be life threatening or necessitate re-transplantation occur in 87% of patients, including pulmonary infections (18.7%), disseminated intravascular coagulation (8.4%), bile leaks or stricture at the site of duct-to-duct anastomosis (13.8%), intra-abdominal abscess (10.2%) or peritonitis (15.1%), renal failure (31.1%), wound complications (11.1%), and cardiac (5.3%) and neurologic (10%) abnormalities.

10. Lymphoma (Hodgkin's and non-Hodgkin's) has been documented in 2.7% of patients secondary to prolonged immunosuppresion.

11. Pathophysiology of the hepatic lesion in rejection is mediated by T-cytotoxic cells directed against class I antigens on ducts, liver cells, and endothelial cells and stimulated by T-helper cells directed against class II antigens on the same cells; antibodies against the recipient cells do not appear to play a part in rejection.

Treatment and Prognosis

1. Immunosuppressive therapy with cyclosporine–steroid protocols is initiated; in addition, in acute rejection, pulsing with monoclonal antilymphocyte antibody (OKT3) and increments in steroid dosages usually result in some improvement. The introduction of immunosuppressive FK506 may decrease the incidence of rejection.

2. Re-transplantation is performed when necessary.

3. Prognosis is slightly better in the pediatric than in the adult age groups.

4. Mortality is higher in disorders associated with cirrhosis (secondary to technical difficulties), recurrence of disease (such as hepatitis B), and neoplasms (recurrence of tumor with metastasis).

5. Before cyclosporine
   (1963–1976):   1-year survival, 33%
                   2-year survival, 20%

   After cyclosporine
   (1980–1984):   1-year survival, 70%
                   2-year survival, 62%
                   5-year survival, 60%

References

Hockerstedt K, Lautenschlager I, Ahonen J, et al. Diagnosis of acute rejection in liver transplantation. J Hepatol 1988;6:217–221.

Maddrey WC, van Thiel DH. Liver transplantation: An overview. Hepatology 1988;8:948–959.

Snover DC, Freese DK, Sharp HL. Liver allograft rejection: An analysis of the use of biopsy in determining outcome of rejection. Am J Surg Pathol 1987;11:1–10.

Snover DC, Sibley RK, Freese DK, et al. Orthotopic liver transplantation: A pathologic study of 63 serial liver biopsies from 17 patients with special reference to the diagnostic features and natural history of rejection. Hepatology 1984;4:1212–1222.

Starzl TE, Iwatsuki S, Gordon RD, et al. Transplantation of the liver. In: Schiff L, Schiff ER, eds. Diseases of the Liver, 6th ed. Philadelphia: J.B. Lippincott, 1987:1255–1266.

Wood RP, Shaw BW, Starzl TE. Extrahepatic complications of liver transplantation. Semin Liver Dis 1985;5:377–384.

Graft-versus-Host Reaction

Major Morphologic Features

1. Portal tracts and parenchyma exhibit a mild lymphocytic infiltration.

2. Epithelial degeneration of interlobular ducts is present:
   a. Vacuolization of cytoplasm
   b. Acidophilic necrosis and individual cell dropout
   c. Hyperchromasia of nuclei
   d. Distortion of duct size and shape

3. *"Endothelialitis"*: Lymphocytes are attached to the endothelium of portal and terminal hepatic veins in a minority of cases.

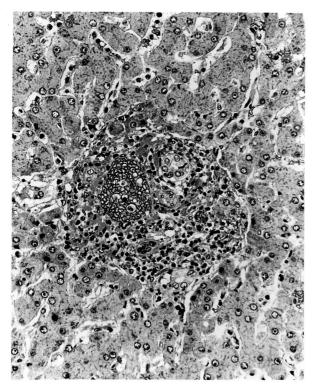

Figure 10–38. Graft-versus-host reaction. The portal tract is slightly expanded as a result of a moderate lymphocytic infiltration and hyperplasia. Bile ducts are present and appear somewhat distorted. The surrounding parenchyma exhibits Kupffer cell hyperplasia and a slight increase in circulating lymphocytes.

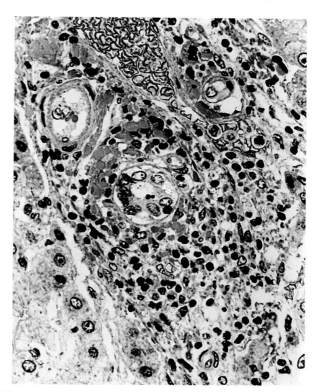

Figure 10–40. Graft-versus-host reaction. The atypical bile duct exhibits a lymphocyte beneath the basement membrane and a single neutrophil within the lumen. Cytoplasmic vacuolization is also present.

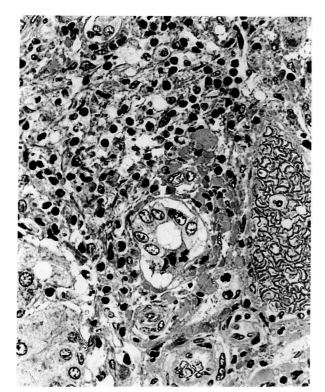

Figure 10–39. Graft-versus-host reaction. The bile duct exhibits marked cytoplasmic vacuolization. Some nuclei show marked shrinkage and hyperchromasia.

Other Features

1. Hepatocytes exhibit acidophilic-type necrosis.
2. Focal hepatocytolysis and Kupffer cell hyperplasia are present.
3. Portal inflammatory cells may spill over into the parenchyma, in some instances resembling "piecemeal" necrosis.
4. Variable degrees of macrovesicular fat may be present.
5. Veno-occlusive changes of terminal hepatic veins have been reported in up to 20% cases.
6. Chronic disease exhibits variable degrees of biliary fibrosis with decreased to absent ducts; biliary cirrhosis has been described.

Differential Diagnosis

1. *Complications of bone marrow transplant:* Common problems relate to the patient's underlying disease that necessitated bone marrow transplant, chemotherapy, and superimposed sepsis in an immunocompromised host. The combination of degenerative duct lesions, minimal mononuclear inflammatory changes, and "endothelialitis" are features most characteristic of graft-versus-host reaction.

Clinical and Biologic Behavior

1. The graft-versus-host reaction occurs after bone marrow grafting and is secondary to donor lymphocytes acting as immunocompetent cells attacking host organ systems, most commonly skin, gastrointestinal tract, and liver.
2. Graft-versus-host reaction has been described with transfusion of granulocytes but is not seen in transplant of kidneys or other organs.
3. Approximately 70% of grafted patients will develop graft-versus-host reaction either alone or complicated with infection; the acute reaction is seen 5 to 50 days post transplant.
4. The risk of developing chronic graft-versus-host reaction rises following the development of acute graft-versus-host reaction and with increasing age of the transplant recipient.
5. Patients present with a desquamative rash, diarrhea, and fever; jaundice occurs in 50% of cases. Mortality is high (60%–70%) in patients undergoing relatively severe reactions.
6. Chronic graft-versus-host reaction (>100 days post transplant) is characterized by severe wasting, skin involvement, and salivary gland injury (Sjögren-like syndrome); biliary fibrosis with decreased ducts and even cirrhosis may eventually occur.
7. Veno-occlusive disease, seen in up to one fifth of the cases, is related in part to pretransplant chemotherapy (e.g., mitomycin C) and/or radiation therapy and possible contribution by the hepatitis non-A, non-B virus.

Treatment and Prognosis

1. In acute graft-versus-host reaction, treatment of infections, use of laminar flow isolation, and immunosuppressive therapy (corticosteroids, antithymocyte globulin) will provide benefit.
2. Transfusion of irradiated blood products at 1500 to 2000 rads to destroy lymphocytes but spare granulocytes and red blood cells will reduce the incidence of acute graft-versus-host reaction.
3. In chronic graft-versus-host reaction, therapy with prednisone alone or in combination with azathioprine, procarbazine, or cyclophosphamide for 9 to 12 months favorably affects the natural course of the disease.
4. Prognosis correlates with severity of clinical disease in affected organ systems; mortality ranges from 7% to 100%.

References

Shulman HM, Sharma P, Amos D, et al. A coded histologic study of hepatic graft-versus-host disease after human bone marrow transplantation. Hepatology 1988;8:463–470.

Sloane JP, Dilly SA. Pathogenesis of graft *versus* host disease. Histopathology 1988;12:105–110.

Snover DC, Weisdorf SA, Ramsay NK, et al. Hepatic graft-versus-host disease: A study of the predictive value of liver biopsy in diagnosis. Hepatology 1984;4:123–130.

Wick MR, Moore SB, Gastineau DA, et al. Immunologic, clinical, and pathologic aspects of human graft-versus-host disease. Mayo Clin Proc 1983;58:603–612.

General References

MacSween RNM. Liver pathology associated with diseases of other organs. In: MacSween RNM, Anthony PP, Scheuer PJ, eds. Pathology of the Liver, 2nd ed. Edinburgh: Churchill Livingstone, 1987:646–688.

Peters RL, Craig JR, eds. Liver Pathology. New York: Churchill Livingstone, 1986.

Scheuer PJ. The liver in systemic diseases, pregnancy and organ transplantation. In: Scheuer PJ, ed. Liver Biopsy Interpretation, 3rd ed. London: Baillière Tindall, 1980:200–232.

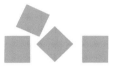

INDEX

Note: Page numbers in italics refer to illustrations; page numbers followed by (t) refer to tables.

Abscess, aspiration of, 108
  bacterial infection and, 107–109, *108*
  cholangiohepatitis and, *48*
  micro-, cholestasis and, 35, *36*
Acetaminophen toxicity, 68–70
  clinical features of, 69–70
  differential diagnosis of, 68–69
  Kupffer cells in, *69*
  macrophages in, *69*
  necrosis due to, *68*
  treatment of, 70
Acetylators, fast, 72
  slow, 72
Acid-fast stain, mycobacteria and, 115, *117*, 117,
  119
  schistosomes and, 132
Acidophil bodies, hepatitis and, *9*
Acinus, 1, *2*
Acquired immunodeficiency syndrome (AIDS). See
  also *Immunodeficiency.*
  Mycobacterium avium–intracellulare and, *117*,
  118
Adenocarcinoma. See also *Cholangiocarcinoma.*
  cystadenoma with, *181*, 182
  metastases from, 180
Adenoma, 175–182
  bile duct, 179–180
    border of, *179*
    clinical features of, 180
    differential diagnosis of, 180
    duct structures of, 179, *179*
    lymphocytic infiltration in, *179*
  liver cell, 175–178
    alcoholic hyalin in, *177*
    bile plugs in, *176*
    capsule of, 175, *177*
    clinical features of, 178
    differential diagnosis of, 175–178
    fatty infiltration in, *177*
    granuloma of, *177*
    hydropic cells in, *176*, *177*
    large cells in, *177*
    nodular hyperplasia vs., 175–178
    oral contraceptives and, 178
    sinusoidal dilatation in, *176*
Aflatoxins, hepatocellular carcinoma and, 192
AIDS. See also *Immunodeficiency.*
  Mycobacterium avium–intracellulare and, *117*,
  118
Alagille's syndrome, 139
  clinical features in, 139

Alanine aminotransferase, 4
Alcohol, collagen stimulation by, 53–54
  liver metabolism of, 53
Alcoholic hyalin, anatomy of, 58
  antibodies to, 58
  biliary cirrhosis and, *42*
  cholestasis and, *38*, 39
  diabetic obesity and, *242*
  diseases manifesting, 238, 239(t)
  drug effects and, 87
  immunoperoxidase stain and, *57*
  Indian childhood cirrhosis and, *163*, 163, 164
  jejunoileal bypass and, 238, 239(t), *240*
  liver cell adenoma and, *177*
  microtubular nature of, 58
  sclerosing hyaline necrosis and, *56*, 56–59, *57*
  Wilson's disease and, *160*
Alcoholic liver disease, cirrhosis and, *61*, 61–63,
  62
  disorders resembling, 238, 239(t)
  fatty liver and, 53–56, *54*, *55*
  foamy degeneration due to, *59*, 60
  inclusions and, 150
  progressive perivenular fibrosis and, *64*, 64–65
  sclerosing hyaline necrosis and, *56*, 56–59, *57*,
  64–65
Alkaline phosphatase, 4
  elevated, paucity of ducts syndrome and, 139
Alkaloids, veno-occlusive disease and, 94
Alpha-fetoprotein, hepatoblastoma and, 198
  hepatocellular carcinoma and, *188*, 190, 191
Amebiasis, 124–126
  abscess of, 107–108, 124–125, *125*
    aspiration of, 126
  clinical features of, 125–126
  differential diagnosis of, 124–125
  pyogenic infection vs., 107
  trophozoites in, 125, *125*, 126
Amyloidosis, 164–167
  clinical features of, 166–167
  differential diagnosis of, 165–166
  eosinophilic deposits of, *165*
  pathogenesis of, *165*, 167
  prognosis in, 167
  staining used in, 165–167
  types of, 164
Andersen's disease, 154(t)
Anemia, sickle cell. See *Sickle cell anemia.*
Angioma, spider, 4
Angiosarcoma, 199–204
  clinical features of, 201